# Drugs Used In Psychiatry

This guide contains color reproductions of some commonly prescribed major psychotherapeutic drugs. This guide mainly illustrates tablets and capsules. A † symbol preceding the name of the drug indicates that other doses are available. Check directly with the manufacturer. *(Although the photos are intended as accurate reproductions of the drug, this guide should be used only as a quick identification aid.)*

P9-DNH-087

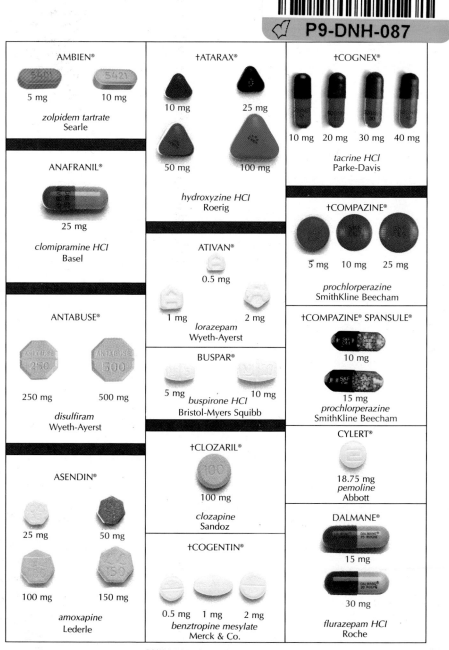

AMBIEN®

5 mg          10 mg

zolpidem tartrate
Searle

ANAFRANIL®

25 mg

clomipramine HCl
Basel

ANTABUSE®

250 mg          500 mg

disulfiram
Wyeth-Ayerst

ASENDIN®

25 mg          50 mg

100 mg          150 mg

amoxapine
Lederle

†ATARAX®

10 mg          25 mg

50 mg          100 mg

hydroxyzine HCl
Roerig

ATIVAN®

0.5 mg

1 mg          2 mg

lorazepam
Wyeth-Ayerst

BUSPAR®

5 mg          10 mg
buspirone HCl
Bristol-Myers Squibb

†CLOZARIL®

100 mg

clozapine
Sandoz

†COGENTIN®

0.5 mg     1 mg     2 mg
benztropine mesylate
Merck & Co.

†COGNEX®

10 mg     20 mg     30 mg     40 mg

tacrine HCl
Parke-Davis

†COMPAZINE®

5 mg     10 mg     25 mg

prochlorperazine
SmithKline Beecham

†COMPAZINE® SPANSULE®

10 mg

15 mg
prochlorperazine
SmithKline Beecham

CYLERT®

18.75 mg
pemoline
Abbott

DALMANE®

15 mg

30 mg

flurazepam HCl
Roche

**WILLIAMS AND WILKINS©**

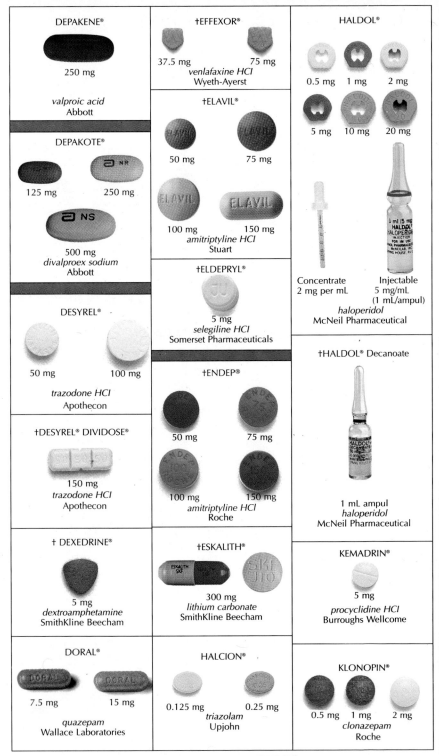

**DEPAKENE®**

250 mg

*valproic acid*
Abbott

**DEPAKOTE®**

125 mg          250 mg

500 mg
*divalproex sodium*
Abbott

**DESYREL®**

50 mg          100 mg

*trazodone HCl*
Apothecon

**†DESYREL® DIVIDOSE®**

150 mg
*trazodone HCl*
Apothecon

**† DEXEDRINE®**

5 mg
*dextroamphetamine*
SmithKline Beecham

**DORAL®**

7.5 mg          15 mg

*quazepam*
Wallace Laboratories

**†EFFEXOR®**

37.5 mg          75 mg
*venlafaxine HCl*
Wyeth-Ayerst

**†ELAVIL®**

50 mg          75 mg

100 mg          150 mg
*amitriptyline HCl*
Stuart

**†ELDEPRYL®**

5 mg
*selegiline HCl*
Somerset Pharmaceuticals

**†ENDEP®**

50 mg          75 mg

100 mg          150 mg
*amitriptyline HCl*
Roche

**†ESKALITH®**

300 mg
*lithium carbonate*
SmithKline Beecham

**HALCION®**

0.125 mg          0.25 mg
*triazolam*
Upjohn

**HALDOL®**

0.5 mg     1 mg     2 mg

5 mg     10 mg     20 mg

Concentrate          Injectable
2 mg per mL          5 mg/mL
                     (1 mL/ampul)
*haloperidol*
McNeil Pharmaceutical

**†HALDOL® Decanoate**

1 mL ampul
*haloperidol*
McNeil Pharmaceutical

**KEMADRIN®**

5 mg
*procyclidine HCl*
Burroughs Wellcome

**KLONOPIN®**

0.5 mg     1 mg     2 mg
*clonazepam*
Roche

**WILLIAMS AND WILKINS©**

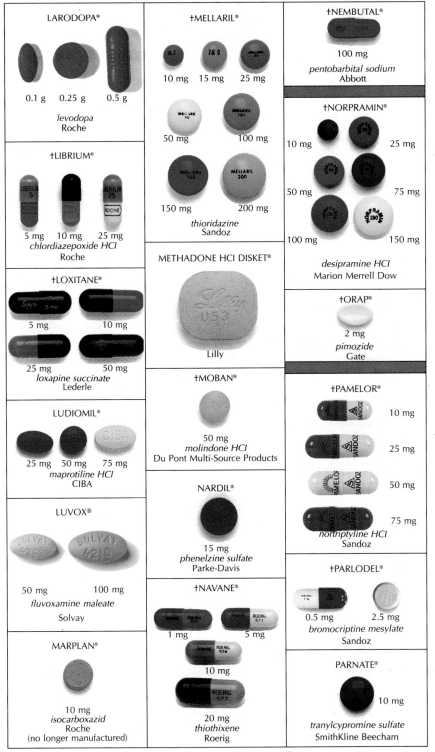

**LARODOPA®**

0.1 g    0.25 g    0.5 g

*levodopa*
Roche

**†LIBRIUM®**

5 mg    10 mg    25 mg

*chlordiazepoxide HCl*
Roche

**†LOXITANE®**

5 mg    10 mg

25 mg    50 mg

*loxapine succinate*
Lederle

**LUDIOMIL®**

25 mg    50 mg    75 mg

*maprotiline HCl*
CIBA

**LUVOX®**

50 mg    100 mg

*fluvoxamine maleate*
Solvay

**MARPLAN®**

10 mg
*isocarboxazid*
Roche
(no longer manufactured)

**†MELLARIL®**

10 mg    15 mg    25 mg

50 mg    100 mg

150 mg    200 mg

*thioridazine*
Sandoz

**METHADONE HCl DISKET®**

Lilly

**†MOBAN®**

50 mg
*molindone HCl*
Du Pont Multi-Source Products

**NARDIL®**

15 mg
*phenelzine sulfate*
Parke-Davis

**†NAVANE®**

1 mg    5 mg

10 mg

20 mg
*thiothixene*
Roerig

**†NEMBUTAL®**

100 mg

*pentobarbital sodium*
Abbott

**†NORPRAMIN®**

10 mg    25 mg

50 mg    75 mg

100 mg    150 mg

*desipramine HCl*
Marion Merrell Dow

**†ORAP®**

2 mg
*pimozide*
Gate

**†PAMELOR®**

10 mg

25 mg

50 mg

75 mg
*nortriptyline HCl*
Sandoz

**†PARLODEL®**

0.5 mg    2.5 mg
*bromocriptine mesylate*
Sandoz

**PARNATE®**

10 mg

*tranylcypromine sulfate*
SmithKline Beecham

**WILLIAMS AND WILKINS©**

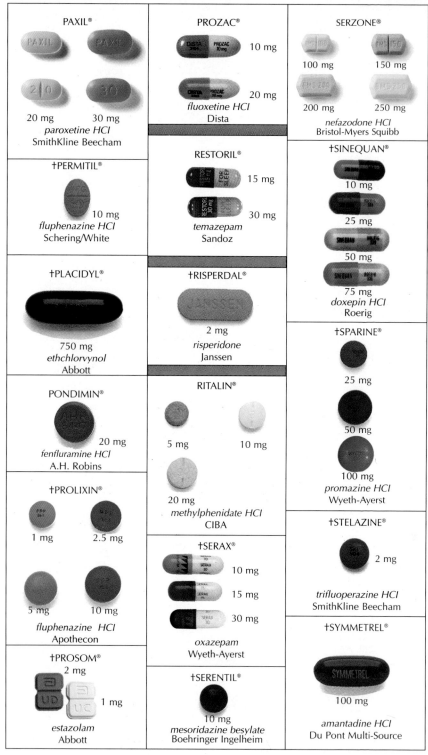

**PAXIL®**

20 mg    30 mg
*paroxetine HCl*
SmithKline Beecham

**†PERMITIL®**
10 mg
*fluphenazine HCl*
Schering/White

**†PLACIDYL®**
750 mg
*ethchlorvynol*
Abbott

**PONDIMIN®**
20 mg
*fenfluramine HCl*
A.H. Robins

**†PROLIXIN®**
1 mg    2.5 mg
5 mg    10 mg
*fluphenazine HCl*
Apothecon

**†PROSOM®**
2 mg
1 mg
*estazolam*
Abbott

**PROZAC®**
10 mg
20 mg
*fluoxetine HCl*
Dista

**RESTORIL®**
15 mg
30 mg
*temazepam*
Sandoz

**†RISPERDAL®**
2 mg
*risperidone*
Janssen

**RITALIN®**
5 mg    10 mg
20 mg
*methylphenidate HCl*
CIBA

**†SERAX®**
10 mg
15 mg
30 mg
*oxazepam*
Wyeth-Ayerst

**†SERENTIL®**
10 mg
*mesoridazine besylate*
Boehringer Ingelheim

**SERZONE®**
100 mg    150 mg
200 mg    250 mg
*nefazodone HCl*
Bristol-Myers Squibb

**†SINEQUAN®**
10 mg
25 mg
50 mg
75 mg
*doxepin HCl*
Roerig

**†SPARINE®**
25 mg
50 mg
100 mg
*promazine HCl*
Wyeth-Ayerst

**†STELAZINE®**
2 mg
*trifluoperazine HCl*
SmithKline Beecham

**†SYMMETREL®**
100 mg
*amantadine HCl*
Du Pont Multi-Source

**WILLIAMS AND WILKINS©**

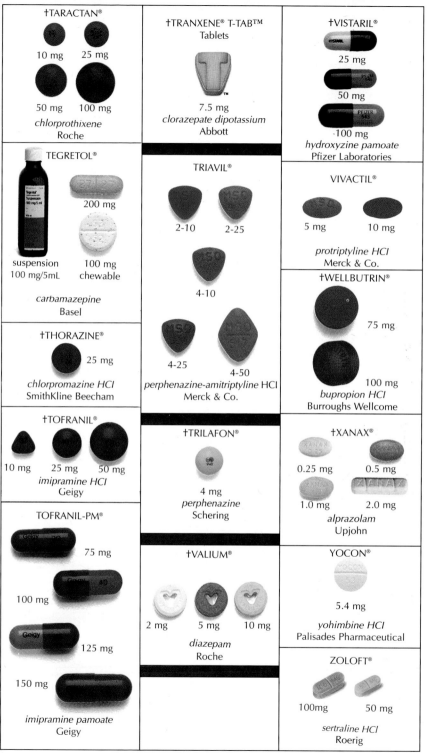

†TARACTAN®
10 mg    25 mg
50 mg    100 mg
chlorprothixene
Roche

TEGRETOL®
200 mg
suspension    100 mg
100 mg/5mL    chewable
carbamazepine
Basel

†THORAZINE®
25 mg
chlorpromazine HCl
SmithKline Beecham

†TOFRANIL®
10 mg    25 mg    50 mg
imipramine HCl
Geigy

TOFRANIL-PM®
75 mg
100 mg
125 mg
150 mg
imipramine pamoate
Geigy

†TRANXENE® T-TAB™
Tablets
7.5 mg
clorazepate dipotassium
Abbott

TRIAVIL®
2-10    2-25
4-10
4-25    4-50
perphenazine-amitriptyline HCl
Merck & Co.

†TRILAFON®
4 mg
perphenazine
Schering

†VALIUM®
2 mg    5 mg    10 mg
diazepam
Roche

†VISTARIL®
25 mg
50 mg
100 mg
hydroxyzine pamoate
Pfizer Laboratories

VIVACTIL®
5 mg    10 mg
protriptyline HCl
Merck & Co.

†WELLBUTRIN®
75 mg
100 mg
bupropion HCl
Burroughs Wellcome

†XANAX®
0.25 mg    0.5 mg
1.0 mg    2.0 mg
alprazolam
Upjohn

YOCON®
5.4 mg
yohimbine HCl
Palisades Pharmaceutical

ZOLOFT®
100mg    50 mg
sertraline HCl
Roerig

**WILLIAMS AND WILKINS**©

# POCKET HANDBOOK OF CLINICAL PSYCHIATRY

*Second Edition*

*Senior Contributing Editor*

# ROBERT CANCRO, M.D., MED D.SC.

Professor and Chairman, Department of Psychiatry,
New York University School of Medicine;
Director, Department of Psychiatry, Tisch Hospital,
the University Hospital of New York University Medical Center,
New York, New York;
Director, Nathan S. Kline Institute for Psychiatric Research,
Orangeburg, New York

# POCKET HANDBOOK OF CLINICAL PSYCHIATRY

## Second Edition

# HAROLD I. KAPLAN, M.D.

Professor of Psychiatry, New York University School of Medicine
Attending Psychiatrist, Tisch Hospital, the University Hospital
of the New York University Medical Center;
Attending Psychiatrist, Bellevue Hospital;
Consultant Psychiatrist, Lenox Hill Hospital,
New York, New York

# BENJAMIN J. SADOCK, M.D.

Professor and Vice Chairman, Department of Psychiatry,
New York University School of Medicine;
Attending Psychiatrist, Tisch Hospital, the University Hospital
of the New York University Medical Center;
Attending Psychiatrist, Bellevue Hospital;
Consultant Psychiatrist, Lenox Hill Hospital,
New York, New York

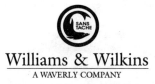

## Williams & Wilkins
### A WAVERLY COMPANY

BALTIMORE • PHILADELPHIA • LONDON • PARIS • BANGKOK
BUENOS AIRES • HONG KONG • MUNICH • SYDNEY • TOKYO • WROCLAW

*Editor:* Susan Gay
*Managing Editor:* Kathleen Courtney Millet
*Production Coordinator:* Barbara J. Felton
*Copy Editor:* John M. Daniel
*Designer:* Wilma E. Rosenberger
*Typesetter:* Automated Graphic Systems

"Kaplan Sadock Psychiatry" with the pyramid logo is a trademark of Williams & Wilkins.

**Notice.** The indications and dosages of all drugs in this book have been recommended in the medical literature and conform to the practices of the general medical community. The medications described do not necessarily have specific approval by the Food and Drug Administration for use in the diseases and dosages for which they are recommended. The package insert for each drug should be consulted for use and dosage as approved by the FDA. Because standards for usage change, it is advisable to keep abreast of revised recommendations, particularly those concerning new drugs.

*Printed in the United States of America*

First Edition, 1990.

**Library of Congress Cataloging-in-Publication Data**

Kaplan, Harold I., .
    Pocket handbook of clinical psychiatry / Harold I. Kaplan, Benjamin J. Sadock. — 2nd ed.
    p. cm.
    Digest companion v. to: Comprehensive textbook of psychiatry/VI/ editors, Harold I. Kaplan, Benjamin J. Sadock. 6th ed. © 1995.
    Includes index.
    ISBN 0-683-04583-0
    1. Psychiatry—Handbooks, manuals, etc.   I. Sadock, Benjamin J.,      II. Comprehensive textbook of psychiatry/VI.   III. Title.
    [DNLM: 1. Mental Disorders—handbooks.   WM 34 K17p 1996]
    RC456.K316   1996
    616.89—dc20
    DNLM/DLC
    for Library of Congress                                                95-37951
                                                                              CIP

*The publishers have made every effort to trace the copyright holders for borrowed material. If they have inadvertently overlooked any, they will be pleased to make the necessary arrangements at the first opportunity.*

97 98 99
2 3 4 5 6 7 8 9 10

*Dedicated to our wives,*
*Nancy Barrett Kaplan*
*and*
*Virginia Alcott Sadock,*
*without whose help and sacrifice*
*this book would not have been possible*

# Preface

This is the second edition of the *Pocket Handbook of Clinical Psychiatry,* which is used by medical students, psychiatric residents, and practicing psychiatrists, who require a ready reference to diagnose and treat the full range of psychiatric disorders in adults and children. The primary care and other nonpsychiatric physicians who encounter and treat patients with emotional disturbances also should find it useful.

Every section has been updated and revised, and new sections have been added. All diagnoses conform to the criteria listed in the newly revised fourth edition of the American Psychiatric Association's *Diagnostic and Statistical Manual of Mental Disorders* (DSM-IV).

With the aid of this compact guide, management of psychiatric illness can readily be commenced, aspects of both psychological and pharmacological treatments can be implemented, and dose ranges and available preparations of various psychotropic medications can be determined.

The *Pocket Handbook* is the digest minicompanion to the much larger and more encyclopedic sixth edition of the *Comprehensive Textbook of Psychiatry* (CTP/VI), edited by the authors. The *Pocket Handbook* is a distillation in that it provides brief summaries of psychiatric disorders, which include key aspects of etiology, epidemiology, clinical picture, and treatment. Psychopharmacological principles and prescribing methods are discussed briefly but thoroughly. Each chapter ends with references to the more detailed relevant sections in CTP/VI. A unique aspect of this book is the colored illustration of all the major psychotropic drugs and other drugs used in psychiatry, denoting both the forms in which they are commercially available and some of their doses to aid convenient recognition and prescription.

The *Pocket Handbook* cannot substitute for a major textbook of psychiatry, such as CTP/VI or its companion, *Kaplan and Sadock's Synopsis of Psychiatry.* It is meant instead to be used as an easily accessible reference by the busy doctor-in-training or clinical practitioner.

Justin Hollingsworth, Justin Hartung, Jennifer Peters, and Lynda Zittel were extraordinarily helpful in the preparation of this book. Others who helped were Peter Kaplan, M.D., Phillip Kaplan, M.D., James Sadock, and Victoria Sadock.

We again want to thank our colleagues who collaborated with us on the first edition of this book: James C.-Y. Chou, M.D., Rebecca M. Jones, M.D., Richard Perry, M.D., Barry Reisburg, M.D., Virginia Sadock, M.D., Matthew B. Smith, M.D., Norman Sussman, M.D., and Henry Weinstein, M.D. Drs. Perry and Sussman were most helpful in updating this edition's sections on child psychiatry and psychopharmacology, respectively. We especially want to acknowledge our debt to Jack Grebb, M.D., our valued coauthor of *Synopsis,* for all his help in all of our projects.

Finally, the authors wish to thank Robert Cancro, M.D., Professor and Chairman of the Department of Psychiatry at New York University (NYU) School of Medicine, who served as Senior Contributing Editor. The authors are deeply grateful for his unwavering support and for the inspiration and leadership he provides to the entire NYU Department of Psychiatry. We are proud to have him as our friend and colleague.

Harold I. Kaplan, M.D.
Benjamin J. Sadock, M.D.

November 1995
New York University Medical Center

# Contents

# 1

## Diagnosis and Classification in Psychiatry

### I. General introduction

A mental disorder is an illness with psychological or behavioral manifestations associated with impaired functioning due to a biological, social, psychological, genetic, physical, or chemical disturbance. It is measured in terms of deviation from some normative concept. Each illness has characteristic signs and symptoms.

Psychiatric disorders are classified according to the fourth edition of the American Psychiatric Association's *Diagnostic and Statistical Manual of Mental Disorders* (DSM-IV). Over 200 illnesses are so classified. The official DSM-IV classification and code numbers (which are used on medical reports and insurance forms) are printed on the front and back pages of this handbook.

The DSM-IV diagnostic system attempts to be reliable (i.e., different observers should obtain the same results) and valid (i.e., it should measure what it is supposed to, e.g., patients diagnosed with schizophrenia really are schizophrenic). DSM-IV uses a descriptive approach, and the characteristic signs and symptoms of each disorder should be present before diagnosis is made. The use of specific criteria increases the reliability of the diagnostic process among clinicians.

In addition to the DSM-IV classification, mental disorders are broadly described as psychotic, neurotic, functional, and organic:

**Psychotic**—loss of reality testing with delusions and hallucinations, e.g., schizophrenia.

**Neurotic**—no loss of reality testing; based on mainly intrapsychic conflicts or life events that cause anxiety; appears as a symptom such as obsession, phobia, compulsion.

**Functional**—no known structural damage or clear-cut etiological factor to account for impairment.

**Organic**—illness caused by a specific agent that causes structural change in the brain; usually associated with cognitive impairment, delirium, or dementia, e.g., Pick's disease. The term "organic" is not used in DSM-IV because it implies that some mental disorders do not have a biological component; however, it still remains in common use.

### II. Classification of disorders

DSM-IV lists 17 major categories of mental disorders; they are defined and classified below.

#### A. Disorders usually first diagnosed in infancy, childhood, or adolescence

1. **Mental retardation.**  Abnormal intellectual functioning; onset during development period; associated with impaired maturation, learning, and social maladjustment; classified according to intelligence quotient (I.Q.) as **mild** (50–55 to 70), **moderate** (35–40 to 50–55), **severe** (20–25 to 35–40), or **profound** (below 20–25).

2. **Learning disorders.**  Maturational deficits in development associated with difficulty in acquiring specific skills in **mathematics**, **writing**, and **reading**.

3. **Motor skills disorder.**  Impairments in the development of motor coordination (called **developmental coordination disorder**). Children with the disorder are often clumsy and uncoordinated.

4. **Communication disorders.**  Developmental impairment resulting in difficulty in producing age-appropriate sentences (**expressive language disorder**), difficulty in using and understanding words (**mixed receptive-expressive language disorder**), difficulty in making expected speech sounds (**phonological disorder**), and disturbances in fluency, rate, and rhythm of speech (**stuttering**).

5. **Pervasive developmental disorders.**  Characterized by autistic, atypical withdrawn behavior, gross immaturity, inadequate development, and failure to develop separate identity from mother; divided into **autistic disorder** (stereotyped behavior usually without speech), **Rett's disorder** (loss of speech and motor skills with decreased head growth), **childhood disintegrative disorder** (loss of acquired speech and motor skills before age 10), **Asperger's disorder** (stereotyped behavior with some ability to communicate), and a **not otherwise specified** (NOS) type.

6. **Attention-deficit and disruptive behavior disorders.**  Characterized by inattention, overaggressiveness, delinquency, destructiveness, hostility, feelings of rejection, negativism, or impulsiveness. Patients usually have no consistent parental discipline or acceptance. Divided into **attention-deficit/hyperactivity disorder** (poor attention span, impulsiveness), **conduct disorder** (delinquency), and **oppositional defiant disorder** (negativism).

7. **Feeding and eating disorders of infancy or early childhood.**  Characterized by disturbed or bizarre feeding and eating habits that usually begin in childhood or adolescence and continue into adulthood. Divided into **pica** (eating nonnutritional substances) and **rumination disorder** (regurgitation).

8. **Tic disorders.**  Characterized by sudden involuntary, recurrent, stereotyped motor movement or vocal sounds. Divided into **Tourette's disorder** (vocal tic and coprolalia), **chronic motor or vocal tic disorder**, and **transient tic disorder**.

9. **Elimination disorders.**  Inability to maintain bowel control (**encopresis**) or bladder control (**enuresis**) because of physiological or psychological immaturity.

10. **Other disorders of infancy, childhood, or adolescence.**  **Selective mutism** (voluntary refusal to speak), **reactive attachment disorder of infancy or early childhood** (severe impairment of ability to relate,

beginning before age 5), **stereotypic movement disorder** (thumb sucking, nail biting, skin picking), and **separation anxiety disorder** (cannot separate from home because of anxiety).

**B. Delirium, dementia, and amnestic and other cognitive disorders.** Disorders characterized by change in brain structure and function resulting in impaired learning, orientation, judgment, memory, and intellectual functions.

**1. Delirium.** Marked by short-term confusion and changes in cognition. There are several causes: a **general medical condition**, e.g., infection, **substance-induced**, e.g., cocaine, opioids, phencyclidine (PCP), **multiple etiologies**, e.g., head trauma and kidney disease, and **delirium NOS**, e.g., sleep deprivation.

**2. Dementia.** Marked by severe impairment in memory, judgment, orientation, and cognition. **Dementia of the Alzheimer's type**—usually occurs in persons over 65 and is manifested by progressive intellectual disorientation and dementia, delusions, or depression; **vascular dementia**—caused by vessel thrombosis or hemorrhage; caused by **other medical conditions,** e.g., human immunodeficiency virus (HIV) disease, head trauma; and miscellaneous group, e.g., Pick's disease, Jakob-Creutzfeldt disease (caused by slow-growing transmittable virus); also may be caused by toxin or medication (**substance-induced**), e.g., gasoline fumes, atropine, or **multiple etiologies** and **NOS.**

**3. Amnestic disorder.** Marked by memory impairment and forgetfulness. Caused by **medical condition** (hypoxia), toxin, or medication, e.g., marijuana, diazepam.

**C. Mental disorders due to a general medical condition.** Signs and symptoms of psychiatric disorders that occur as a direct result of medical disease. Includes disorders caused by syphilis, encephalitis, abscess, cardiovascular disease or trauma, epilepsy, intracranial neoplasm, endocrine disorders, pellagra, avitaminosis, systemic infection (e.g., typhoid, malaria), and degenerative central nervous system (CNS) diseases (e.g., multiple sclerosis). May produce **catatonic disorder,** e.g., immobility from stroke, or **personality change,** e.g., due to brain tumor. Also may produce delirium, dementia, amnestic disorder, psychotic disorder, mood disorder, anxiety disorder, sexual dysfunction, and sleep disorder.

**D. Substance-related disorders.**

**1. Substance use disorders.** Dependence on or **abuse** of any psychoactive drug (previously called drug addiction). Covers patients addicted to or dependent on such drugs as **alcohol, nicotine** (tobacco), and **caffeine.** Patients may be dependent on or abuse opium, opium alkaloids, and their derivatives; synthetic analgesics with morphinelike effects, such as PCP; barbiturates; other hypnotics, sedatives, or anxiolytics; **cocaine;** *Cannabis sativa* (hashish, marijuana); psychostimulants, such as **amphetamines; hallucinogens;** and **inhalants.**

**2. Substance-induced disorders.** Psychoactive drugs and other substances may cause **intoxication** and **withdrawal** syndromes in addition to **delirium, persisting dementia, persisting amnestic disorder, psy-**

chotic disorder, mood disorder, anxiety disorder, sexual dysfunction, and sleep disorder.

3. **Alcohol-related disorders.** Subclass of substance-related disorders that includes **alcohol intoxication** (simple drunkenness), **intoxication delirium** (from being drunk for several days), **alcohol withdrawal**, **withdrawal delirium** (includes delirium tremens [DTs]), **alcohol-induced psychotic disorder** (includes alcohol hallucinosis—differentiated from DTs by clear sensorium), **alcohol-induced persisting amnestic disorder** (Korsakoff's syndrome—often preceded by Wernicke's encephalopathy, a neurological condition of ataxia, ophthalmoplegia, and confusion, or may coexist [Wernicke-Korsakoff syndrome]), and **alcohol-induced persisting dementia** (differentiated from Wernicke's and Korsakoff's syndromes by multiple cognitive deficits). **Mood disorder**, **anxiety disorder**, and **sleep disorder** induced by alcohol may also occur.

E. **Schizophrenia and other psychotic disorders.** Covers disorders manifested by disturbances of thinking and misinterpretation of reality, often with delusions and hallucinations.

1. **Schizophrenia.** Characterized by changes in affect (ambivalent, constricted, and inappropriate responsiveness, loss of empathy with others), behavior (withdrawn, aggressive, bizarre), and thinking (distortion of reality, sometimes with delusions and hallucinations). Schizophrenia includes five types: (1) **disorganized** (hebephrenic) **type**— disorganized thinking, giggling, shallow and inappropriate affect, silly and regressive behavior and mannerisms, frequent somatic complaints, and occasional transient and unorganized delusions and hallucinations; (2) **catatonic type**—the excited subtype is characterized by excessive and sometimes violent motor activity, and the withdrawn subtype is characterized by generalized inhibition, stupor, mutism, negativism, waxy flexibility, and in some cases a vegetative state; (3) **paranoid type**—schizophrenia characterized by persecutory or grandiose delusions and sometimes by hallucinations or excessive religiosity, and the patient is often hostile and aggressive; (4) **undifferentiated type**— disorganized behavior with prominent delusions and hallucinations; and (5) **residual type**—patients with signs of schizophrenia, after a psychotic schizophrenic episode, who are no longer psychotic. (**Postpsychotic depressive disorder of schizophrenia** can occur during the residual phase.)

2. **Delusional (paranoid) disorder.** Psychotic disorder in which there are persistent delusions, e.g., **erotomanic, grandiose, jealous, persecutory, somatic, unspecified.** Paranoia is a rare condition characterized by the gradual development of an elaborate delusional system with grandiose ideas; it has a chronic course; the rest of the personality remains intact.

3. **Brief psychotic disorder.** Psychotic disorder of less than 4 weeks' duration brought on by an external stressor.

4. **Schizophreniform disorder.** Similar to schizophrenia with delusions, hallucinations, and incoherence but that lasts less than 6 months.

5. **Schizoaffective disorder.** Characterized by a mixture of schizophrenic symptoms and pronounced elation (**bipolar type**) or depression (**depressive type**).

6 **Shared psychotic disorder.** Same delusion occurs in two persons, one of whom is less intelligent or more dependent on the other (also known as shared paranoid disorder, *folie à deux*).

7. **Psychotic disorder due to a general medical condition.** Hallucinations or delusions that result from medical illness, e.g., temporal lobe epilepsy, avitaminosis, meningitis.

8. **Substance-induced psychotic disorder.** Symptoms of psychosis caused by psychoactive or other substances, e.g., hallucinogens, cocaine.

9. **Psychotic disorder NOS.** (Also known as atypical psychosis.) Psychotic features that are related to (1) a specific culture (*koro*—found in South and East Asia, fear of shrinking penis), (2) a certain time or event (postpartum psychosis—48–72 hours after childbirth), or (3) a unique set of symptoms (Capgras's syndrome—patients think they have a double).

F. **Mood disorders.** (Previously called affective disorders.) Characterized by a disorder of depression that dominates the patient's mental life and is responsible for diminished function. Mood disorders may be caused by a **medical condition**, or by psychoactive drugs (cocaine) or medication (antineoplastic agents, reserpine).

1. **Bipolar disorders.** Marked by severe mood swings between depression and elation and by remission and recurrence. **Bipolar I**—full manic or mixed episode, usually with major depressive episode; **bipolar II**—major depressive episode and hypomanic episode (less intense than mania) without manic or mixed episode; **cyclothymic disorder**—less severe type of bipolar disorder.

2. **Depressive disorders.** Major depressive disorder—severely depressed mood, mental and motor retardation, apprehension, uneasiness, perplexity, agitation, guilty feelings, suicidal ideation, usually recurrent. **Dysthymic disorder**—less severe form of depression usually caused by identifiable event or loss (also called depressive neurosis). **Postpartum** depression occurs within 1 month after childbirth. **Seasonal pattern** depression (also called seasonal affective disorder [SAD]) occurs most often during winter months.

G. **Anxiety disorders.** Characterized by massive and persistent anxiety (**generalized anxiety disorder**), often to the point of panic (**panic disorder**) and fears of going outside the home (**agoraphobia**); fear of specific situations or objects (**specific phobia**) or of performance and public speaking (**social phobia**); involuntary and persistent intrusions of thoughts, desires, urges, or actions (**obsessive-compulsive disorder**). Includes **posttraumatic stress disorder** (PTSD)—follows extraordinary life stress (war, catastrophe) and characterized by anxiety, nightmares, agitation, and sometimes depression; **acute stress disorder** is similar to PTSD but lasts for 4 weeks or less. May also be due to (1) a **medical condition,** e.g., hyperthyroidism, or (2) a **substance,** e.g., cocaine.

**H. Somatoform disorders.** Marked by preoccupation with the body and fears of disease. Classified into **somatization disorder**—multiple somatic complaints without organic pathology; **conversion disorder** (hysteria, Briquet's syndrome)—disorder in which the special senses or voluntary nervous system is affected, causing blindness, deafness, anosmia, anesthesias, paresthesias, paralysis, ataxias, akinesias, or dyskinesias; patients often show inappropriate lack of concern and may derive some benefits from their actions; **hypochondriasis** (hypochondriacal neurosis)—condition marked by preoccupation with the body and persistent fears of presumed disease; **pain disorder**—preoccupation with pain in which psychological factors play a part; **body dysmorphic disorder**—unrealistic concern that part of the body is deformed.

**I. Factitious disorders.** Characterized by the intentional production or feigning of psychological symptoms, physical symptoms, or both to assume sick role (also called Munchausen's syndrome).

**J. Dissociative disorders.** Characterized by sudden, temporary change in consciousness or identity. **Dissociative** (psychogenic) **amnesia**—loss of memory without organic cause; **dissociative** (psychogenic) **fugue**—unexpected wandering from home; **dissociative identity disorder** (multiple personality disorder)—person has two or more separate identities; **depersonalization disorder**—feeling that things are unreal.

**K. Sexual and gender identity disorders.** Divided into paraphilias, gender identity disorders, and sexual dysfunctions. **Paraphilias** cover persons whose sexual interests are primarily directed toward objects rather than people, toward sexual acts not usually associated with coitus, or toward coitus performed under bizarre circumstances. Included are **exhibitionism, fetishism, frotteurism, pedophilia, sexual masochism, sexual sadism, transvestic fetishism** (cross-dressing), and **voyeurism**.

Sexual dysfunctions cover disorders of **desire (hypoactive sexual desire disorder, sexual aversion disorder), arousal (female sexual arousal disorder**, i.e., anorgasmia, **male erectile disorder**, i.e., impotence), **orgasm (female orgasmic disorder**, i.e., anorgasmia, **male orgasmic disorder**, i.e., delayed or retarded ejaculation, **premature ejaculation**), and **sexual pain (dyspareunia, vaginismus)**. Sexual dysfunction may be due to a **medical condition** (multiple sclerosis) or **substance abuse** (amphetamine).

Gender identity disorders (including transsexualism) are characterized by persistent discomfort with one's biological sex and the desire to lose one's sex characteristics, e.g., castration.

**L. Eating disorders.** Characterized by marked disturbance in eating behavior. Includes **anorexia nervosa** (loss of body weight, refusal to eat) and **bulimia nervosa** (binge eating with or without vomiting).

**M. Sleep disorders.** Covers (1) **dyssomnias,** in which the person has sleep problems, cannot fall asleep (**insomnia**), or sleeps too much (**hypersomnia**); (2) **parasomnias,** such as **nightmares, sleepwalking,** or **sleep terror disorder** (person wakes up in an immobilized state of terror); (3) **narcolepsy** (sleep attacks with loss of muscle tone [cataplexy]); (4) **breathing-related sleep disorders** (snoring, apnea); and (5) **circadian rhythm sleep disorder**

(daytime sleepiness, jetlag). Sleep disorders can also be caused by **medical disease**, e.g., Parkinson's disease, and **substance** abuse, e.g., alcoholism.

N. **Impulse-control disorders (not elsewhere classified).** Covers disorders in which persons cannot control impulses and act out. Subtypes include **intermittent explosive disorder** (aggression), **kleptomania** (stealing), **pyromania** (fire setting), **trichotillomania** (hair pulling), and **pathological gambling**.

O. **Adjustment disorder.** Maladaptive reaction to a clearly defined life stress. Divided into subtypes depending on symptoms—**with anxiety, depressed mood, mixed anxiety and depressed mood, disturbance of conduct,** and **mixed disturbance of emotions and conduct**.

P. **Personality disorder.** Disorders characterized by deeply ingrained, generally lifelong maladaptive patterns of behavior that are usually recognizable at adolescence or earlier.

1. **Paranoid personality disorder.** Characterized by unwarranted suspicion, hypersensitivity, jealousy, envy, rigidity, excessive self-importance, and a tendency to blame and ascribe evil motives to others.

2. **Schizoid personality disorder.** Characterized by shyness, oversensitivity, seclusiveness, avoidance of close or competitive relationships, eccentricity, no loss of capacity to recognize reality, daydreaming, and an inability to express hostility and aggression.

3. **Schizotypal personality disorder.** Similar to schizoid, but the person exhibits slight losses of reality testing and odd beliefs and is aloof and withdrawn.

4. **Obsessive-compulsive personality disorder.** Characterized by excessive concern with conformity and standards of conscience; patient may be rigid, overconscientious, overdutiful, overinhibited, and unable to relax. (Three Ps—punctual, parsimonious, precise.)

5. **Histrionic personality disorder.** Characterized by emotional instability, excitability, overreactivity, vanity, immaturity, dependency, and self-dramatization that is attention-seeking and seductive.

6. **Avoidant personality disorder.** Characterized by low energy, easy fatigability, lack of enthusiasm, inability to enjoy life, and oversensitivity to stress.

7. **Antisocial personality disorder.** Covers persons in conflict with society. Persons are incapable of loyalty; are selfish, callous, irresponsible, impulsive, and unable to feel guilt or learn from experience; have a low level of frustration tolerance; and have a tendency to blame others.

8. **Narcissistic personality disorder.** Characterized by grandiose feelings, sense of entitlement, lack of empathy, envy, manipulativeness, and need for attention and admiration.

9. **Borderline personality disorder.** Characterized by instability, impulsiveness, chaotic sexuality, suicidal acts, self-mutilation, identity problems, and feelings of emptiness and boredom.

10. **Dependent personality disorder.** Characterized by passive and submissive behavior; person is unsure of himself or herself and becomes entirely dependent on others.

**Q. Other conditions that may be a focus of clinical attention.** Includes conditions in which there is no mental disorder, but the problem is the focus of diagnosis or treatment.

1. **Psychological factors affecting physical condition.** Disorders characterized by physical symptoms caused or affected by emotional factors; usually involve a single organ system with autonomic nervous system control or input. Examples are atopic dermatitis, backache, bronchial asthma, hypertension, migraine, ulcer, irritable colon, and colitis.

2. **Medication-induced movement disorders.** Disorders caused by medications, especially dopamine receptor antagonists, e.g., chlorpromazine (Thorazine). Includes **parkinsonism, neuroleptic malignant syndrome** (muscle rigidity, hypothermia), **acute dystonia** (muscle spasm), **acute akathisia** (restlessness), **tardive dyskinesia** (choreiform movements), and **postural tremor.**

3. **Relational problems.** Impaired social interaction within a relational unit. Includes **parent-child problem**, spouse or **partner problem,** and **sibling problem.** May also result when one member is mentally or physically ill, and the other is stressed as a result.

4. **Problems related to abuse or neglect.** Includes **physical abuse** and **sexual abuse** of children and adults.

**R. Additional conditions that may be a focus of clinical attention.** Conditions in which persons have problems not severe enough to warrant a psychiatric diagnosis but that interfere with functioning. Classified into **adult** and **child or adolescent antisocial behavior** (repeated criminal acts), **borderline intellectual functioning** (I.Q. 71–84), **malingering** (voluntary production of symptoms), **noncompliance with treatment, occupational** or **academic problem, phase of life problem** (parenthood, unemployment), **bereavement, age-related cognitive decline** (normal forgetfulness of old age), **identity problem** (career choice, sexual orientation), **religious or spiritual problem**, and **acculturation problem** (immigration).

**S. Other categories.** In addition to the diagnostic categories listed above, other categories of illness are listed in DSM-IV that require further study before becoming an official part of DSM. Those include the following:

1. **Postconcussional disorder.** Cognitive impairment, headache, sleep problems, dizziness, change in personality occurring after head injury.

2. **Mild neurocognitive disorder.** Disturbances in memory, comprehension, attention as a result of medical disease, e.g., electrolyte imbalance, hypothyroidism, early stages of multiple sclerosis.

3. **Caffeine withdrawal.** Fatigue, depression, anxiety after cessation of coffee intake.

4. **Postpsychotic depressive disorder of schizophrenia.** A depressive episode, which may be prolonged, arising in the aftermath of a schizophrenic illness.

5. **Simple deteriorative disorder (simple schizophrenia).** Characterized by oddities of conduct, inability to meet demands of society, blunting of affect, loss of volition, and social impoverishment. Delusions and hallucinations are not evident. See Chapter 7.

6. **Minor depressive disorder, recurrent brief depressive disorder, and premenstrual dysphoric disorder.** **Minor depressive disorder** is associated with mild symptoms, such as worry and overconcern with minor autonomic symptoms (tremor and palpitations). **Recurrent brief depressive disorder** is characterized by recurrent episodes of depression, each of which lasts less than 2 weeks (typically 2–3 days) and each of which ends with complete recovery. **Premenstrual dysphoric disorder** occurs 1 week before menses (luteal phase) with depressed mood, anxiety, irritability, lethargy, sleep disturbances. See Chapter 9.

7. **Mixed anxiety-depressive disorder.** Characterized by symptoms of both anxiety and depression, neither of which predominates (sometimes called neurasthenia).

8. **Factitious disorder by proxy.** Also known as Munchausen syndrome by proxy; parents feign illness in their children. See Chapter 11.

9. **Dissociative trance disorder.** Marked by temporary loss of sense of personal identity and awareness of the surroundings; patient acts as if taken over by another personality, spirit, or force. See Chapter 12.

10. **Binge-eating disorder.** Variant of bulimia nervosa, characterized by recurrent episodes of binge eating without self-induced vomiting and laxative abuse.

11. **Depressive personality disorder and passive-aggressive personality disorder.** These personality disorders are classified in the NOS category of personality disorders. See Chapter 18.

---

*For more detailed discussion of this topic, see Classification of Mental Disorders, Chap 11, pp 671–704 in CTP/VI.*

# 2

## Psychiatric Examination: History, Mental Status, and Clinical Signs and Symptoms

### I. General introduction

Patient interviewing is the core skill in medicine and psychiatry, and communication between doctor and patient is the basis of good medical practice. The purpose of the interview is to (1) obtain historical perspective of the patient's life, (2) establish rapport and a therapeutic alliance, (3) develop mutual trust and confidence, (4) understand present functioning, (5) make a diagnosis, and (6) establish a treatment plan.

### II. Clinical interview techniques

A. Arrange for a comfortable, private setting.

B. Introduce yourself, greet the patient by name, tell the purpose of the interview.

C. Put the patient at ease, establish rapport by showing personal qualities of empathy and sensitivity.

D. Do not make value judgments.

E. Carefully observe the patient's nonverbal behavior, posture, mannerisms, and physical appearance.

F. Avoid excessive note-taking.

G. Keep the interview active. Do not argue or get angry.

H. Use language consistent with the patient's intelligence.

I. Length of interview: 15–90 minutes depending on the patient's status (average time, 45–60 minutes); less time with delirious or uncooperative patients; more time with verbal, cooperative patients.

J. Use open-ended questions for neurotic, verbal, high intelligence quotient (I.Q.) patients, e.g., "Tell me more about that." Use structured and closed-ended questions when interview time is limited or the patient suffers from psychosis, delirium, or dementia (closed-ended questions usually require a yes-or-no answer). Avoid suggesting answers, e.g., "You feel depressed, don't you?" (Table 2–1). Some situations require special types of interviews (Table 2–2).

K. The psychiatric examination consists of two parts: the history and the mental status. An outline of the psychiatric history and mental status follows. Sample questions and suggestions about the findings are given. To ensure a systematic approach, all topics should eventually be covered, although the order should not be followed rigidly.

TABLE 2-1
**PROS AND CONS OF OPEN- AND CLOSED-ENDED QUESTIONS**

| Aspect | Broad, Open-Ended Questions | Narrow, Closed-Ended Questions |
|---|---|---|
| Genuineness | *High*<br>They produce spontaneous formulations | *Low*<br>They lead the patient |
| Reliability | *Low*<br>They may lead to nonreproducible answers | *High*<br>Narrow focus; but they may suggest answers |
| Precision | *Low*<br>Intent of question is vague | *High*<br>Intent of question is clear |
| Time efficiency | *Low*<br>Circumstantial elaborations | *High*<br>May invite yes/no answers |
| Completeness of diagnostic coverage | *Low*<br>Patient selects the topic | *High*<br>Interviewer selects the topic |
| Acceptance by patient | *Varies*<br>Most patients prefer expressing themselves freely; others become guarded and feel insecure | *Varies*<br>Some patients enjoy clear-cut checks; others hate to be pressed into a yes/no format |

Table from Othmer E, Othmer SC: *The Clinical Interview Using DSM-IV.* American Psychiatric Press, Washington, DC, 1989, p 48. Used with permission.

TABLE 2-2
**SPECIAL SITUATIONS AND TYPES OF INTERVIEWS**

| | |
|---|---|
| **Withdrawn patient** | Be active, structure interview. Pay attention to nonverbal clues, body movements. Change subject if patient has difficulty in discussing certain areas. |
| **Family interview** | Focus attention on identified patient's problem. Ask how each member reacts—angry, interested, frightened, anxious, who wants to help. |
| **Depression** | Elicit suicidal ideation if present; does patient have a plan? Try to raise self-esteem by commenting positively on accomplishments. |
| **Aggressive patient** | Do not be close in closed room. Sit near door for quick exit. Have security guard nearby or in room. Set limits. If patient seems too agitated, terminate interview immediately. |
| **Psychosomatic patient** | Do not discuss somatic symptoms as "in your head." Assure patient that complaint is "real." |
| **Delusional patient** | Do not challenge delusions directly; you may tell patients that you do not agree with their thinking but that you understand their belief system. |
| **Mania** | Try to set limits. Tell patient you need specific information, e.g., who is in your family, and later you will talk about other areas. Be firm but not belligerent. |
| **Drug-assisted interview** | 10% sodium amobarbital (Amytal) intravenously at 1 mL/minute. After 150–500 mg, patient gets drowsy and is willing to answer queries. Used in catatonia, mutism, amnesia. Patient confusion suggests an organic condition. Benzodiazepines, e.g., diazepam (Valium), may also be used to induce narcosis. |

## III. Psychiatric history

The psychiatric history is the chronological story of the patient's life from birth to present (also called anamnesis).

| Topics | Questions/Comments |
|---|---|
| **Identifying data:** Name, age, race, sex, marital status, religion, education, address, phone number, occupation, source of referral, source of information if patient cannot cooperate. | This may be recorded while writing up the interview. |
| **Chief complaint (CC):** Brief statement in patient's own words of why patient is in the hospital or is being seen in consultation. | "Why are you coming to see a psychiatrist?" "What brought you to the hospital?" "What seems to be the problem?" Record answers verbatim. |
| **History of present illness (HPI):** Development of symptoms from time of onset to present; relation of life events, conflicts, stressors; drugs; change from previous level of functioning. | Record in patient's own words as much as possible. Get history of previous hospitalizations and treatment. |
| **Previous psychiatric and medical disorders:** Psychiatric disorders; psychosomatic, medical, neurological illnesses (e.g., craniocerebral trauma, convulsions). | Ascertain extent of illness, treatment, medications, outcomes, hospitals, doctors. Determine whether illness serves some additional purpose (secondary gain). |
| **Personal history:**<br>  **Birth and infancy** | To the extent known by the patient, ascertain mother's pregnancy and delivery, planned or unwanted pregnancy, developmental landmarks—standing, walking, talking, temperament. |
|   **Childhood** | Feeding habits, toilet training, personality (shy, outgoing), general conduct and behavior, relationship with parents or caregivers, peers. Separations, nightmares, bedwetting, fears. |
|   **Adolescence** | Peer and authority relationships, school history, grades, emotional problems, drug use, age of puberty. |
|   **Adulthood** | Work history, choice of career, marital history, children, education, finances, military history, religion. |

**Sexual history:** Sexual development, masturbation, anorgasmia, impotence, premature ejaculation, paraphilia, sexual orientation, general attitudes and feelings.

"Are there or have there been any problems or concerns about your sex life?" "How did you learn about sex?"

**Family history:** Psychiatric, medical, and genetic illnesses in mother, father, siblings; age of parents and occupations; if deceased, date and cause. Feelings about each family member, finances.

Get medication history of family (medications effective in family members for similar disorders may be effective in patient). "Describe your living conditions." "Did you have your own room?"

## IV. Mental status

The mental status is a cross section of the patient's psychological life and represents the sum total of the psychiatrist's observations and impressions at the moment. It also serves for future comparison to follow the progress of the patient.

### Topics

### Questions

**General appearance:** Note appearance, gait, dress, grooming (neat or unkempt), posture, gestures, facial expressions. Does patient appear older or younger than stated age?

Introduce yourself and direct patient to take a seat. In the hospital, bring your chair to bedside, do not sit on the bed. *Suggestions:* Unkempt and disheveled in organic or medical disorder; pinpoint pupils in narcotic addiction; withdrawal and stooped posture in depression.

**Motoric behavior:** Level of activity— psychomotor agitation or psychomotor retardation—tics, tremors, automatisms, mannerisms, grimacing, stereotypes, negativism, apraxia, echopraxia, waxy flexibility; emotional appearance—anxious, tense, panicky, bewildered, sad, unhappy; voice—faint, loud, hoarse; eye contact.

You may ask about obvious mannerisms, e.g., "I notice that your hand still shakes; can you tell me about that?" *Suggestions:* Fixed posturing, odd behavior in schizophrenia. Hyperactive with stimulant (cocaine) abuse and in mania. Psychomotor retardation in depression; tremors with anxiety. Eye contact is normally made approximately half the time during the interview.

**Attitude during interview:** How patient relates to examiner—irritable, aggressive, seductive, guarded, defensive, indifferent, apathetic, cooperative, sarcastic.

Comment about attitude. "You seem irritated about something; is that an accurate observation?" *Suggestions:* Suspiciousness in paranoia; seductive in hysteria; apathetic in medical illness or dementia.

**Mood:** Steady or sustained emotional state—gloomy, tense, hopeless, ecstatic, resentful, happy, bashful, sad, exultant, elated, euphoric, depressed, apathetic, anhedonic, fearful, suicidal, grandiose, nihilistic.

"How do you feel?" "How are your spirits?" "Do you have thoughts that life is not worth living or that you want to harm yourself?" "Do you have plans to take your own life?" "Do you want to die?"
*Suggestions:* Suicidal ideas in 25% of depressives; elation in mania.

**Affect:** Feeling tone associated with idea—labile, blunt, appropriate to content, inappropriate, flat, *la belle indifférence.*

Observe nonverbal signs of emotion, body movement, facies, rhythm of voice (prosody).
*Suggestions:* Changes in affect usual with schizophrenia: loss of prosody in organic or medical disorder, catatonia.

**Speech:** Slow, fast, pressured, garrulous, spontaneous, taciturn, stammering, stuttering, slurring, staccato. Pitch, articulation, aphasia, coprolalia, echolalia, incoherent, logorrhea, mute, paucity, stilted.

Ask patient to say "Methodist Episcopalian" to test for dysarthria.
*Suggestions:* Manic patients show pressured speech; paucity of speech in depression; uneven or slurred speech in organic illness.

**Perceptual disorders:** Hallucinations—olfactory, auditory, haptic (tactile), gustatory, visual; illusions; hypnopompic or hypnagogic experiences; feelings of unreality, déjà vu, *déjà entendu,* macropsia.

"Do you ever see things or hear voices?" "Do you have strange experiences as you fall asleep or upon awakening?" "Has the world changed in any way?"
*Suggestions:* Visual hallucinations suggest schizophrenia. Tactile hallucinations suggest cocainism, delirium tremens (DTs).

**Thought content:** Delusions—persecutory (paranoid), grandiose, infidelity, somatic, sensory, thought broadcasting, thought insertion, ideas of reference, ideas of unreality, phobias, obsessions, compulsions, ambivalence, autism, dereism, blocking, suicidal or homicidal preoccupation, conflicts, nihilistic ideas, hypochondriasis, depersonalization, derealization, flight of ideas, *idée fixe,* magical thinking, neologisms.

"Do you feel people want to harm you?" "Do you have special powers?" "Is anyone trying to influence you?" "Do you have strange body sensations?" "Are there thoughts that you can't get out of your mind?" "Do you think about the end of the world?" Ask about fantasies and dreams.
*Suggestions:* Are delusions congruent with mood (grandiose delusions with elated mood) or incongruent? Mood-incongruent delusions point to schizophrenia. Illusions are common in delirium.

**Thought process:** Goal-directed ideas, loosened associations, illogical, tangential, relevant, circumstantial, rambling, ability to abstract, flight of ideas, clang associations, perseveration.

Ask meaning of proverbs to test abstraction, e.g., "People in glass houses should not throw stones." Concrete answer is, "Glass breaks." Abstract answers deal with projection, morality, criticism. Ask similarity between bird and butterfly (both alive), bread and cake (both food). *Suggestions:* Loose associations point to schizophrenia; flight of ideas, to mania; inability to abstract, to schizophrenia, brain damage.

**Sensorium:** Level of consciousness— alert, clear, confused, clouded, comatose, stuporous; orientation to time, place, person; cognition.

"What place is this?" "What is today's date?" "Do you know who I am?" "Do you know who you are?" *Suggestions:* Delirium or dementia shows clouded or wandering sensorium. Orientation to person remains intact longer than orientation to time or place.

**Memory:**
  **Remote memory**
  **(long-term memory)**

"Where were you born?" "Where did you go to school?" "Date of marriage?" "Birthdays of children?" "What were last week's newspaper headlines?" *Suggestions:* Patients with dementia of the Alzheimer's type retain remote memory longer than recent memory. Hypermnesia is seen in paranoid personality. Gaps in memory may be localized or filled in with confabulatory details.

  **Recent memory**

"Where were you yesterday?" "What did you eat at your last meal?" In organic brain disease, recent memory loss (amnesia) usually occurs before remote memory loss.

  **Immediate memory**
  **(short-term memory)**

Ask patient to repeat six digits forward, then backward (normal response). Ask patient to try to remember three nonrelated items; test patient after 5 minutes. *Suggestions:* Loss of memory occurs with organicity, dissociative disorder, conversion disorder. Anxiety can impair immediate retention and recent memory. Anterograde memory loss (amnesia) occurs after taking certain drugs, e.g., benzodiazepines.

**Concentration and calculation:** Ability to pay attention, distractibility, ability to do simple math.

Ask patient to count from 1 to 20 rapidly; do simple calculations (2 × 3, 4 × 9); do serial 7 test, i.e., subtract 7 from 100 and keep subtracting 7. "How many nickels in $1.35?"
*Suggestions:* Rule out organic cause versus anxiety or depression (pseudodementia).

**Information and intelligence:** Use of vocabulary, level of education, fund of knowledge.

"Distance from New York City to Los Angeles." "Name some vegetables." "What is the largest river in the United States?"
*Suggestions:* Check educational level to judge results. Rule out mental retardation, borderline intellectual functioning.

**Judgment:** Ability to understand relationships between facts and to draw conclusions; response in social situations.

"What is the thing to do if you find an envelope in the street that is sealed, stamped, and addressed?"
*Suggestions:* Impaired in organic brain disease, schizophrenia, borderline intellectual functioning, intoxication.

**Insight level:** Realizing that there is physical or mental problem; denial of illness, ascribing blame to outside factors; recognizing need for treatment.

"Do you think you have a problem?" "Do you need treatment?" "What are your plans for the future?"
*Suggestions:* Impaired in delirium, dementia, frontal lobe syndrome, psychosis, borderline intellectual functioning.

## V. Medical and neurological examination

Some psychiatric disorders may have an organic or medical cause, e.g., depression secondary to meningioma. Neurological or medical examination may be indicated in those situations. See Chapter 27 for laboratory tests used in psychiatry, e.g., magnetic resonance imaging.

## VI. Recording results of the history and the mental status

By the end of examination, you must be able to judge (1) presence or absence of psychosis, (2) any organic or medical disorders, and (3) whether the patient is suicidal or homicidal (in addition to diagnosis).

Record every case on an axis, which is a class of information. There are five axes in DSM-IV. Assess and comment on each axis.

**Axis I: Clinical syndromes**—list the mental disorder here, e.g., schizophrenia, bipolar disorder. Other conditions that may be a focus of clinical attention (except borderline intellectual functioning) are also listed on Axis I. (These are problems not sufficiently severe to warrant to a psychiatric diagnosis, e.g., relational problems, bereavement.)

TABLE 2–3
**GLOBAL ASSESSMENT OF FUNCTIONING (GAF) SCALE**

Consider psychological, social, and occupational functioning on a hypothetical continuum of mental health–illness. Do not include impairment in functioning due to physical (or environmental) limitations.

**Code** (**Note:** Use intermediate codes when appropriate, e.g., 45, 68, 72.)

100   **Superior functioning in a wide range of activities, life's problems never seem to get out of hand,**
91   **is sought out by others because of his or her many positive qualities. No symptoms.**

90   **Absent or minimal symptoms** (e.g., mild anxiety before an exam), **good functioning in all areas,**
|   **interested and involved in a wide range of activities, socially effective, generally satisfied with life,**
81   no more than everyday problems or concerns (e.g., an occasional argument with family members).

80   **If symptoms are present, they are transient and expectable reactions to psychosocial stressors**
|   (e.g., difficulty concentrating after family argument); **no more than slight impairment in social,**
71   **occupational, or school functioning** (e.g., temporarily falling behind in schoolwork).

70   **Some mild symptoms** (e.g., depressed mood and mild insomnia) **OR some difficulty in social,**
|   **occupational, or school functioning** (e.g., occasional truancy, or theft within the household), but
61   generally functioning pretty well, has some meaningful interpersonal relationships.

60   **Moderate symptoms** (e.g., flat affect and circumstantial speech, occasional panic attacks) **OR**
|   **moderate difficulty in social, occupational, or school functioning** (e.g., few friends, conflicts with
51   peers or coworkers).

50   **Serious symptoms** (e.g., suicidal ideation, severe obsessional rituals, frequent shoplifting) **OR any**
|   **serious impairment in social, occupational, or school functioning** (e.g., no friends, unable to keep
41   a job).

40   **Some impairment in reality testing or communication** (e.g., speech is at times illogical, obscure,
|   or irrelevant) **OR major impairment in several areas, such as work or school, family relations,**
|   **judgment, thinking, or mood** (e.g., depressed man avoids friends, neglects family, and is unable
31   to work; child frequently beats up younger children, is defiant at home, and is failing at school).

30   **Behavior is considerably influenced by delusions or hallucinations OR serious impairment in com-**
|   **munication or judgment** (e.g., sometimes incoherent, acts grossly inappropriately, suicidal preoccu-
21   pation) **OR inability to function in almost all areas** (e.g., stays in bed all day; no job, home, or friends).

20   **Some danger of hurting self or others** (e.g., suicide attempts without clear expectation of death;
|   frequently violent; manic excitement) **OR occasionally fails to maintain minimal personal hygiene**
11   (e.g., smears feces) **OR gross impairment in communication** (e.g., largely incoherent or mute).

10   **Persistent danger of severely hurting self or others** (e.g., recurrent violence) **OR persistent inability**
1   **to maintain minimal personal hygiene OR serious suicidal act with clear expectation of death.**

0   Inadequate information.

Used with permission, APA.

**Axis II: Personality disorders and mental retardation**—mental retardation and personality disorders are listed here. Defense mechanisms and personality traits may also be listed here. Diagnoses on Axis I and Axis II can coexist. The Axis I or Axis II condition that is responsible for bringing the patient to the psychiatrist or hospital is called the principal or main diagnosis.

**Axis III: Physical disorders or conditions**—if the patient has a physical disorder, e.g., cirrhosis, list that here.

**Axis IV: Psychosocial and environmental problems**—describe current stress in the patient's life: divorce, injury, death of a loved one.

**Axis V: Global assessment of functioning (GAF)**—rate the highest level of social, occupational, and psychological functioning of the patient according to Table 2–3 (GAF scale). Use the 12 months prior to the current evaluation as a reference point. Rate from 1 (lowest) to 100 (highest) or 0 (inadequate information).

A sample DSM-IV diagnosis could look like this:

| | |
|---|---|
| Axis I | Schizophrenia, catatonic type |
| Axis II | Borderline personality disorder |
| Axis III | Hypertension |
| Axis IV | Psychosocial problem: death of mother |
| Axis V | Current global assessment of functioning: 30 (behavior influenced by dementia) |

Table 2–4 shows the DSM-IV multiaxial evaluation form, which is useful as a template on which to record the diagnosis. Table 2–5 shows how to record diagnoses using a nonaxial format.

After diagnosis, there are four other areas to be covered:

1. **Psychodynamic formulation**—determine the defense mechanisms used to control anxiety and summarize psychological factors, including precipitating events that account for illness. Table 2–6 presents a glossary of defense mechanisms and coping styles.
2. **Differential diagnosis**—list other mental and physical disorders that have to be ruled out.
3. **Prognosis**—describe the course of the illness and expected outcome based on history, mental status, and good or bad prognostic factors.
4. **Treatment plan**—describe type of treatment, i.e., psychotherapy, drug therapy, behavior modification, hospitalization; counseling by psychologist, social worker, vocational guidance counselor. Assess patient's cooperativeness, reliability, judgment, insight, and intelligence and their impact on treatment.

## VII. Definitions of signs and symptoms found in mental status examination

**Abstraction:** Ability to separate a quality from an object and to think or to perform symbolically, e.g., *boat* is concrete, *sailing* is abstract; impaired in brain dysfunction, schizophrenia.

**Affect:** Subjective feeling tone that accompanies an idea or mental representation; objective behavioral component described as blunted (severely reduced), flat (absent), restricted (reduced), appropriate (harmonious), inappropriate (out of harmony), and labile (unstable); one of Bleuler's four As (impaired in schizophrenia).

**Aggression:** Hostile or angry feelings, thoughts, or actions directed toward an object or person; seen in mania, impulse-control disorders, e.g., intermittent explosive disorders.

**Agitation:** Tension state in which anxiety is manifested in psychomotor area with hyperactivity and general perturbation; seen in depression, schizophrenia, mania.

**Ambivalence:** Coexistence of opposing attitudes or emotions, e.g., love and hate, toward a given person or thing at the same time; one of Bleuler's four As (seen in schizophrenia).

**Amnesia:** Loss of memory manifested by total or partial inability to recall past experiences; seen in brain dysfunction, amnestic disorder, dissociative disorders, e.g., dissociative fugue.

TABLE 2–4
**MULTIAXIAL EVALUATION REPORT FORM**

The following form is offered as one possibility for reporting multiaxial evaluations. In some settings, this form may be used exactly as is; in other settings, the form may be adapted to satisfy special needs.

*AXIS I: Clinical Disorders*
    *Other Conditions That May Be a Focus of Clinical Attention*

Diagnostic code                        DSM-IV name

\_\_\_ \_\_\_ \_\_\_ . \_\_\_ \_\_\_      _____

\_\_\_ \_\_\_ \_\_\_ . \_\_\_ \_\_\_      _____

\_\_\_ \_\_\_ \_\_\_ . \_\_\_ \_\_\_      _____

*AXIS II: Personality Disorders*
    *Mental Retardation*

Diagnostic code                        DSM-IV name

\_\_\_ \_\_\_ \_\_\_ . \_\_\_ \_\_\_      _____

\_\_\_ \_\_\_ \_\_\_ . \_\_\_ \_\_\_      _____

*AXIS III: General Medical Conditions*

ICD-9-CM code                       ICD-9-CM name

\_\_\_ \_\_\_ \_\_\_ . \_\_\_ \_\_\_      _____

\_\_\_ \_\_\_ \_\_\_ . \_\_\_ \_\_\_      _____

\_\_\_ \_\_\_ \_\_\_ . \_\_\_ \_\_\_      _____

*AXIS IV: Psychosocial and Environmental Problems*

*Check:*
☐ **Problems with primary support group** *Specify:* _____
☐ **Problems related to the social environment** *Specify:* _____
☐ **Educational problems** *Specify:* _____
☐ **Occupational problems** *Specify:* _____
☐ **Housing problems** *Specify:* _____
☐ **Economic problems** *Specify:* _____
☐ **Problems with access to health care services** *Specify:* _____
☐ **Problems related to interaction with the legal system/crime** *Specify:* _____
☐ **Other psychosocial and environmental problems** *Specify:* _____

*AXIS V: Global Assessment of Functioning Scale*      Score: \_\_\_ \_\_\_ \_\_\_

                                              Time frame: _____

        **Anterograde (AA):** Loss of immediate, short-term memory; occurs after trauma, drug intake, transient ischemic attack.

        **Localized:** Loss of memory for an isolated event; not a total loss of memory; also referred to as **lacunar amnesia** and **patch amnesia**; seen in brain lesions, anxiety, fugue.

        **Retrograde (RA):** Loss of past, remote, long-term memory; occurs in dementia.

     **Anhedonia:** Absence of pleasure in acts that normally are pleasurable; most common symptom is depression.

     **Anxiety:** Feeling of dread, impending doom; seen in anxiety disorders, schizophrenia, mood disorders.

     **Apathy:** Lack of feeling, emotion, interest, or concern; common in depression.

TABLE 2–5
**NONAXIAL FORMAT**

Clinicians who do not wish to use the multiaxial format may simply list the appropriate diagnoses. Those choosing this option should follow the general rule of recording as many coexisting mental disorders, general medical conditions, and other factors that are relevant to the care and treatment of the individual. The principal diagnosis or the reason for visit should be listed first.

The examples listed below illustrate the reporting of diagnosis in a format that does not use the multiaxial system.

**Example 1:**
Major depressive disorder, single episode, severe without psychotic features
Alcohol abuse
Dependent personality disorder
  Frequent use of denial

**Example 2:**
Dysthymic disorder
Reading disorder
Otitis media, recurrent

**Example 3:**
Mood disorder due to hypothyroidism, with depressive features
Hypothyroidism
Chronic angle-closure glaucoma
  Histrionic personality features

**Example 4:**
Partner relational problems

Used with permission, APA.

**Aphasia:** Impaired or absent communication by speech, writing, or signs, due to dysfunction of brain centers in the dominant hemisphere.

**Ataxia:** Inability to coordinate muscles in the execution of voluntary movement; seen in cerebellar lesions, tardive dyskinesia.

**Autistic thinking:** Form of subjective thinking with total disregard of reality; one of Bleuler's four As (seen in schizophrenia).

**Automatism:** Condition in which a person engages in activity without conscious knowledge of doing so.

**Blocking:** Sudden cessation in the train of thought or in the midst of a sentence; also known as **thought deprivation**; common in schizophrenia.

**Catalepsy:** Inordinate maintenance of postures or physical attitudes; synonymous with **flexibilitas cerea** or **waxy flexibility**; seen in catatonic type of schizophrenia.

**Cataplexy:** Temporary paralysis or immobilization and collapse caused by strong emotions; part of narcolepsy.

**Catatonia:** Type of schizophrenia characterized by periods of physical rigidity, negativism, excitement, and stupor.

  **Catatonic excitement:** Marked agitation, impulsivity, and aggressive behavior.

  **Catatonic rigidity:** Rigid posturing and stereotypical behavior.

**Circumstantiality:** Thought and speech associated with unnecessary detail that is usually relevant to a question and that ultimately leads to an answer; seen in schizophrenia, obsessive-compulsive disorder.

**Clang association:** Association, i.e., relationship, based on similarity of sound, without regard for differences in meaning; common in mania.

**Clouding of consciousness:** Impairment of orientation, perception, and attention; seen in brain dysfunctions.

TABLE 2–6
## GLOSSARY OF SPECIFIC DEFENSE MECHANISMS AND COPING STYLES

**acting out**   The individual deals with emotional conflict or internal or external stressors by actions rather than reflections or feelings. This definition is broader than the original concept of the acting out of transference feelings or wishes during psychotherapy and is intended to include behavior arising both within and outside the transference relationship. Defensive acting out is not synonymous with ''bad behavior'' because it requires evidence that the behavior is related to emotional conflicts.

**affiliation**   The individual deals with emotional conflict or internal or external stressors by turning to others for help or support. This involves sharing problems with others but does not imply trying to make someone else responsible for them.

**altruism**   The individual deals with emotional conflict or internal or external stressors by dedication to meeting the needs of others. Unlike the self-sacrifice sometimes characteristic of reaction formation, the individual receives gratification either vicariously or from the response of others.

**anticipation**   The individual deals with emotional conflict or internal or external stressors by experiencing emotional reactions in advance of, or anticipating consequences of, possible future events and considering realistic, alternative responses or solutions.

**autistic fantasy**   The individual deals with emotional conflict or internal or external stressors by excessive daydreaming as a substitute for human relationships, more effective action, or problem solving.

**denial**   The individual deals with emotional conflict or internal or external stressors by refusing to acknowledge some painful aspect of external reality or subjective experience that would be apparent to others. The term *psychotic denial* is used when there is gross impairment in reality testing.

**devaluation**   The individual deals with emotional conflict or internal or external stressors by attributing exaggerated negative qualities to self or others.

**displacement**   The individual deals with emotional conflict or internal or external stressors by transferring a feeling about, or a response to, one object onto another (usually less threatening) substitute object.

**dissociation**   The individual deals with emotional conflict or internal or external stressors with a breakdown in the usually integrated functions of consciousness, memory, perception of self or the environment, or sensory/motor behavior.

**help-rejecting complaining**   The individual deals with emotional conflict or internal or external stressors by complaining or making repetitious requests for help that disguise covert feelings of hostility or reproach toward others, which are then expressed by rejecting the suggestions, advice, or help that others offer. The complaints or requests may involve physical or psychological symptoms or life problems.

**humor**   The individual deals with emotional conflict or external stressors by emphasizing the amusing or ironic aspects of the conflict or stressor.

**idealization**   The individual deals with emotional conflict or internal or external stressors by attributing exaggerated positive qualities to others.

**intellectualization**   The individual deals with emotional conflict or internal or external stressors by the excessive use of abstract thinking or the making of generalizations to control or minimize disturbing feelings.

**isolation of affect**   The individual deals with emotional conflict or internal or external stressors by the separation of ideas from the feelings originally associated with them. The individual loses touch with the feelings associated with a given idea (e.g., a traumatic event) while remaining aware of the cognitive elements of it (e.g., descriptive details).

**omnipotence**   The individual deals with emotional conflict or internal or external stressors by feeling or acting as if he or she possesses special powers or abilities and is superior to others.

**passive aggression**   The individual deals with emotional conflict or internal or external stressors by indirectly and unassertively expressing aggression toward others. There is a facade of overt compliance masking covert resistance, resentment, or hostility. Passive aggression often occurs in response to demands for independent action or performance or the lack of gratification of dependent wishes but may be adaptive for individuals in subordinate positions who have no other way to express assertiveness more overtly.

**projection**   The individual deals with emotional conflict or internal or external stressors by falsely attributing to another his or her own acceptable feelings, impulses, or thoughts.

**projective identification**   As in projection, the individual deals with emotional conflict or internal or external stressors by falsely attributing to another his or her own unacceptable feelings, impulses, or thoughts. Unlike simple projection, the individual does not fully disavow what is projected. Instead, the individual remains aware of his or her own affects or impulses but misattributes them as justifiable reactions to the other person. Not infrequently, the individual induces the very feelings in others that were first mistakenly believed to be there, making it difficult to clarify who did what to whom first.

*continued on next page*

TABLE 2–6 *(continued)*
**GLOSSARY OF SPECIFIC DEFENSE MECHANISMS AND COPING STYLES**

**rationalization**   The individual deals with emotional conflict or internal or external stressors by concealing the true motivations for his or her own thoughts, actions, or feelings through the elaboration of reassuring or self-serving but incorrect explanations.

**reaction formation**   The individual deals with emotional conflict or internal or external stressors by substituting behavior, thoughts, or feelings that are diametrically opposed to his or her own unacceptable thoughts or feelings (this usually occurs in conjunction with their repression).

**repression**   The individual deals with emotional conflict or internal or external stressors by expelling disturbing wishes, thoughts, or experiences from conscious awareness. The feeling component may remain conscious, detached from its associated ideas.

**self-assertion**   The individual deals with emotional conflict or stressors by expressing his or her feelings and thoughts directly in a way that is not coercive or manipulative.

**self-observation**   The individual deals with emotional conflict or stressors by reflecting on his or her own thoughts, feelings, motivation, and behavior, and responding appropriately.

**splitting**   The individual deals with emotional conflict or internal or external stressors by compartmentalizing opposite affect states and failing to integrate the positive and negative qualities of the self or others into cohesive images. Because ambivalent affects cannot be experienced simultaneously, more balanced views and expectations of self or others are excluded from emotional awareness. Self and object images tend to alternate between polar opposites: exclusively loving, powerful, worthy, nurturant, and kind—or exclusively bad, hateful, angry, destructive, rejecting, or worthless.

**sublimation**   The individual deals with emotional conflict or internal or external stressors by channeling potentially maladaptive feelings or impulses into socially acceptable behavior (e.g., contact sports to channel angry impulses).

**suppression**   The individual deals with emotional conflict or internal or external stressors by intentionally avoiding thinking about disturbing problems, wishes, feelings, or experiences.

**undoing**   The individual deals with emotional conflict or internal or external stressors by words or behavior designed to negate or to make amends symbolically for unacceptable thoughts, feelings, or actions.

Used with permission, APA.

**Cognition:** Quality of knowing, including perceiving, recognizing, judging, sensing, reasoning, and imagining; impaired in brain dysfunction, mental retardation, cognitive disorders.

**Coma:** Most profound degree of stupor in which all consciousness is lost and all voluntary activity ceases; organically based.

**Compulsion:** Irresistible impulse to perform an irrational act; seen in impulse-control and obsessive-compulsive disorders.

**Confabulation:** Fabrication of stories in response to questions about situations or events that are not recalled.

**Conflict:** Mental struggle that arises from simultaneous operation of opposing impulses, drives, or external (environmental) or internal demands; called *intrapsychic* when conflict is between forces within the personality, *extrapsychic* when conflict is between the self and the environment.

**Confusional state:** Disturbed orientation with respect to time, place, or person.

**Consciousness:** Awareness of one's own internal thoughts and feelings and ability to recognize external environment; impaired in brain dysfunction, delirium, and dissociative fugue and other dissociative states.

**Coprolalia:** Involuntary utterance of vulgar or obscene words; seen in Tourette's disorder.

***Déjà entendu:*** Feeling that one is hearing or perceiving what one has heard before; seen in anxiety disorders, fatigue.

**Déjà vu:** Feeling that one is seeing or experiencing what one has seen before; seen in anxiety disorders, fatigue.

**Delusion:** False belief, i.e., one not shared by others, that is firmly maintained, even though contradicted by social reality; most common in schizophrenia.

**Grandiose delusion:** Belief that one is possessed of greatness, i.e., **megalomania**; such ideas are referred to as **delusions of grandeur**; seen in schizophrenia, mania, tertiary syphilis; a variation is that someone of high social status is deeply in love with the person, usually a woman—also called **erotomania, Clérembault's syndrome,** and **delusional loving.**

**Induced delusion:** Hallucination aroused in one person by another; also called *folie á deux.*

**Infidelity delusion:** False belief that a loved one is unfaithful, e.g., **amorous paranoia.**

**Persecutory (paranoid) delusion:** Excessive or irrational suspiciousness and distrustfulness of others, characterized by systematized delusions of persecution; seen in paranoid schizophrenia.

**Somatic delusion:** Belief that patient's body or parts of the body are diseased or distorted.

**Depersonalization:** Feeling of having lost one's personal identity and of being different, strange, or unreal; part of dissociative disorders.

**Depression:** Feeling tone characterized by sadness, apathy, pessimism, and a sense of loneliness; part of major depressive and other mood disorders.

**Derealization:** Feeling of changed reality; environment is strange or unreal; common in anxiety and dissociative disorders.

**Dereism:** Mental activity not in accordance with reality, logic, or experience.

**Disorientation:** Loss of awareness of position of self in relation to space, time, or other persons; confusion.

**Distractibility:** Condition in which the patient changes from topic to topic in accordance with stimuli from within and from without; seen in mania.

**Dysarthria:** Difficulty in speech production due to incoordination of speech apparatus.

**Dyskinesia:** Any disturbance of movement.

**Echolalia:** Imitative repetition of speech of another; seen in schizophrenia.

**Echopraxia:** Imitative repetition of movements of another; sometimes seen in catatonic schizophrenia.

**Ecstasy:** State of elation beyond reason and control; trance state of overwhelming emotion, e.g., religious fervor.

**Elation:** Affect consisting of feelings of euphoria, triumph, intense self-satisfaction, or optimism.

**Euphoria:** Exaggerated feeling of physical or emotional well-being, usually of psychological origin; seen in brain dysfunctions, drug-induced and other states.

**Exaltation:** Excessively intensified sense of well-being; seen in mania.

**Fear:** Unpleasant emotional and physiological response to recognized sources of danger (to be distinguished from anxiety).

**Flight of ideas:** Rapid shifting from one topic to another; also called **topical flight**; themes can sometimes be followed; part of manic episode.

**Grandiosity:** Feelings of great importance; absurd exaggeration; seen in mania, schizophrenia.

**Hallucination:** Sensory perception for which there is no external stimulus; seen in schizophrenia, toxic psychoses.

**Auditory hallucination:** Associated with sound; most common in schizophrenia.

**Gustatory hallucination:** Associated with taste.

**Haptic hallucination:** Associated with sensation of touch; common in DTs, cocainism (cocaine intoxication).

**Hypnagogic hallucination:** Occurs upon awakening.

**Lilliputian hallucination:** Hallucinated object appears reduced in size; also called **microptic hallucination**; seen in toxic psychoses.

**Visual hallucination:** Associated with sight.

**Hypermnesia:** Exaggerated memory; ability to recall material not ordinarily available to memory process.

**Hypochondriasis:** Somatic overconcern with and morbid attention to details of body functioning; exaggeration of any symptom.

**Ideas of reference:** Incorrect interpretation of casual incidents and external events as directly referring to oneself; may become intense enough to constitute delusions.

**Ideas of unreality:** Thoughts that events are artificial, illusory, unpredictable, or do not exist; seen in schizophrenia, anxiety disorders, dissociative disorders.

*Ideé fixe:* Fixed idea; describes a compulsive drive, an obsessive idea, or a delusion.

**Illusion:** Erroneous perception; false response to a sensory stimulus; seen in schizophrenia, toxic psychoses.

**Incoherence:** Quality or state of being loose; lacking cohesion.

**Insight:** Knowledge of objective reality of a situation; person is aware of a mental problem.

**Intelligence quotient (I.Q.):** Numerical rating determined through psychological testing that indicates approximate relationship of person's mental age (MA) to chronological age (CA); expressed mathematically as I.Q. $= (MA/CA) \times 100$.

**Intoxication:** State due to recent ingestion or presence in the body of a chemical agent, causing maladaptive behavior because of its effects on the central nervous system.

**Judgment:** Ability to recognize true relation of ideas; capacity to draw correct conclusions from experience; impaired in schizophrenia, brain dysfunction.

*La belle indifférence:* Literally means beautiful indifference; condition of certain patients with conversion disorders who show an inappropriate lack of concern about their disabilities.

**Logorrhea:** Uncontrollable, excessive talking; seen in mania, schizophrenia.

**Loosening of associations:** Various disturbances of associations that render speech (and thought) inexact, vague, diffuse, unfocused; one of Bleuler's four As (seen in schizophrenia).

**Macropsia:** False perception that objects are larger than they really are; seen in drug intoxication.

**Magical thinking:** Conviction that thinking equates with doing; characterized by lack of realistic relation between cause and effect; occurs in dreams, children, primitive peoples, and patients under a variety of conditions; seen in obsessive-compulsive disorder.

**Mannerism:** Gesture or other form of expression peculiar to a given person; seen in schizophrenia.

**Memory:** Ability, process, or act of remembering or recalling; ability to reproduce what has been learned or experienced.

**Immediate (short-term) memory:** Refers to immediate retention, i.e., events of the past few moments; also known as **working memory** and **buffer memory**.

**Recent memory:** Refers to events over past few days.

**Remote (long-term) memory:** Refers to events in distant past.

**Mood:** Feeling tone, particularly as experienced internally by a person.

**Mood-congruent:** In harmony; mood-appropriate; ideas consistent with mood; common in bipolar disorder.

**Mood-incongruent:** Mood-inappropriate; ideas out of harmony with mood; common in schizophrenia.

**Mutism:** Inability to speak; common in catatonic schizophrenia, fugue states.

**Negativism:** Opposition of resistance, either covert or overt, to outside suggestions or advice; may be seen in schizophrenia.

**Neologism:** New word created by patient, which is often a blend of other words; seen in schizophrenia.

**Nihilism:** Feelings of nonexistence and hopelessness; may assume delusional proportions; common in depression.

**Obsession:** Idea, emotion, or impulse that repetitively and insistently forces itself into consciousness, although it is unwelcome; part of obsessive-compulsive disorder.

**Orientation:** Awareness of one's self in relation to time, place, or person; lost in brain dysfunction, delirium.

**Panic:** Sudden, overwhelming anxiety of such intensity that it produces terror and physiological changes.

**Paucity of speech:** Limited use of speech; seen in autistic disorder, catatonic schizophrenia, major depressive disorder.

**Perseveration:** Involuntary, excessive continuation or recurrence of a response or activity, most often verbal; seen in schizophrenia, e.g., perseverative speech.

**Phobia:** A morbid fear associated with extreme anxiety; part of specific and social phobias and agoraphobia.

**Psychomotor retardation:** Slowed psychic activity, motor activity, or both; seen in depression, catatonic schizophrenia. Opposite can also occur, i.e., psychomotor agitation.

**Stereotypy:** Constant, almost mechanical, repetition of any action; common in schizophrenia.

**Stilted speech:** Formal, stiff speech pattern.

**Stupor:** State in which a person does not react to or is unaware of the surroundings (in catatonic schizophrenic stupor the unawareness is more apparent than real); due to neurological or psychiatric disorders.

**Thought broadcasting:** Delusion about thoughts being aired to the outside world; one of Schneider's first rank symptoms (seen in schizophrenia).

**Thought disorder:** Disturbance of speech, communication, or content of thought, e.g., delusions, ideas of reference, poverty of thought, flight of ideas, perseveration, loosening of associations; can be caused by a functional mental disorder or a medical condition; characteristic of schizophrenia.

**Thought insertion:** Delusion that thoughts are placed into the mind by outside influences. One of Schneider's first rank symptoms (seen in schizophrenia).

**Tic:** Sudden involuntary muscle movement; seen in tic disorders.

**Verbigeration:** Stereotypy of seemingly meaningless repetition of words or sentences.

**Word salad:** Mixture of words and phrases that lack comprehensive meaning or logical coherence; commonly seen in schizophrenic states.

---

*For more detailed discussion of this topic, see Strauss GD: The Psychiatric Interview, History, and Mental Status Examination, Sec 9.1, p 521; Kaplan HI, Sadock BJ: Psychiatric Report, Sec 9.2, p 531; Kaplan HI, Sadock BJ: Typical Signs and Symptoms of Psychiatric Illness, Sec 9.3, p 535; Marder SR: Psychiatric Rating Scales, Sec 9.8, p 619; Yager J, Gitlin MJ: Clinical Manifestations of Psychiatric Disorders, Chap 10, p 637; Sadock BJ, Kaplan HI: Classification of Mental Disorders, Sec 11.1, p 671, in CTP/VI.*

---

# 3

## Delirium, Dementia, Amnestic and Other Cognitive Disorders, and Mental Disorders Due to Medical Conditions

### I. General introduction

Delirium, dementia, amnestic disorder, and other cognitive disorders are often grouped together as organic mental disorders. *Organic* implies brain dysfunction. In DSM-IV the disorders previously classified as organic mental disorders have been divided into three major categories: (1) delirium, dementia, and amnestic and other cognitive disorders, (2) mental disorders due to a general medical condition, and (3) substance-related disorders.

### II. Clinical evaluation

**A. History.** May be time-consuming and require information from others. Need information about premorbid condition.

**B. Physical.** Emphasize neurological system, but do not overlook other systems.

**C. Mental status.** Carefully evaluate cognition but not to the point of missing other information, especially appearance and general behavior, mood, affect, and thought content and process.

**D. Cognitive evaluation.** Screening tests by psychiatrists are nonspecific but sensitive to a wide range of impairments. Develop a routine. Suspicious findings usually warrant an extensive cognitive evaluation.

**E. Nonspecific signs of brain dysfunction**

1. Intellectual, memory, and cognitive impairment (paucity of thoughts, lack of intellectual flexibility, perseveration, poor judgment).
2. Change in personality.
3. Disinhibition (inappropriateness or exacerbation of underlying personality traits).
4. Poverty of speech with decreased vocabulary and use of clichés.
5. Prominent visual hallucinations.
6. Mood initially may be depressed, anxious, and labile, but it may progress to apathy.
7. Affect may be shallow or flat.

**F. Lab tests**

1. Psychometric assessment (psychological testing)—more sensitive to organicity; standardized; can utilize probabilities in interpretation; requires patient cooperation. Psychologist needs to be told where to focus his or her assessment.

TABLE 3-1
**DSM-IV DIAGNOSTIC CRITERIA FOR DELIRIUM DUE TO A GENERAL MEDICAL CONDITION**

A. Disturbance of consciousness (i.e., reduced clarity of awareness of the environment) with reduced ability to focus, sustain, or shift attention.
B. A change in cognition (such as memory deficit, disorientation, language disturbance) or the development of a perceptual disturbance that is not better accounted for by a preexisting, established, or evolving dementia.
C. The disturbance develops over a short period of time (usually hours to days) and tends to fluctuate during the course of the day.
D. There is evidence from the history, physical examination, or laboratory findings that the disturbance is caused by the direct physiological consequences of a general medical condition.

Used with permission, APA.

TABLE 3-2
**DSM-IV DIAGNOSTIC CRITERIA FOR SUBSTANCE INTOXICATION DELIRIUM**

A. Disturbance of consciousness (i.e., reduced clarity of awareness of the environment) with reduced ability to focus, sustain, or shift attention.
B. A change in cognition (such as memory deficit, disorientation, language disturbance) or the development of a perceptual disturbance that is not better accounted for by a preexisting, established, or evolving dementia.
C. The disturbance develops over a short period of time (usually hours to days) and tends to fluctuate during the course of the day.
D. There is evidence from the history, physical examination, or laboratory findings of either (1) or (2):
   (1) The symptoms in criteria A and B developed during substance intoxication
   (2) Medication use is etiologically related to the disturbance

Used with permission, APA.

2. Skull x-ray, electroencephalogram (EEG), computed tomography (CT), magnetic resonance imaging (MRI), lumbar puncture, brain scan, and angiography, as indicated.

## III. Delirium

**A. Definition.**  Acute reversible mental disorder characterized by confusion and some impairment of consciousness; generally associated with emotional lability, hallucinations or illusions, and inappropriate, impulsive, irrational, or violent behavior.

**B. Diagnosis, signs, and symptoms.**  Delirium is diagnosed according to etiology: delirium due to a medical condition (Table 3–1), substance-induced delirium (substance intoxication delirium [Table 3–2] and withdrawal delirium), and delirium not otherwise specified (NOS).

**C. Epidemiology.**  Common among hospitalized patients—about 10% in all hospitalized patients, 20% in postburn patients, 30% in intensive care unit (ICU) patients, 30% in hospitalized acquired immune deficiency syndrome (AIDS) patients. Very young and elderly patients are more susceptible to delirium. Patients with a history of delirium or brain damage are more likely to have an episode of delirium than the general population.

**D. Etiology.**  There are multiple causes, including infection, fever, metabolic imbalance, hepatic or renal disease, endocrine dysfunctions, thiamine deficiency, substance intoxication and withdrawal, postoperative states, severe blood loss, cardiac arrhythmias and heart failure, hypertensive encephalopathy, head trauma, seizures, side effects of many medications, certain focal brain lesions (right parietal lobe and medial surface of occipital lobe), and sensory deprivation, e.g., blindness, deafness. Delirium may be thought of as a common pathway for any brain insult.

**E. Lab tests.**   Delirium is a medical emergency that demands identification of the cause as rapidly as possible. If the likely cause is not apparent, then a complete medical workup should be immediate. Even if an apparent cause is identified, there may be multiple causes. The workup should include vital signs, complete blood count (CBC) with differential, erythrocyte sedimentation rate (ESR), complete blood chemistries, liver and renal function tests, urinalysis, urine toxicology, electrocardiogram (EKG), chest x-ray, CT scan of head, and lumbar puncture (if indicated). The EEG often shows diffuse slowing throughout or focal areas of hyperactivity.

**F. Differential diagnosis**

   1. **Dementia.**   See Table 3–3.
   2. **Schizophrenia and mania.**   Usually do not have the rapidly fluctuating course of delirium, nor do they impair the level of consciousness or significantly impair cognition.
   3. **Dissociative disorders.**   May show spotty amnesia but lack the global cognitive impairment and abnormal psychomotor and sleep patterns of delirium.

**G. Course and prognosis.**   The course is usually rapid. The delirium may spontaneously clear. Delirium may also rapidly progress to death or permanent dementia, if untreated. If the underlying cause is treated, there may be a rapid recovery. Some residual deficits may persist, however.

TABLE 3–3
**CLINICAL DIFFERENTIATION OF DELIRIUM AND DEMENTIA**

|  | Delirium | Dementia |
| --- | --- | --- |
| History | Acute disease | Chronic disease |
| Onset | Rapid | Insidious (usually) |
| Duration | Days–weeks | Months–years |
| Course | Fluctuating | Chronically progressive |
| Level of consciousness | Fluctuating | Normal |
| Orientation | Impaired, at least periodically | Intact initially |
| Affect | Anxious, irritable | Labile but not usually anxious |
| Thinking | Often disordered | Decreased amount |
| Memory | Recent memory is markedly impaired | Both recent and remote are impaired |
| Perception | Hallucinations common (especially visual) | Hallucinations less common (except sundowning) |
| Psychomotor | Retarded, agitated, or mixed | Normal |
| Sleep | Disrupted sleep-wake cycle | Less disruption of sleep-wake cycle |
| Attention and awareness | Prominently impaired | Less impaired |
| Reversibility | Often reversible | Majority not reversible |

*Note:* Demented patients are more susceptible to delirium, and delirium superimposed on dementia is common.

**H. Treatment.** Identify the cause and reverse it. Correct metabolic abnormalities; ensure proper hydration, electrolyte balances, and nutrition; optimize the sensory environment for the patient, e.g., decreased stimuli for a delirium tremens patient and appropriate increased stimulation for a patient delirious from sensory deprivation. Low doses of a high-potency antipsychotic may be used for agitation, e.g., haloperidol (Haldol) 2–5 mg orally or intramuscularly every 4 hours as needed. Benzodiazepines, e.g., lorazepam (Ativan) 1–2 mg orally or intramuscularly every 4 hours as needed, can also be used for agitation or insomnia, especially in a patient who may be at risk for seizures, e.g., a patient suffering from alcohol withdrawal or withdrawal from sedative-hypnotics.

## IV. Dementia

**A. Definition.** Mental disorder characterized by general impairment in intellectual functioning, frequently characterized by failing memory, difficulty with calculations (acalculia), distractibility, alterations in mood and affect, impairment in judgment and abstraction, reduced facility with language, and disturbance of orientation. Although generally irreversible because of underlying progressive degenerative brain disease, dementia may be reversible if the cause can be treated.

**B. Diagnosis, signs, and symptoms.** The major defects in dementia involve orientation, memory, perception, intellectual functioning, and reasoning. There can be marked change in personality, affect, and behavior.

Dementia is diagnosed according to its etiology: dementia of the Alzheimer's type (DAT), vascular dementia, dementia due to other general medical conditions (Table 3–4), substance-induced persisting dementia, dementia due to multiple etiologies, and dementia NOS.

TABLE 3–4
**DIAGNOSTIC CRITERIA FOR DEMENTIA DUE TO OTHER GENERAL MEDICAL CONDITIONS**

A. The development of multiple cognitive deficits manifested by both
   1. Memory impairment (impaired ability to learn new information or to recall previously learned information)
   2. One (or more) of the following cognitive disturbances:
      a. Aphasia (language disturbance)
      b. Apraxia (impaired ability to carry out motor activities despite intact motor function)
      c. Agnosia (failure to recognize or identify objects despite intact sensory function)
      d. Disturbance in executive functioning (i.e., planning, organizing, sequencing, abstracting)
B. The cognitive deficits in criteria A1 and A2 each cause significant impairment in social or occupational functioning and represent a significant decline from a previous level of functioning.
C. There is evidence from the history, physical examination, or laboratory findings that the disturbance is the direct physiological consequence of one of the general medical conditions listed below.
D. The deficits do not occur exclusively during the course of a delirium.

**Dementia due to HIV disease**
**Dementia due to head trauma**
**Dementia due to Parkinson's disease**
**Dementia due to Huntington's disease**
**Dementia due to Pick's disease**
**Dementia due to Creutzfeldt-Jakob disease**
**Dementia due to . . .** *(indicate the general medical condition not listed above)*
   For example, normal-pressure hydrocephalus, hypothyroidism, brain tumor, vitamin B$_{12}$ deficiency, intracranial radiation
**Coding note:** Also code the general medical condition on Axis III.

Used with permission, APA.

TABLE 3–5
**ETIOLOGIES OF DEMENTIA**

| | |
|---|---|
| **Tumor** | **Physiological** |
| Primary cerebral[a] | Epilepsy[a] |
| **Trauma** | Normal pressure hydrocephalus[a] |
| Hematomas[a] | **Metabolic** |
| Posttraumatic dementia[a] | Vitamin deficiencies[a] |
| **Infection (chronic)** | Chronic metabolic disturbances[a'] |
| Metastatic[a] | Chronic anoxic states[a] |
| Syphilis | Chronic endocrinopathies[a] |
| Creutzfeldt-Jakob disease[b] | **Degenerative dementias** |
| AIDS dementia complex[c] | Alzheimer's disease[b] |
| **Cardiac/vascular** | Pick's disease (dementias of frontal lobe type)[b] |
| Single infarction[a] | Parkinson's disease[a] |
| Multiple infarction[b] | Progressive supranuclear palsy[c] |
| Large infarction | Idiopathic cerebral ferrocalcinosis (Fahr's disease)[c] |
| Lacunar infarction | Wilson's disease[a] |
| Binswanger's disease (subcortical | **Demyelinating** |
| arteriosclerotic encephalopathies) | Multiple sclerosis[c] |
| Hemodynamic type[a] | **Drugs and toxins** |
| **Congenital/hereditary** | Alcohol[a] |
| Huntington's disease[c] | Heavy metals[a] |
| Metachromatic leukodystrophy[c] | Carbon monoxide poisoning[a] |
| **Primary psychiatric** | Medications[a] |
| Pseudodementia[c] | Irradiation[a] |

[a]Variable or mixed pattern.
[b]Predominantly cortical pattern.
[c]Predominantly subcortical pattern.

Table from Caine ED, Grossman H, Lyness JM: Delirium, dementia, and amnestic and other cognitive disorders and mental disorders due to a general medical condition. In *Comprehensive Textbook of Psychiatry*, ed 6, HI Kaplan, BJ Sadock, eds, Williams & Wilkins, Baltimore, 1995, p 734.

C. **Epidemiology.**   Primarily a syndrome of the elderly. About 5% of Americans over the age of 65 have severe dementia, and 15% have mild dementia. About 20% of Americans over the age of 80 have severe dementia. Increasing age is the most important risk factor. One fourth of demented patients have some treatable illness. One tenth of all dementias are reversible.

D. **Etiology.**   See Table 3–5. Most common cause is Alzheimer's disease followed by vascular disease (mixed forms are also common). Human immunodeficiency virus (HIV) infection, including AIDS, is also a common cause (1% of dementias).

E. **Lab tests.**   First identify a potentially reversible cause for the dementia; then identify other treatable medical conditions that may otherwise worsen the dementia (cognitive decline is often precipitated by other medical illness). The workup should include vital signs, CBC with differential, ESR, complete blood chemistries, serum $B_{12}$ and folate levels, liver and renal function tests, thyroid function tests, urinalysis, urine toxicology, EKG, chest x-ray, CT scan or MRI of head, and lumbar puncture.

F. **Differential diagnosis**

1. **Age-related cognitive decline (normal aging).**   Associated with a decreased ability to learn new material and a slowing of thought processes due to normal aging. In addition, there is a syndrome of benign senescent forgetfulness, which does not show a progressively deteriorating course.

TABLE 3–6
**DEMENTIA VERSUS DEPRESSION**

| Feature | Dementia | Pseudodementia |
|---|---|---|
| Age | Usually elderly | Nonspecific |
| Onset | Vague | Days to weeks |
| Course | Slow, worse at night | Rapid, even through day |
| History | Systemic illness or drugs | Mood disorder |
| Awareness | Unaware, unconcerned | Aware, distressed |
| Organic signs | Often present | Absent |
| Cognition[a] | Prominent impairment | Personality changes |
| Mental status examination | Consistent, spotty deficits | Variable deficits in different modalities |
| | Approximates, confabulates, perseverates | Apathetic, ''I don't know'' |
| | Emphasizes trivial accomplishments | Emphasizes failures |
| | Shallow or labile mood | Depressed |
| Behavior | Appropriate to degree of cognitive impairment | Incongruent with degree of cognitive impairment |
| Cooperation | Cooperative but frustrated | Uncooperative with little effort |
| CT and EEG | Abnormal | Normal |

[a]Benzodiazepines and barbiturates worsen cognitive impairments in the demented patient, whereas they help the depressed patient to relax.

**2. Depression.** Depression in the elderly may present as symptoms of cognitive impairment, which has led to the term "pseudodementia." The apparently demented patient is really depressed and responds well to antidepressant drugs or electroconvulsive therapy (ECT). Many demented patients also become depressed as they begin to comprehend their progressive cognitive impairment. In patients with both dementia and depression, a treatment trial with antidepressants or ECT is often warranted. Table 3–6 differentiates dementia from depression.

**3. Delirium.** Also characterized by global cognitive impairment. Demented patients often have a superimposed delirium. Dementia tends to be chronic and lacks the prominent features of rapid fluctuations, sudden onset, impaired attention, changing level of consciousness, psychomotor disturbance, acutely disturbed sleep-wake cycle, and prominent hallucinations or delusions that characterize delirium.

**G. Course and prognosis.** Dementia may be progressive, remitting, or stable. Because about 10% of dementias are reversible—e.g., hypothyroidism, central nervous system (CNS) syphilis, subdural hematoma, $B_{12}$ deficiency, uremia, and hypoxia—the course in these cases depends on the speed with which the cause is reversed. If the cause is reversed too late, there may be residual deficits with a subsequently stable course if there has not been extensive brain damage. For dementia with no identifiable cause, e.g., DAT, the course is likely to be one of slow deterioration. The patient may become lost in familiar places, later lose the ability to handle money, even later fail to recognize family members, and eventually become incontinent of stool and urine.

**H. Treatment.** Treatment is generally supportive. Ensure proper treatment of any concurrent medical problems. Maintain proper nutrition, exercise, and activities. Provide an environment that provides frequent cues for orientation to day, date, place, and time. As functioning decreases, nursing home placement may be necessary. Often, cognitive impairment may become worse at night (sundowning). Some nursing homes have successfully developed a schedule of night-time activities to help manage this problem.

1. **Psychological.**   Supportive therapy, group therapy, and referral to organizations for families of demented patients can help them to cope and to feel less frustrated and helpless.

2. **Pharmacological.**   In general, barbiturates and benzodiazepines should be avoided, since they can worsen cognition. For agitation, low doses of an antipsychotic are effective, e.g., haloperidol 2 mg orally or intramuscularly, or thioridazine (Mellaril) 25–50 mg orally. Some clinicians suggest a short-acting benzodiazepine for sleep, e.g., triazolam (Halcion) 0.25 mg orally, but this may cause further memory deficits the next day.

## V. DAT

A. **Definition.**   A progressive dementia in which all known reversible causes have been ruled out. Two types—with late onset (onset after age 65) and with early onset (onset before or at age 65).

B. **Diagnosis, signs, and symptoms.**   See Table 3–7.

C. **Epidemiology.**   DAT accounts for 50–60% of all dementias. May affect as much as 5% of persons over age 65 and 15–25% of persons age 85 or older. DAT may be more common in women, but this may be due to women's longer life expectancy. Relatives of DAT patients are more likely than the general population to develop DAT. There is a high concordance rate among twins. Some forms of DAT run in families, and in these families DAT follows a pattern of autosomal dominant transmission. DAT in one family has been linked to an anomaly on chromosome 21.

The relation between DAT and Down's syndrome has further supported genetic hypotheses of DAT. All Down's syndrome patients who live into the third decade of life develop the characteristic brain histopathological abnormalities found in DAT patients.

Rates of DAT are lower in nonindustrialized countries, but this may be an artifact of their lower level of medical care and thus decreased sensitivity in making the diagnosis.

D. **Etiology.**   Hypothetical risk factors include maternal age at birth, exposure to aluminum, history of head trauma, deficiencies of brain choline, autoimmunity, and others. A viral theory exists but lacks scientific support (two other dementing diseases—*kuru* and Creutzfeldt-Jakob disease—have been shown to be caused by transmissible viruses). None of these hypotheses has been clearly proven for DAT. The only known risk factor is increasing age.

E. **Pathology.**   The characteristic neuropathological changes first described by Alois Alzheimer are neurofibrillary tangles, senile plaques, and granulova-cuolar degenerations. These changes can also appear with normal aging, but they are always present in brains of DAT patients. They are most prominent in the amygdala, hippocampus, cortex, and basal forebrain. A definitive diagnosis of Alzheimer's disease can only be made histopathologically. The aluminum toxicity theory of etiology is based on the fact that these pathologi-

TABLE 3–7
**DSM-IV DIAGNOSTIC CRITERIA FOR DEMENTIA OF THE ALZHEIMER'S TYPE**

A. The development of multiple cognitive deficits manifested by both
   (1) memory impairment (impaired ability to learn new information or to recall previously learned information)
   (2) one (or more) of the following cognitive disturbances:
      (a) aphasia (language disturbance)
      (b) apraxia (impaired ability to carry out motor activities despite intact motor function)
      (c) agnosia (failure to recognize or identify objects despite intact sensory function)
      (d) disturbance in executive functioning (i.e., planning, organizing, sequencing, abstracting)
B. The cognitive deficits in criteria A1 and A2 each cause significant impairment in social or occupational functioning and represent a significant decline from a previous level of functioning.
C. The course is characterized by gradual onset and continuing cognitive decline.
D. The cognitive deficits in criteria A1 and A2 are not due to any of the following:
   (1) other central nervous system conditions that cause progressive deficits in memory and cognition (e.g., cerebrovascular disease, Parkinson's disease, Huntington's disease, subdural hematoma, normal-pressure hydrocephalus, brain tumor)
   (2) systemic conditions that are known to cause dementia (e.g., hypothyroidism, vitamin $B_{12}$ or folic acid deficiency, niacin deficiency, hypercalcemia, neurosyphilis, HIV infection)
   (3) substance-induced conditions
E. The deficits do not occur exclusively during the course of a delirium
F. The disturbance is not better accounted for by another Axis I disorder (e.g., major depressive disorder, schizophrenia)

*Code* based on type of onset and predominant features:
  **With early onset:** if onset is at age 65 years or below
  **With delirium:** if delirium is superimposed on the dementia
  **With delusions:** if delusions are the predominant feature
  **With depressed mood:** if depressed mood (including presentations that meet full symptom criteria for a major depressive episode) is the predominant feature; a separate diagnosis of mood disorder due to a general medical condition is not given
  **Uncomplicated:** if none of the above predominates in the current clinical presentation
  **With late onset:** if onset is after age 65 years
  **With delirium:** if delirium is superimposed on the dementia
  **With delusions:** if delusions are the predominant feature
  **With depressed mood:** if depressed mood (including presentations that meet full symptom criteria for a major depressive episode) is the predominant feature. A separate diagnosis of mood disorder due to a general medical condition is not given.
  **Uncomplicated:** if none of the above predominates in the current clinical presentation

*Specify* if:
  **With behavioral disturbance**

**Coding note:** Also code Alzheimer's disease on Axis III.

Used with permission, APA.

cal structures in the brain contain high amounts of aluminum. Clinical diagnosis of DAT should only be considered either possible or probable Alzheimer's disease.

Other abnormalities that have been found in DAT patients include diffuse cortical atrophy on CT or MRI, enlarged ventricles, and decreased brain acetylcholine metabolism. The finding of low levels of acetylcholine explains why these patients are highly susceptible to anticholinergic effects of medication and has led to development of choline replacement strategies for treatment.

## F. Course and prognosis

1. Usually insidious onset in a person's 50s or 60s; slowly progressive.
2. Aphasia, apraxia, and agnosia often present after several years.
3. Patient may later develop motor and gait disturbances; may become bedridden.
4. Mean survival is 8 years; ranges from 1 to 20 years.

G. **Treatment.** Tacrine (Cognex) has been approved by the Food and Drug Administration (FDA) as a treatment for Alzheimer's disease. The drug is a moderately long-acting inhibitor of cholinesterase activity, and well controlled trials have shown a clinically significant improvement in 20–25% of patients who take it. Because of the cholinomimetic activity of the drug, some patients cannot tolerate it because of side effects. Some patients have to discontinue tacrine because of elevations in liver enzymes.

## VI. Vascular dementia

A. **Definition.** Dementia due to cerebrovascular disease. Dementia usually progresses in a stepwise fashion with each recurrent infarct. Patients will notice one specific moment when their functioning became worse and will improve slightly over subsequent days until their next infarct. Neurological signs are common. Impaired cognition may be patchy, with some areas intact.

B. **Diagnosis, signs, and symptoms.** See Table 3–8.

C. **Epidemiology.** Accounts for 15–30% of all dementia; most common in persons 60–70 years of age. Less common than DAT. More common in men than in women. Onset is at an earlier age than with DAT. Risk factors include hypertension, heart disease, and other risk factors for stroke.

D. **Lab tests.** CT scan or MRI will show infarcts.

E. **Differential diagnosis**

  1. **DAT.** Vascular dementia may be difficult to differentiate from DAT. Obtain a good history of the course of the disease, noting whether the onset was abrupt, whether the course was insidious or stepwise, and

---

TABLE 3–8
**DSM-IV DIAGNOSTIC CRITERIA FOR VASCULAR DEMENTIA**

A. The development of multiple cognitive deficits manifested by both
  (1) memory impairment (impaired ability to learn new information or to recall previously learned information)
  (2) one (or more) of the following cognitive disturbances:
      (a) aphasia (language disturbance)
      (b) apraxia (impaired ability to carry out motor activities despite intact motor function)
      (c) agnosia (failure to recognize or identify objects despite intact sensory function)
      (d) disturbance in executive functioning (i.e., planning, organizing, sequencing, abstracting)
B. The cognitive deficits in criteria A1 and A2 each cause significant impairment in social or occupational functioning and represent a significant decline from a previous level of functioning.
C. Focal neurological signs and symptoms (e.g., exaggeration of deep tendon reflexes, extensor plantar response, pseudobulbar palsy, gait abnormalities, weakness of an extremity) or laboratory evidence indicative of cerebrovascular disease (e.g., multiple infarctions involving cortex and underlying white matter) that are judged to be etiologically related to the disturbance.
D. The deficits do not occur exclusively during the course of a delirium.

*Code* based on predominant features:
  **With delirium:** if delirium is superimposed on the dementia
  **With delusions:** if delusions are the predominant feature
  **With depressed mood:** if depressed mood (including presentations that meet full symptom criteria for a major depressive episode) is the predominant feature. A separate diagnosis of mood disorder due to a general medical condition is not given.
  **Uncomplicated:** if none of the above predominates in the current clinical presentation

*Specify* if:
  **With behavioral disturbance**

**Coding note:** Also code cerebrovascular condition on Axis III.

Used with permission, APA.

whether neurological impairment was present. Identify vascular disease risk factors and obtain brain image. If a patient has features of both vascular dementia and DAT, then the diagnosis should be dementia due to multiple etiologies.

2. **Depression.**   Vascular dementia patients may also become depressed, as described above in patients with pseudodementia. Depression is unlikely to produce focal neurological findings. If present, depression should be diagnosed and treated.

3. **Strokes and transient ischemic attacks (TIAs).**   Generally do not lead to a progressively demented patient. TIAs are brief episodes of focal neurological dysfunction lasting less than 24 hours (usually 5–15 minutes). A completed-stroke patient may have some cognitive deficits, but unless there is a massive loss of brain tissue, a single stroke generally will not cause dementia.

F. **Treatment.**   The treatment is to identify and reverse the cause of the strokes. Hypertension, diabetes, and cardiac disease must be treated. Nursing home placement may be necessary if impairment is severe. Treatment is supportive and symptomatic. Antidepressant or antipsychotic medication and benzodiazepines can be used, but the brain-damaged patients may develop adverse effects from any psychoactive drug.

## VII. Pick's disease

This relatively rare primary degenerative dementia is clinically similar to DAT. However, the frontal lobe is prominently involved, and frontal signs of disinhibited behavior may present early. Reactive gliosis is found in frontal and temporal lobes. Diagnosis often is made at autopsy, although CT or MRI can show prominent frontal lobe involvement.

## VIII. Creutzfeldt-Jakob disease

This rapidly progressive degenerative dementing disease is caused by a transmissible slow virus (although new findings reveal that it may have a genetic origin). Onset usually occurs in a patient's 40s or 50s. The very first signs of this disease may be vague somatic complaints or unspecified feelings of anxiety. Other signs include ataxia, extrapyramidal signs, choreoathetosis, and dysarthria. Usually fatal within 2 years of diagnosis. CT scan shows atrophy in cortex and cerebellum. There is a characteristic EEG in later stages. There is no known treatment.

## IX. Huntington's disease

A. **Definition.**   A genetic autosomal dominant disease with complete penetrance (chromosome 4) characterized by choreoathetoid movement and dementia. A person with one parent with Huntington's disease has a 50% chance of developing the disease.

B. **Diagnosis.**   Onset usually occurs in a patient's 30s to 40s (the patient frequently already has children). Choreiform movements usually present first and become progressively more severe. Dementia presents later, often with psychotic features. Dementia may first be described by the patient's family as a personality change. Look for a family history.

**C. Associated psychiatric symptoms and complications**
1. 25% personality changes.
2. 25% schizophreniform.
3. 50% mood.
4. 25% begin with sudden-onset dementia.
5. 90% of patients develop dementia.

**D. Epidemiology.**  Incidence is 2–6 cases a year per 100,000 persons. Over 1,000 cases have been traced to two brothers who immigrated to Long Island, New York from England. Incidence is equal in men and women.

**E. Pathophysiology.**  Atrophy of brain with extensive involvement of the basal ganglia and the caudate nucleus in particular.

**F. Differential diagnosis.**  When choreiform movements first present, they are often misinterpreted as inconsequential habit spasms or tics. Up to 75% of patients with Huntington's disease are initially misdiagnosed with a primary psychiatric disorder. Features distinguishing it from DAT are the high incidence of depression and psychosis and the classic choreoathetoid movement disorder.

**G. Course and prognosis.**  The course is progressive and usually leads to death 15–20 years after diagnosis. Suicide is common.

**H. Treatment.**  Institutionalization may be needed as chorea progresses. Symptoms of insomnia, anxiety, and depression can be relieved with benzodiazepines and antidepressants. Psychotic symptoms can be treated with high-potency antipsychotics. Genetic counseling is the most important intervention.

**X. Parkinson's disease**

**A. Definition.**  An idiopathic movement disorder with onset usually late in life, characterized by bradykinesia, resting tremor, pill-rolling tremor, mask-like faces, cogwheel rigidity, and shuffling gait. Intellectual impairment is common, and 40–80% of patients become demented. Depression is extremely common.

**B. Epidemiology.**  Annual prevalence in the Western hemisphere is 200 cases per 100,000 persons.

**C. Etiology.**  Unknown for most patients. There are decreased cells in substantia nigra, decreased dopamine, and degeneration of dopaminergic tracts. Parkinsonism can be caused by repeated head trauma and a contaminant of an illicitly made synthetic heroin, N-methyl-4-phenyl-1,2,3,6 tetrahydropyridine (MPTP).

**D. Treatment.**  L-dopa (levodopa [Larodopa]) is a dopamine precursor and is often combined with carbidopa, a dopa decarboxylase inhibitor, to increase brain dopamine levels. Amantadine (Symadine) has also been used synergistically with L-dopa. Some surgeons have tried implanting adrenal medulla tissue into the brain to produce dopamine with some favorable results. Depression is treatable with antidepressants or ECT.

**XI. Other dementias**

See Table 3–5. Other dementias include those due to Wilson's disease, supranuclear palsy, normal pressure hydrocephalus (dementia, ataxia, incontinence), and brain tumors.

Systemic causes of dementia: thyroid disease, pituitary diseases (Addison's and Cushing's diseases), liver failure, dialysis, nicotinic acid deficiency (pellagra causes the three Ds: dementia, dermatitis, diarrhea), $B_{12}$ deficiency, folate deficiency, infections, heavy metal intoxication, chronic alcohol abuse.

## XII. Amnestic disorder

**A. Definition.**   Impaired recent, short-term, and long-term memory attributed to a specific organic etiology, i.e., drug or medical disease. Patient is normal in other areas of cognition.

**B. Diagnosis, signs, and symptoms.**   Amnestic disorders are diagnosed according to their etiology: Amnestic disorder due to a general medical condition (Table 3–9), substance-induced persisting amnestic disorder, and amnestic disorder NOS.

**C. Etiology.**   See Table 3–10. Most common form is due to thiamine deficiency associated with alcohol dependence. May also result from head trauma, surgery, hypoxia, infarction, and herpes simplex encephalitis. Typically, any process that damages certain diencephalic and medial temporal structures (e.g., mammillary bodies, fornix, hippocampus) can cause the disorder.

TABLE 3–9
**DSM-IV DIAGNOSTIC CRITERIA FOR AMNESTIC DISORDER DUE TO A GENERAL MEDICAL CONDITION**

A. The development of memory impairment as manifested by impairment in the ability to learn new information or the inability to recall previously learned information.
B. The memory disturbance causes significant impairment in social or occupational functioning and represents a significant decline from a previous level of functioning.
C. The memory disturbance does not occur exclusively during the course of a delirium or a dementia.
D. There is evidence from the history, physical examination, or laboratory findings that the disturbance is the direct physiological consequence of a general medical condition (including physical trauma).

*Specify* if:
   **Transient:** if memory impairment lasts for 1 month or less
   **Chronic:** if memory impairment lasts for more than 1 month

**Coding note:** Include the name of the general medical condition on Axis I, e.g., amnestic disorder due to head trauma; also code the general medical condition on Axis III.

Used with permission, APA.

TABLE 3–10
**MAJOR CAUSES OF AMNESTIC DISORDERS**

| | |
|---|---|
| **Systemic medical conditions** | Hypoxia (including nonfatal hanging attempts |
| Thiamine deficiency (Korsakoff's syndrome) | and carbon monoxide poisoning) |
| Hypoglycemia | Transient global amnesia |
| | Electroconvulsive therapy |
| **Primary brain conditions** | Multiple sclerosis |
| Seizures | |
| Head trauma (closed and penetrating) | **Substances** |
| Cerebral tumors (especially thalamic and | Alcohol |
| temporal lobe) | Neurotoxins |
| Cerebrovascular diseases (especially thalamic | Benzodiazepines (and other sedative- |
| and temporal lobe) | hypnotics) |
| Surgical procedures on the brain | Many over-the-counter preparations |
| Encephalitis due to herpes simplex | |

**D. Differential diagnosis.**   Amnesia also is a part of delirium and dementia, but these disorders involve impairments in many other areas of cognition. Factitious disorders may simulate amnesia, but the amnestic deficits will be inconsistent. Patients with dissociative disorders are more likely to have lost their orientation to self and may have more selective memory deficits than do patients with amnestic disorders. Dissociative disorders are also often associated with emotionally stressful life events involving money, the legal system, or troubled relationships.

**E. Treatment.**   Identify the cause and reverse it if possible; otherwise, institute supportive medical procedures, e.g., fluids, blood pressure maintenance.

## XIII. Transient global amnesia

A. Abrupt episodes of profound amnesia in all modalities.
B. Patient is fully alert, distant memory is intact.
C. Usually occurs in late middle age or old age.
D. Usually lasts several hours.
E. Patient is bewildered and confused after an episode and may repeatedly ask others about what happened.
F. Usually associated with cerebrovascular disease, but also with episodic medical conditions, e.g., seizures.

## XIV. Mental disorders due to a general medical condition

The disorders are characterized by a medical condition (e.g. cerebrovascular disease, head trauma) that directly causes psychiatric symptoms (e.g., catatonia, depression, anxiety). (The medical condition is coded on Axis III.) Causes include endocrinopathies, deficiency states, connective tissue diseases, CNS disorders, and toxic effects of medication. Some disorders due to a general medical condition include amnestic, psychotic, mood, anxiety, and sleep disorders; personality change; and sexual dysfunction due to a general medical condition. Similar to functional diagnoses except that prominent symptoms are due to a specific organic factor; patient is normal in other areas of cognition.

## XV. Other conditions and disorders

### A. Personality change due to a general medical condition

1. Clear, persistent change in personality.
2. Several types:
    **a. Labile type**—affective instability, irritability, anxiety.
    **b. Disinhibited type**—impaired social judgment, sexual acting out.
    **c. Aggressive type**—inappropriate outbursts or aggression.
    **d. Apathetic type**—apathy and indifference.
    **e. Paranoid type**—suspiciousness or paranoid ideation.
    **f. Other, combined, and unspecified types.**
3. Etiologies usually involve structural brain damage.

### B. Systemic lupus erythematosus (SLE)

1. One of the collagen vascular diseases with direct CNS involvement (others include polyarteritis nodosa and temporal arteritis).
2. Mental symptoms are common (60%) and may occur early.

3. No characteristic form or pattern.
4. Delirium is the most common mental syndrome.
5. Psychotic depression is more common than schizophrenialike features.
6. May progress to dementia.
7. Seizures are common (50%), including grand mal and temporal lobe types.
8. A variety of movement disorders.

**C. Migraine**
1. Associated psychiatric symptoms and complications
   a. 10% memory change.
   b. 6% delirium.
   c. 6% hallucinations.
   d. 6% body image change.
   e. 4% depression.
2. Chronic migraine produces social-vocational disability and depression.
3. High intelligence, obsessive features.
4. Lifetime prevalence for the entire population is 20–25%.
5. More common in women.
6. Some family patterns.
7. Severe, dull, throbbing headache usually occurs upon awakening; often unilateral.
8. Gradual in onset, lasts hours to days.
9. Aura is common with visual hallucination, somatic hallucinations, paresthesias.
10. Precipitated by certain foods, stress, temperature changes.
11. Associated autonomic instability (nausea, vomiting, paroxysmal atrial tachycardia).
12. Etiology may be vasodilation or vasoconstriction, but autonomic dysfunction is also possible.
13. Treatment with analgesics, opioids, hydroxyzine, ergot alkaloids, anti-inflammatory drugs.
14. Propranolol (Inderal) is used in prophylaxis.
15. Sumatriptan (Imitrex) for acute attacks with aura (classic migraine) or without. (Do not use with hemiplegic or basilar migraines.)
16. Psychotherapy important—separate etiology from treatment, use a rehabilitation model for impaired functioning and symptom control, deal directly with secondary gain. Biofeedback, hypnosis, relaxation techniques, and behavior modification also are helpful.
17. Common differential is tension headaches, which are bilateral, day-long, and without prodrome.

**D. Multiple sclerosis**
1. More common in Northern hemisphere.
2. Psychiatric changes are common (75%).
3. Depression is common early in course.
4. Later, with frontal lobe involvement, disinhibition and maniclike symptoms occur, including euphoria.
5. Intellectual deterioration is common (60%), ranging from mild memory loss to dementia.

TABLE 3–11
**CLINICAL FEATURES DISTINGUISHING SEIZURES AND PSEUDOSEIZURES[a]**

| Feature | Seizure | Pseudoseizure |
| --- | --- | --- |
| Aura | Common stereotyped | Rare |
| Timing | Nocturnal common | Only when awake |
| Incontinence | Common | Rare |
| Cyanosis | Common | Rare |
| Postictal confusion | Yes | No |
| Body movement | Tonic or clonic | Nonstereotyped and asynchronous |
| Self-injury | Common | Rare |
| EEG | May be abnormal | Normal |
| Affected by suggestion | No | Yes |
| Secondary gain | No | Yes |

[a]Note that some patients with organic seizure disorders may also have pseudoseizures.

6. Psychosis is reported, but rates are unclear.
7. Hysteria is common, especially late in disease.
8. Symptoms are exacerbated by physical or emotional trauma.
9. MRI is needed for workup.

### E.  Epilepsy

1. Ictal and postictal confusional syndromes.
2. Prevalence of psychosis in epilepsy is 7%.
3. Epilepsy is 3–7 times more common in psychotic patients.
4. Lifetime prevalence of psychosis in epileptics is 10%.
5. Seizures versus pseudoseizures (Table 3–11).
6. Temporal lobe epilepsy (TLE)
   a. TLE type is the most likely to produce psychiatric symptoms.
   b. Often involves schizophrenialike psychosis.
   c. Often difficult to distinguish from schizophrenia with aggressiveness.
   d. Varied and complex auras that may masquerade as functional illness, e.g., hallucinations, depersonalization, derealization.
   e. Automatisms, autonomic effects, and visceral sensations, e.g., epigastric aura, stomach churning, salivation, flushing, tachycardia, dizziness.
   f. Altered perceptual experiences, e.g., distortions, hallucinations, depersonalization, feeling remote, feeling something has a peculiar significance, déjà vu, *jamais vu.*
   g. Hallucinations of taste and smell are common and may be accompanied by lip smacking or pursing, chewing, or tasting and swallowing movements.
   h. Subjective disorders of thinking and memory.
   i. Strong affective experiences, most commonly fear and anxiety.

### F.  Brain tumors

1. Neurological signs, headache, nausea, vomiting, seizures, visual loss, papilledema, virtually any psychiatric symptoms are possible.
2. Symptoms often are due to raised intracranial pressure or mass effects rather than direct effects of tumor.
3. Suicidal ideation is present in 10% of patients, usually during headache paroxysms.

4. Although rare in a psychiatric practice, most patients with brain tumors have psychiatric symptoms.
    a. Slow tumors ! personality change.
    b. Rapid tumors ! cognitive change.
5. Frontal lobe tumors—depression, inappropriate affect, disinhibition, dementia, impaired coordination, psychotic symptoms. Often misdiagnosed as primary degenerative dementia; neurological signs often are absent.
6. Temporal lobe tumors—anxiety, depression, hallucinations (especially gustatory and olfactory), TLE symptoms, schizophrenialike psychosis.
7. Parietal lobe tumors—fewer psychiatric symptoms (anosognosia, apraxia, aphasia); may be mistaken for hysteria.

## G. Head trauma

1. Wide range of acute and chronic clinical pictures.
2. Duration of disorientation is an approximate guide to prognosis.
3. Brain imaging shows classic *contrecoup* lesion, edema acutely.
4. Acute—amnesia (posttraumatic amnesia often resolves abruptly), agitation, withdrawn behavior, psychosis (acute posttraumatic psychosis), delirium.
5. Chronic—amnesia, psychosis, mood disorder, personality change, and (rarely) dementia.
6. Factors affecting course—mental constitution, premorbid personality, epilepsy (very strongly affects work ability), environment, litigation, emotional repercussion of injury, response to intellectual losses, and amount and location of brain damage.
7. Generally, the patient's coping mechanisms may affect the eventual course much more than the actual amount of brain damage will.

## H. Herpes encephalitis (herpes simplex virus).

Neuropsychiatric disorder caused by CNS infection by the herpes simplex virus. Symptoms often involve anosmia, olfactory and gustatory hallucinations, personality changes, and bizarre and psychotic behavior; onset usually is sudden or rapid. (Microcephaly, mental retardation, intracranial calcification, and ocular abnormalities may result from infection during birth.)

1. **Lab tests.** EEG abnormalities in the acute stage include slowing (diffuse or focal) and high-voltage sharp waves in the temporal regions. CT, MRI, and SPECT often reveal structural changes or reduced blood flow in the temporal lobes and the orbitofrontal regions.
2. **Treatment.** Arabinosyladenine reduces mortality and morbidity if initiated early.

## I. Heavy metal poisoning

1. **Lead.** Abdominal colic, lead neuropathy, lead encephalopathy. May present suddenly as delirium, seizures, elevated blood pressure, impaired memory and concentration, headache, tremor, deafness, transient aphasia, and hemianopsia. Chronic headache, depression, weakness, vertigo, hyperesthesia for visual and auditory stimuli. Treatment with calcium lactate, milk, chelating agents.
2. **Mercury.** Mad Hatter's syndrome (thermometers, photoengravers, ore workers, fingerprinters, chemical workers, repairers of electric

meters, felt hat industry)—gastritis, bleeding gums, excessive salivation, coarse tremor with coarse jerky movements. Presents as nervous, timid, and shy, blushes easily; embarrasses in social situations; irritable and quarrelsome; loses temper easily.

**3. Manganese.**   (Ore workers, dry batteries, bleaching, welding.) Headache; asthenia; torpor; hypersomnia; impotence; uncontrollable laughter and crying; impulses to run, dance, sing, or talk; may commit senseless crimes. Parkinsonism develops later.

**4. Arsenic.**   (Fur and glass industries, insecticides.) Long-term exposure—dermatitis, conjunctivitis, lacrimation, anorexia, headache, vertigo, apathy, drowsiness, intellectual impairment, peripheral neuritis. May eventually present as Korsakoff's psychosis.

**5. Thallium.**   (From pesticides.) Tingling, abdominal pain, vomiting, headache, tachycardia, gastritis, offensive breath, alopecia, ataxia, paresthesias, peripheral neuropathy, retrobulbar neuritis, tremor, chorea, athetosis, myoclonic jerking, impaired consciousness, depression, seizures, delirium.

---

*For a more detailed discussion of this topic, see Reichman WE: Neuropsychiatric Aspects of Cerebrovascular Disorders and Tumors, Sec 2.2, p 187; Mendez MF: Neuropsychiatric Aspects of Epilepsy, Sec 2.3, p 198; Capruso DX, Levin HS: Neuropsychiatric Aspects of Head Trauma, Sec 2.4, p 207; Rabins PV, McMahon FJ: Neuropsychiatric Aspects of Multiple Sclerosis and Other Demyelinating Disorders, Sec 2.6, p 231; Van Gorp WG, Cummings JL: Neuorpsychiatric Aspects of Infectious Disorders, Sec 2.7, p 235; Stern RA, Prange AJ: Neuropsychiatric Aspects of Endocrine Disorders, Sec 2.8, p 241; Singer EJ: Neuropsychiatric Aspects of Headache, Sec 2.9, p 251; Caine ED, Grossman H, Lyness JM: Delirium, Dementia, and Amnestic and Other Cognitive Disorders and Mental Disorders Due to a General Medical Condition, Chap 12, p 705; Matsuyama SS: Genetics of Dementia, Sec 49.3, p 2527; Small GW: Alzheimer's Disease and Other Dementing Disorders, Sec 49.6a, p 2562, in CTP/VI.*

---

# 4

# Neuropsychiatric Aspects of HIV and AIDS

## I. General considerations

Acquired immune deficiency syndrome (AIDS) was first reported in 1981. In the United States, over 400,000 active cases of AIDS have already been diagnosed. At least two types of the human immunodeficiency virus (HIV) have been identified, HIV-1 and HIV-2. HIV-1 is the causative agent for the vast majority of HIV-related diseases. Estimates place the number of Americans infected with the retrovirus at 1–2 million, most of whom are predicted to develop AIDS. HIV is transmitted between persons by means of bodily fluids, such as blood and semen, and can be transmitted through sexual activity, through intravenous (IV) use of contaminated syringes and blood transfusions, and from mother to fetus during pregnancy.

Data strongly suggest that treatment of asymptomatic HIV-positive patients, i.e., patients who have not yet developed full-blown AIDS, with such drugs as azidothymidine (AZT) (Zidovudine) decreases the emergence of symptoms of AIDS. Therefore, early screening is crucial. Possible indications for HIV testing are outlined in Table 4–1.

Some patients are so concerned about the possibility of having contracted the AIDS virus that the patient and physician may feel it necessary to perform the test even if no risk factors are apparent.

HIV testing must be accompanied by informed pretest and posttest counseling. Physicians must know that tremendous psychological stress can accompany HIV testing. Some of the major issues involved in pretest counseling are listed in Table 4–2.

Pretest counseling anticipates the potential reactions of patients on receiving test results. Patients should be informed that at some testing centers only the

TABLE 4–1
**POSSIBLE INDICATIONS FOR HUMAN IMMUNODEFICIENCY VIRUS (HIV) TESTING**

1. Patients who belong to a high-risk group: (1) men who have had sex with another man since 1977, (2) intravenous drug abusers since 1977, (3) hemophiliacs or other patients who have received blood or blood product transfusions not screened for HIV since 1977, (4) sexual partners of people from any of these groups, (5) sexual partners of people with known HIV exposure—people with cuts, wounds, sores, or needlesticks whose lesions have had direct contact with HIV-infected blood
2. Patients who request testing; not all patients will admit to the presence of risk factors (e.g., because of shame, fear)
3. Patients with symptoms of AIDS or HIV infection
4. Women belonging to a high-risk group who are planning pregnancy or who are pregnant
5. Blood, semen, or organ donors
6. Patients with dementia in a high-risk group

Table adapted from Rosse RB, Giese AA, Deutsch SI, Morihisa JM: *Laboratory & Diagnostic Testing in Psychiatry.* American Psychiatric Press, Washington, DC, 1989, p 54. Used with permission.

TABLE 4–2
**PRETEST HIV COUNSELING**

1. Discuss meaning of a positive result and clarify distortions (e.g., the test detects exposure to the AIDS virus; it is not a test for AIDS)
2. Discuss the meaning of a negative result (e.g., seroconversion requires time, recent high-risk behavior might require follow-up testing)
3. Be available to discuss the patient's fears and concerns (unrealistic fears might require appropriate psychological intervention)
4. Discuss why the test is necessary (not all patients will admit to high-risk behaviors)
5. Explore the patient's potential reactions to a positive result (e.g., ``I'll kill myself if I'm positive.'') Take appropriate necessary steps to intervene in a potentially catastrophic reaction
6. Explore past reactions to severe stresses
7. Discuss the confidentiality issues relevant to the testing situation (e.g., is it an anonymous or a nonanonymous setting). Inform the patient of other possible testing options wherein the counseling and testing can be done completely anonymously (e.g., where the result would not be made a permanent part of a hospital chart). Discuss who might have access to the test results
8. Discuss with the patient how being seropositive can potentially affect social status (e.g., health and life insurance coverage, employment, housing)
9. Explore high-risk behaviors and recommend risk-reducing interventions
10. Document discussions in chart
11. Allow the patient time to ask questions

Table from Rosse RB, Giese AA, Deutsch SI, Morihisa JM: *Laboratory & Diagnostic Testing in Psychiatry.* American Psychiatric Press, Washington, DC, 1989, p 55. Used with permission.

TABLE 4–3
**POSTTEST HIV COUNSELING**

1. Interpretation of test result: Clarify distortion (e.g., ``a negative test still means you could contact the virus in the future—it does not mean you are immune from AIDS''). Ask questions of the patient about his or her understanding and emotional reaction to test result
2. Recommendations for prevention of transmission (careful discussion of high-risk behaviors and guidelines for prevention of transmission)
3. Recommendations on the follow-up of sexual partners and needle contacts
4. If test is positive, recommendations against donating blood, sperm, or organs and against sharing razors, toothbrushes, and anything else that might have blood on it
5. Referral for appropriate psychological support: HIV-positive persons often need to have available a mental health team (assess need for inpatient versus outpatient care; consider individual or group supportive therapy). Common themes include shock of diagnosis, fear of death and social consequences, grief over potential losses, and dashed hope for good news. Also look for depression, hopelessness, anger, frustration, guilt, and obsessional themes. Activate supports available to patient (e.g., family, friends, community services).

Table from Rosse RB, Giese AA, Deutsch SI, Morihisa JM: *Laboratory & Diagnostic Testing in Psychiatry.* American Psychiatric Press, Washington, DC, 1989, p 58. Used with permission.

patient knows the result, and physicians should be aware that the medical record is not always confidential. Records can be subpoenaed and become a part of public record; insurance companies can occasionally gain access to a patient's file. The patient should be informed prior to testing whether the testing center requires the physician to inform sexual partners of positive test results.

Some of the issues involved in posttest counseling, when a patient who has been tested for HIV is informed of the result, are described in Table 4–3.

## II. Central nervous system (CNS) clinical manifestations

See Table 4–4. HIV-infected patients are commonly reported to have CNS involvement, even in the absence of other signs or symptoms of AIDS. When AIDS is present, approximately 60% of patients exhibit neurological symptoms; pathological involvement of the brain has been reported in 75–90% of patients at autopsy.

TABLE 4-4
**DISEASES AFFECTING CNS IN PATIENTS WITH AIDS**

**Primary viral diseases**
  HIV encephalopathy
  Atypical aseptic meningitis
  Vacuolar myelopathy
**Secondary viruses** (encephalitis, myelitis, retinitis, vasculitis)
  Cytomegalovirus
  Herpes simplex virus types 1 and 2
  Herpes varicella-zoster virus
  Papovavirus (PML)
**Nonviral infections** (encephalitis, meningitis, abscess)
  *Toxoplasma gondii*
  *Cryptococcus neoformans*
  *Candida albicans*
  *Histoplasma capsulatum*
  *Aspergillus fumigatus*
  *Coccidiodes immitis*
  *Acremonium albamensis*
  *Rhizopus species*
  *Mycobacterium avium-intracellulare*
  *Mycobacterium tuberculosis hominis*
  *Mycobacterium kansasii*
  *Listeria monocytogenes*
  *Nocardia asteroides*
**Neoplasms**
  Primary CNS lymphoma
  Metastatic systemic lymphoma
  Metastatic Kaposi's sarcoma
**Cerebrovascular diseases**
  Infarction
  Hemorrhage
  Vasculitis
**Complications of systemic therapy**

Table from Beckett A: The neurobiology of human immunodeficiency virus infection. In *American Psychiatric Press Review of Psychiatry*, vol 9. A Tasman, SM Goldfinger, CA Kaufman, eds. American Psychiatric Press, Washington, DC, 1990, p 595. Used with permission.

Mental disorders associated with HIV infection include dementia, mood disorder, and personality change due to a general medical condition. Psychiatric conditions associated with HIV infection include depression, acute psychosis, and mania. Diseases that occasionally cause dementia in patients with AIDS include cerebral toxoplasmosis, cryptococcal meningitis, and primary brain lymphoma. A distinct neurological entity, HIV encephalopathy (previously known as AIDS dementia complex) is the most common neurological problem in AIDS. HIV-1 is believed to be the direct cause of this syndrome. The major clinical manifestations of HIV encephalopathy are outlined in Table 4–5.

HIV encephalopathy may occur before AIDS is diagnosed. Clinicians initially may mistake the patient's social withdrawal, apathy, psychomotor retardation, and deficits in concentration or memory as depression. HIV encephalopathy may present suddenly after the use of psychoactive drugs or other stress, although careful questioning of the patient's family or friends usually reveals that the onset was not as acute as it appeared. The prognosis of dementia due to HIV disease is poor. Of patients who develop dementia, 50–75% die within 6 months.

## III. Psychiatric syndromes

  **A. Dementia.**   Causes include HIV, as well as CNS infections, CNS neoplasms, CNS abnormalities caused by systemic disorders and endocrinopathies, and adverse CNS responses to drugs.

TABLE 4–5
**CLINICAL MANIFESTATIONS OF HIV ENCEPHALOPATHY**[a]

| Common | Occasional | Uncommon |
|---|---|---|
| Absence of will (abulia) | Motor deficits | Aphasia |
| Apathy | Psychiatric problems | Apraxia |
| Decreased memory | Seizures | Decreased level of consciousness |
| Inability to concentrate | | |
| Mild headaches | | |
| Psychomotor retardation | | |
| Social withdrawal | | |

[a]HIV encephalopathy was previously called "AIDS dementia complex"; however, HIV-related encephalopathy and dementia can develop in patients who do not meet the diagnostic criteria for AIDS.

Table adapted from Bredesen DE, Ho DD, Vinters H, Daar ES: The acquired immunodeficiency syndrome (AIDS) dementia complex (clinical conference). Ann Intern Med, *111*:401, 1989. Used with permission.

**B. Delirium.**   Can result from the same variety of causes that lead to dementia in HIV-infected patients. Delirium is probably underdiagnosed.

**C. Anxiety disorders.**   Patients with HIV infection may have any of the anxiety disorders, but generalized anxiety disorder, posttraumatic stress disorder, and obsessive-compulsive disorder are particularly common.

**D. Adjustment disorder.**   Adjustment disorder with anxiety or depressed mood reportedly occurs in 5–20% of HIV-infected patients.

**E. Depressive disorders.**   The range of HIV-infected patients reported to meet the diagnostic criteria for depressive disorders is 4–40%.

**F. Substance abuse.**   Patients may be tempted to use drugs regularly in an attempt to deal with depression or anxiety.

**G. Suicide.**   Suicide ideation and suicide attempts may be increased in patients with HIV infection and AIDS. The risk factors for suicide are having friends who died from AIDS-related causes; recent notification of HIV seropositivity, i.e., having a positive HIV antibody test result; relapses; difficult social issues relating to homosexuality; inadequate social and financial support; and presence of dementia or delirium.

**H. Worried well.**   Persons in high-risk groups who, although they are seronegative and disease-free, are anxious or have an obsession about contracting the virus. Symptoms can include generalized anxiety, panic attacks, obsessive-compulsive disorder, and hypochondriasis. Repeated negative serum test results can reassure some patients. For those who cannot be reassured, supportive or insight-oriented therapy may be indicated.

## IV. Treatment

**A. Prevention.**   All persons at any risk for HIV infection should be informed about safe-sex practices and the need to avoid sharing contaminated hypodermic needles. Preventive strategies are complicated by the complex societal values surrounding sexual acts, sexual orientation, birth control, and substance abuse.

**Safe sex**—a common question that physicians should be prepared to answer is, "What is safe and unsafe sex?" Patients should be advised that if they are HIV-positive or if a new sexual partner's history is unknown to them and there is any reason for concern, the guidelines listed in Table 4–6 should be followed.

TABLE 4–6
**AIDS SAFE SEX GUIDELINES**

**Remember:** Any activity that allows for exchange of body fluids of one person and the mouth, anus, vagina, bloodstream, cuts, or sores of another person is considered *unsafe* at this time.

*Safe-Sex Practices*
Massage, hugging, body-to-body rubbing
Dry social kissing
Masturbation
Acting out sexual fantasies (that do not include any unsafe sex practices)
Using vibrators or other instruments (provided they are not shared)

*Low-Risk Sex Practices* (these activities are not considered completely safe)
French (wet) kissing (without mouth sores)
Mutual masturbation
Vaginal and anal intercourse using a condom
Oral sex, male (fellatio) using a condom
Oral sex, female (cunnilingus), with barrier
External contact with semen or urine provided there are no breaks in the skin

*Unsafe-Sex Practices*
Vaginal or anal intercourse without a condom
Semen, urine, or feces in the mouth or vagina
Unprotected oral sex (fellatio or cunnilingus)
Blood contact of any kind
Sharing sex instruments or needles

Table from Moffatt B, Spiegel J, Parrish S, Helquist M: *AIDS: A Self-Care Manual.* IBS Press, Santa Monica, CA, 1987, p 125. Used with permission.

**B. Medical therapy.** Treatment of medical complications should be vigorous and involve a broad range of agents (Table 4–7). In addition, a regimen of agents with activity against HIV should be instituted (Table 4–8). AZT is an inhibitor of reverse transcriptase and has been shown to slow the course of the disease in many patients and to prolong the survival of some patients. The use of AZT is often limited by associated severe adverse affects, although other antiretroviral drugs are being used clinically, e.g., dideoxyinosine (ddI) (Didanosine).

**C. Pharmacological.** When the CNS is involved, especially when organic psychiatric symptoms are present (e.g., anxiety, psychosis, or depression), appropriate psychotropic medications are indicated. Small doses of antipsychotics, e.g., trifluoperazine (Stelazine) and haloperidol (Haldol), may be useful in controlling agitation. Antidepressants, particularly those with few anticholinergic side effects, help in treating depression. If brain damage is present, drugs with anticholinergic effects must be used cautiously to prevent an atropine psychosis. Some clinicians have had positive results treating depressed AIDS patients with small doses of amphetamine. Benzodiazepines often are useful for anxiety or insomnia, although they may exacerbate cognitive symptoms. Small doses of sedating antipsychotics, e.g., 25 mg of thioridazine (Mellaril), or antihistamines may then be used. Lithium (Eskalith) may be useful in persons with manic symptoms, but renal function and lithium concentrations must be carefully monitored if there is renal impairment from the illness. Suicidal depression is common in advanced cases; antidepressant medication and close supervision of the patient, including psychiatric hospitalization with suicidal precautions, may be necessary. Approximately 60% of AIDS patients develop some type of cognitive disor-

TABLE 4–7
**TREATMENT OF OPPORTUNISTIC INFECTIONS**[a]

| Infection | Treatment | Dosage[b] |
|-----------|-----------|-----------|
| Pneumocystis carinii | Sulfamethoxazole-trimethoprim | 20 mg/kg/day of trimethoprim 100 mg/kg/day of sulfamethoxazole |
| | or | |
| | Pentamidine isethionate | 4 mg/kg/day IV |
| Cryptococcal meningitis | Amphotericin B | 0.4–0.6 mg/kg/day IV |
| | and | |
| | Flucytosine | 100 mg/kg/day |
| Toxoplasmosis | Sulfadiazine sodium | 4 g/day po |
| | and | |
| | Pyrimethamine | 25–50 mg/day po |
| Mycobacterium avium-intracellulare | No clearly active agent | |
| Cryptosporidiosis | No clearly active agent | |
| Oral candidiasis | Clotrimazole troche | 5 troches/day |
| | or | |
| | Nystatin swish | 5,000 U qid |
| | or | |
| | Ketoconazole | 200–400 mg bid |
| Esophageal candidiasis | Ketoconazole | 200 mg bid |
| Cytomegalovirus | 9-(2-hydroxy-1-(hydroxymethol) ethoxymethyl) guanine | Dose not established (investigational) |
| Herpes simplex | Acyclovir sodium | 200 mg five times daily |
| Herpes zoster (disseminated) | Acyclovir sodium | 10 mg/kg/day IV 800 mg five times daily po |

[a]IV indicates administered intravenously; po, by mouth; qid. four times daily; U, units.
[b]A syndrome called AIDS-related complex (ARC) has been described in patients who do not have an opportunistic infection. Such patients are seropositive and present with weight loss, fever, night sweats, generalized lymphadenopathy, chronic fatigue, and depression.

Table from Kaplan LD, Wofsy C, Volberding P: Treatment of patients with acquired immunodeficiency syndrome and associated manifestations. JAMA, 257:1367, 1987. Used with permission.

TABLE 4–8
**AGENTS WITH ACTIVITY AGAINST HIV**

| Agent | Mechanism of Action | Major Toxicity |
|-------|--------------------|----------------|
| Suramin sodium | Inhibits reverse transcriptase | Fever, rash, fatigue, adrenal insufficiency, renal insufficiency, hepatic failure |
| Ribavirin | Guanosine analogue interferes with 5' capping of viral mRNA | Hemolytic anemia |
| HPA-23 | Inhibits reverse transcriptase | Thrombocytopenia |
| Phosphonoformate | Inhibits reverse transcriptase | Renal failure |
| Azidothymidine (AZT) | Inhibits reverse transcriptase, DNA chain terminator | Headache, leukopenia, macrocytic anemia |
| α-Interferon | Interferes with assembly of viral proteins | Flulike symptoms, fatigue, weight loss, neutropenia |
| AL721 | Extracts cholesterol from cellular membranes | No data |
| 2', 3'-Dideoxynucleosides | Chain terminators of DNA synthesis | No data |

Table from Kaplan LD, Wofsy C, Volberding P: Treatment of patients with acquired immunodeficiency syndrome and associated manifestations. JAMA, 257:1367, 1987. Used with permission.

TABLE 4–9
**SOMATIC TREATMENT OF PSYCHIATRIC SIGNS AND SYMPTOMS ASSOCIATED WITH AIDS**

| Psychiatric Signs and Symptoms | Treatment | Comment |
|---|---|---|
| Anxiety<br>Insomnia | Anxiolytics<br>Antihistamines | Benzodiazepines are useful but may exacerbate cognitive symptoms; low doses of sedating antipsychotics, e.g., thioridazine (Mellaril), or antihistamines (diphenhydramine (Benadryl)) may be helpful |
| Severe anxiety<br>Cognitive disorder with agitation<br>Psychotic episode | Antipsychotics | Chlorpromazine (Thorazine) equivalents of 50–200 mg/day (may need lower dosages than generally used due to presence of brain damage) |
| Major depressive disorder | Antidepressants | Those drugs with few anticholinergic side effects are favored to decrease possibility of atropine psychosis; low-dose amphetamines have been used |
| Mania | Lithium | Renal function must be carefully monitored |

der, e.g., dementia; the usual measures of medical, environmental, and social support should be instituted in these situations (Table 4–9).

**D. Psychotherapy.**    The role of both individual and group psychotherapy is important. The psychiatrist can help patients deal with feelings of guilt regarding behavior that is disapproved of by other segments of society and that has contributed to developing AIDS. Many patients infected with HIV feel that they are being punished for a deviant lifestyle. Difficult health care decisions, e.g., whether to participate in an experimental drug trial, as well as terminal care and life support systems, should be explored. In addition, all infected persons must be educated concerning safe sexual practices. Involving the patient's spouse or lover often is warranted. Treatment of homosexual and bisexual persons with AIDS often involves helping the patients come out to their families and deal with the possible issues of rejection, guilt, shame, and anger.

Treatment of IV drug users involves discussing the patient's continued use of IV drugs. The possible ill effects of drug abuse on a patient's health needs to be weighed against the effect of adding drug withdrawal to an AIDS patient's existing problems. Educating patients about the danger of sharing contaminated needles is of utmost importance.

*For more detailed discussion of this topic, see Van Gorp WG, Cummings JL: Neuropsychiatric Aspects of Infectious Disorders, Sec 2.7, p 235; Grant I, Atkinson JH Jr: Psychiatric Aspects of Acquired Immune Deficiency Syndrome, Sec 29.2, p 1669; Hinken GH: Van Gorp WF, Satz P: Neuropsychological and Neuropsychiatric Aspects of HIV Infection in Adults, Sec 29.2a, p 1669, in CTP/VI.*

# 5

# Substance-Related Disorders

## I. General introduction

Substance abuse occurs in all segments of all societies. The proper evaluation of any patient requires an assessment of substance use. Substance abuse results in decreased work and school performance, accidents, intoxication while working, absenteeism, violent crime, and theft. Adolescents are the most vulnerable age group for developing substance abuse problems. Men are more at risk than women.

**A. Evaluation.** Substance-abusing patients are often difficult to detect and evaluate. Not easily categorized, they almost always underestimate the amount of substance used, are prone to use denial, are often manipulative, and often fear the consequences of acknowledging the problem. Because these patients may be unreliable, it is necessary to obtain information from other sources, such as family members.

When dealing with these patients, clinicians must present clear, firm, and consistent limits, which will be tested frequently. Such patients usually require a confrontational approach. Although clinicians may feel angered by being manipulated, they should not act on these feelings.

Substance abuse frequently coexists with other psychiatric conditions, such as depressive or anxiety disorders. These conditions, however, are difficult to properly evaluate in the presence of ongoing substance abuse, which itself causes symptoms. Substance abuse is frequently associated with personality disorders, e.g., antisocial, borderline, narcissistic. Depressed, anxious, or psychotic patients may self-medicate with either prescribed or nonprescribed substances. Substance-induced disorders should always be considered in the evaluation of depression, anxiety, or psychosis.

**1. Toxicology**

Urine or blood test is useful in confirming suspected substance use. The two types of tests are screening and confirmatory. Screening tests are sensitive but not specific (many false positives). Confirm positive screening results with a specific confirmatory test for an identified drug. Although most drugs are well detected in urine, some are best detected in blood, e.g., barbiturates or alcohol. Absolute blood concentrations can sometimes be useful, e.g., a high concentration in the absence of clinical signs of intoxication would imply tolerance. Urine toxicology is usually positive for up to 2 days after taking most drugs.

**2. Physical examination**

    a. Carefully consider whether concomitant medical conditions are substance-related. Look specifically for the following:

        **i. Subcutaneous or intravenous abusers**—acquired immune deficiency syndrome (AIDS), scars from intravenous (IV) or subcutaneous injection, abscesses, infections from contaminated injections, bacterial endocarditis, drug-induced or infectious hepatitis, thrombophlebitis, tetanus.

ii. **Cocaine, heroin, or other drug snorters**—deviated or perforated nasal septum, nasal bleeding, rhinitis.

iii. **Cocaine freebasers, crack, marijuana, or other drug smokers, and inhalant abusers**—bronchitis, asthma, chronic respiratory conditions.

b. Determine the pattern of abuse. Is it continuous or episodic? When, where, and with whom is the substance taken? Is the abuse recreational or confined to certain social contexts? Find out how much of the patient's life is associated with obtaining, taking, withdrawing from, and recovering from substances. How much do the substances affect the patient's social and work functioning? How does he or she get and pay for the substances? Always specifically describe the substance and route of administration rather than the category, i.e., use "intravenous heroin withdrawal" rather than "opioid withdrawal." If describing polysubstance abuse, list all substances. Substance abusers typically abuse multiple substances.

**B. Diagnoses.**   See Table 5–1.

**C. Treatment.**   See Table 5–2. In general, the management of intoxication involves observation for possible overdose, evaluation for possible polysubstance intoxication and concomitant medical conditions, and supportive treatment, such as protecting the patient from injury. The treatment of abuse or dependence involves abstinence and long-term treatment.

1. **Period of abstinence.**   Anything that improves abstinence should be used.

2. **Long-term treatment lasting at least 6 months.**   Relapse is common. A variety of methods, including individual therapy, group therapy, self-help groups (such as Alcoholics Anonymous, Narcotics Anonymous), therapeutic communities, family groups (such as Al-anon), and chemical maintenance (methadone [Dolophine], disulfiram [Antabuse], naltrexone [Trexan]), as well as a variety of philosophical approaches, including addictive, medical, and moral (or inspirational) models may all help. Find what works for each patient.

**D. Definitions**

1. **Intoxication.**   See Table 5–3. Maladaptive behavior associated with recent drug ingestion. The effects of intoxication of any drug can vary widely among persons and depend on such factors as dose, circumstances, and underlying personality.

2. **Withdrawal.**   See Table 5–3. Psychoactive substance-specific syndrome following cessation of heavy use (implies tolerance and indicates dependence).

3. **Tolerance.**   Need for more of a substance to become intoxicated or the same amount of a drug producing decreased effect with continued use.

4. **Abuse.**   A maladaptive pattern of substance use resulting in repeated problems and adverse consequences, e.g., use in hazardous situations, legal, social, occupational problems.

TABLE 5–1
**DSM-IV DIAGNOSES ASSOCIATED WITH CLASS OF SUBSTANCES**

| | Dependence | Abuse | Intoxication | Withdrawal | Intoxication Delirium | Withdrawal Delirium | Dementia | Amnestic Disorder | Psychotic Disorders | Mood Disorders | Anxiety Disorders | Sexual Dysfunctions | Sleep Disorders |
|---|---|---|---|---|---|---|---|---|---|---|---|---|---|
| Alcohol | X | X | X | X | I | W | P | P | I/W | I/W | I/W | I | I/W |
| Amphetamines | X | X | X | X | I | — | — | — | I | I/W | I | I | I/W |
| Caffeine | | | X | | | | | | | | I | | I |
| Cannabis | X | X | X | | I | | | | I | | I | | |
| Cocaine | X | X | X | X | I | | | | I | I/W | I/W | I | I/W |
| Hallucinogens | X | X | X | | I | | | | I[a] | I | I | | |
| Inhalants | X | X | X | | I | | P | | I | I | I | | |
| Nicotine | X | | | X | | | | | | | | | |
| Opioids | X | X | X | X | I | | | | I | I | | I | I/W |
| Phencyclidine | X | X | X | | I | | | | I | I | I | | |
| Sedatives, hypnotics, or anxiolytics | X | X | X | X | I | W | P | P | I/W | I/W | W | I | I/W |
| Polysubstance | X | | | | | | | | | | | | |
| Other | X | X | X | X | I | W | P | P | I/W | I/W | I/W | I | I/W |

[a] Also Hallucinogen persisting perception disorder (flashbacks).

**Note:** X, I, W, I/W, or P indicates that the category is recognized in DSM-IV. In addition, I indicates that the specifier "with onset during intoxication" may be noted for the category (except for intoxication delirium); W indicates that the specifier "with onset during withdrawal" may be noted for the category (except for withdrawal delirium); and I/W indicates that either "with onset during intoxication" or "with onset during withdrawal" may be noted for the category. P indicates that the disorder is "persisting."

Used with permission, APA.

TABLE 5–2
**PSYCHOACTIVE DRUG-RELATED CONDITIONS AND TREATMENTS**

| Drug | Behavioral Effects | Physical Effects | Lab Findings | Treatment |
|---|---|---|---|---|
| Opioids: opium, morphine, heroin, meperidine, methadone, pentazocine | Euphoria, drowsiness, anorexia, decreased sex drive, hypoactivity, change in personality | Miosis, pruritus, nausea, bradycardia, constipation, needle tracks in arms, legs, groin | Detected in blood up to 24 hours after last dose | For gradual withdrawal: methadone 5–10 mg every 6 hr for 24 hr, then decrease dose for 10 days. For overdose: naloxone 0.4 mg IM every 20 minutes for 3 doses; keep airway open; give O₂ |
| Amphetamine and other sympathomimetics (including cocaine) and amphetamine-like substances | Alertness, loquaciousness, euphoria, hyperactive, irritability, aggressiveness, agitation, paranoid trends, impotence, visual and tactile hallucinations | Mydriasis, tremor, halitosis, dry mouth, tachycardia, hypertension, weight loss, arrhythmias, fever, convulsions, perforated nasal septum (with snorting) | Detected in blood and urine | For agitation: diazepam IM or PO 5–10 mg every 3 hr; for tachyarrhythmias: propanolol (Inderal) 10–20 mg PO every 4 hr; vitamin C 0.5 gm qid PO may increase urinary excretion by acidifying urine |
| Hallucinogens: LSD, psilocybin (mushrooms), mescaline (peyote), DET, DMT, DOM or STP, MDA | 8–12 hr duration with flashback after abstinence, visual hallucinations, paranoid ideation, false sense of achievement and strength, suicidal or homicidal tendencies, depersonalization, derealization | Mydriasis, ataxia, hyperemic conjunctiva, tachycardia, hypertension | None | Emotional support (talking down); for mild agitation: diazepam 10 mg IM or PO every 2 hr for 4 doses; for severe agitation: haloperidol 1–5 mg IM and repeat every 6 hr prn. May have to continue haloperidol 1–2 mg per day PO for weeks to prevent flashback syndrome. Phenothiazines may be used only with LSD. **Caution:** phenothiazines can produce *fatal* results if used with other hallucinogens (eg, DET, DMT) especially if they are adulterated with strychnine or belladonna alkaloids |

| Substance | Signs/Symptoms | Laboratory | Treatment |
|---|---|---|---|
| PCP and phencyclidine-like substances (including ketamine, TCP) | 8–12 hr duration (about 2 hr for ketamine), hallucinations, paranoid ideation, labile mood, loose associations (may mimic schizophrenia), catatonia, violent behavior, convulsions | Detected in urine up to 5 days after ingestion | Phenothiazines contraindicated for first week after ingestion; for violent delusions: haloperidol 1–4 mg IM or PO every 2–4 hr until patient is calm |
| CNS depressants: barbiturates, methaqualone (illegal), meprobamate, benzodiazepines, glutethimide | Drowsiness, confusion, inattentiveness | Detected in blood | For barbiturates: Substitute 30 mg liquid phenobarbital for every 100 mg barbiturates abused and give in divided doses every 6 hr and then decrease by 20% every other day; may also substitute diazepam for barbiturate abused. Give 10 mg every 2–4 hr for 24 hr and then reduce dose. For benzodiazepines: gradual reduction of diazepam every other day over 10-day period |
| Volatile hydrocarbons and petroleum derivatives; glue, benzene, gasoline, varnish thinner, lighter fluid, aerosols | Euphoria, clouded sensorium, slurred speech, ataxia, hallucinations in 50% of cases, psychoses, permanent brain damage if used daily over 6 mo | Relevant to determine tissue damage (SGOT) | For agitation: haloperidol 1–5 mg every 6 hr until calm; avoid epinephrine because of myocardial sensitization |
| | Odor on breath, tachycardia with possible ventricular fibrillation, possible damage of brain, liver, kidneys, myocardium | | |
| Other inhalants: nitrous oxide | Euphoria, drowsiness, ataxia, confusion | None | Hypoxia is treated with $O_2$ inhalation |
| | Analgesia, respiratory depression, hypotension | | |
| Alcohol | Poor judgment, loquaciousness, mood change, aggression, impaired attention, amnesia | Blood level between 100 and 200 mg/dL | For delirium: diazepam 5–10 mg IM or PO every 3 hr, IM vitamin B complex, hydration. For hallucinosis: haloperidol 1–4 mg every 6 hr IM or PO |
| | Nystagmus, flushed face, ataxia, slurred speech | | |
| Belladonna alkaloids (found in OTC medications and morning glory seeds); stramonium, homatropine, atropine, scopolomine, hyoscyamine | Hot skin, erythema, weakness, thirst, blurred vision, confusion, excitement, delirium, stupor, coma (anticholinergic delirium) | None | Antidote is physostigmine 2 mg IV every 20 min; IV should be controlled at no more than 1 mg/min; watch for copious salivary secretion because of anticholinesterase activity. Propranolol for tachyarrhythmias |
| | Dry mouth and throat, mydriasis, twitching, dysphagia, light sensitivity, pyrexia, hypertension followed by shock, urinary retention | | |

Table adapted from *Desk Reference on Drug Misuse and Abuse*, New York State Medical Society, New York, 1964.

TABLE 5–3
**SIGNS AND SYMPTOMS OF SUBSTANCE INTOXICATION AND WITHDRAWAL**

| Substance | Intoxication | Withdrawal |
|---|---|---|
| Opioid | Drowsiness<br>Slurred speech<br>Impaired attention or memory<br>Analgesia<br>Anorexia<br>Decreased sex drive<br>Hypoactivity | Craving for drug<br>Nausea, vomiting<br>Muscle aches<br>Lacrimation, rhinorrhea<br>Pupillary dilation<br>Piloerection<br>Sweating<br>Diarrhea<br>Fever<br>Insomnia<br>Yawning |
| Amphetamine or cocaine | Perspiration, chills<br>Tachycardia<br>Pupillary dilation<br>Elevated blood pressure<br>Nausea, vomiting<br>Tremor<br>Arrhythmia<br>Fever<br>Convulsions<br>Anorexia, weight loss<br>Dry mouth<br>Impotence<br>Hallucinations<br>Hyperactivity<br>Irritability<br>Aggressiveness<br>Paranoid ideation | Dysphoria<br>Fatigue<br>Sleep disorder<br>Agitation<br>Craving |
| Sedative, hypnotic, or anxiolytic | Slurred speech<br>Incoordination<br>Unsteady gait<br>Impaired attention or memory | Nausea, vomiting<br>Malaise, weakness<br>Autonomic hyperactivity<br>Anxiety, irritability<br>Increased sensitivity to light and sound<br>Coarse tremor<br>Marked insomnia<br>Seizures |

5. **Dependence.**  Psychological or physical need to continue taking the substance. Dependence on a drug may be physical, psychological, or both. **Psychological dependence,** also referred to as habituation, is characterized by a continuous or intermittent craving for the substance. **Physiological (physical) dependence** is characterized by **tolerance,** a need to take the substance to prevent the occurrence of a withdrawal or abstinence syndrome. **Note:** The presence of withdrawal symptoms upon abstinence usually implies dependence. Other than for short-term treatment of withdrawal symptoms, the distinction between abuse and dependence is of limited clinical significance.

6. **Addiction.**  A nonscientific term that implies psychological dependence, drug-seeking behavior, physical dependence and tolerance, and associated deterioration of physical and mental health. It still appears despite its official removal from the medical nosology.

## II. Opioids

Lifetime risk of opioid dependence or abuse is 0.7% in the United States, which has an estimated 500,000 addicts (with half in New York City). Opioids include opium derivatives, as well as synthetic drugs: opium, morphine, diacetyl-morphine (heroin, smack, horse), methadone, codeine, oxycodone (Percodan, Percocet), hydromorphone (Dilaudid), levorphanol (Levo-Dromoran), pentazo-cine (Talwin), meperidine (Demerol), propoxyphene (Darvon), among others. Table 5–4 lists the durations of action of opioids.

**A. Route of administration.** Depends on the drug. Opium is smoked. Her-oin is typically injected (IV or subcutaneously) or inhaled (snorted) nasally, and may be combined with stimulants for IV injection (speedball). Pharma-ceutically available opioids are typically taken orally, but some are also injectable. Heroin is exclusively a drug of abuse and is most commonly abused by patients of lower socioeconomic status, who often engage in criminal activities to pay for drugs.

**B. Dose.** Often is difficult to determine by history for two reasons. First, the abuser has no way of knowing the concentration of the heroin he or she has bought and may underestimate the amount (which can lead to accidental overdose if the person suddenly gets one bag containing 15% heroin when the typical amount is 5%). Second, the abuser may overstate the dosage in an attempt to get more methadone.

**C. Intoxication**

   1. **Objective signs and symptoms.** Central nervous system (CNS) depression, decreased gastrointestinal (GI) motility, respiratory depres-sion, analgesia, nausea and vomiting, slurred speech, hypotension, brady-cardia, pupillary constriction, seizures (in overdose). Tolerant patients still will have pupillary constriction and constipation.

   2. **Subjective signs and symptoms.** Euphoria (heroin intoxication described as a total body orgasm), at times anxious dysphoria, tran-quility, decreased attention and memory, drowsiness, and psychomotor retardation.

**D. Overdose.** Can be a medical emergency and is usually accidental. Can result from incorrect estimation of dose or erratic pattern of use in which person has lost previous tolerance to drug. Often caused by combined use with other CNS depressants, e.g., alcohol or sedative-hypnotics. Clinical signs include pinpoint pupils, respiratory depression, CNS depression.

   1. **Treatment**
      a. Intensive care unit (ICU) admission and support vital functions, e.g., IV fluids.
      b. Immediate IV naloxone (Narcan), an opioid antagonist—0.8 mg (0.01 mg per kg for neonates) IV and wait 15 minutes.

TABLE 5–4
**DURATION OF ACTION OF OPIOIDS**

| Drug | Duration of Action (in Hours) |
| --- | --- |
| Heroin | 3–4 |
| Meperidine | 2–4 |
| Morphine, hydromorphone | 4–5 |
| Methadone | 12–24 |
| Propoxyphene | 12 |
| Pentazocine | 2–3 |

    c. If no response, give 1.6 mg IV and wait 15 minutes.

    d. If still no response, give 3.2 mg IV and suspect another diagnosis.

    e. If successful, continue at 0.4 mg every hour IV.

**2.** Always consider possible polysubstance overdose. A patient successfully treated with naloxone may wake up briefly only to succumb to a subsequent overdose from another slower-acting drug, e.g., sedative-hypnotic, taken simultaneously. Remember that naloxone will precipitate rapid withdrawal symptoms. It has a short half-life and must be administered continuously until the opioid has been cleared (up to 3 days for methadone). Babies born to opioid-abusing mothers may experience intoxication, overdose, or withdrawal.

**E. Withdrawal.** Seldom a medical emergency. Clinical signs are flulike and include drug craving, anxiety, lacrimation, rhinorrhea, yawning, sweating, insomnia, hot and cold flashes, muscle aches, abdominal cramping, dilated pupils, piloerection, tremor, restlessness, nausea and vomiting, diarrhea, and increased vital signs. Intensity depends on previous dose and on rate of decrease. Less intense with drugs that have long half-lives, such as methadone; more intense with drugs that have short half-lives, such as meperidine. Patients have severe craving for opioid drugs and will demand and manipulate for opioids. Beware of fakers and look for piloerection, dilated pupils, tachycardia, hypertension. If objective signs are absent, do not give opioids for withdrawal. The goal of detoxification is to minimize withdrawal symptoms (in order to prevent the patient from abandoning treatment) while steadily decreasing opioid dose. Untreated opioid withdrawal results in no serious medical sequelae in otherwise healthy people.

**1. Detoxification.** If objective withdrawal signs are present, give methadone 10 mg. If withdrawal persists after 4–6 hours, give an additional 5–10 mg, which may be repeated every 4–6 hours. Total dose in 24 hours equals the dose for the second day (seldom more than 40 mg). Give twice a day or every day and decrease dosage by 5 mg a day for heroin withdrawal; methadone withdrawal may require slower detoxification. Pentazocine-dependent patients should be detoxified on pentazocine because of its mixed opioid receptor agonist and antagonist properties. Many nonopioid drugs have been tried for opioid detoxification, but the only promising one is clonidine (Catapres), which is a centrally acting $\alpha_2$-agonist that effectively relieves the nausea, vomiting, and diarrhea associated with opioid withdrawal (it is not effective for most other symptoms). Give 0.1–0.2 mg every 3 hours as needed, not to exceed 0.8 mg a day. Titrate dose according to symptoms. When dosage is stabilized, taper over 2 weeks. Hypotension is a side effect. Clonidine is short acting and not a narcotic.

    The general approach in withdrawal is one of support, detoxification, and progression to methadone maintenance or abstinence. Patients dependent on multiple drugs, e.g., an opioid and a sedative-hypnotic, should be maintained on a stable dosage of one drug while being detoxified from the other. Naltrexone (a long-acting oral opioid antagonist) can be used with clonidine to expedite detoxification. After detoxification, oral naltrexone has been effective in helping to maintain abstinence for up to 2 months.

2. **Methadone maintenance.**  The main long-term treatment for opiate dependence, methadone maintenance is a slow, extended detoxification. Most patients can be maintained on daily dosages of 60 mg or less. Although often criticized, methadone maintenance programs do decrease rates of heroin use. A sufficient methadone dosage is necessary; use of plasma methadone concentrations may help to determine appropriate dosage.

3. **Therapeutic communities.**  Residential programs that emphasize abstinence and group therapy in a structured environment, e.g., Phoenix House.

## III. Sedatives, hypnotics, and anxiolytics

The major complication of sedative, hypnotic, or anxiolytic intoxication is overdose with associated CNS and respiratory depression. Although mild intoxication is not in itself dangerous (unless the patient is driving or operating machinery), the possibility of a covert overdose must always be considered. Sedative, hypnotic, or anxiolytic intoxication is similar to alcohol intoxication, but idiosyncratic aggressive reactions are uncommon. These drugs are often taken with other CNS depressants, e.g., alcohol, which can produce additive effects. Withdrawal is dangerous and can lead to delirium or seizures.

Sedatives, hypnotics, and anxiolytics are the most commonly prescribed psychoactive drugs. Lifetime prevalence of abuse or dependence is 1.1%. Sedative-hypnotics are taken orally. Usually, dependence develops only after at least several months of daily use, but persons vary widely in this respect. Because most of these drugs have legitimate uses, they have become part of the establishment, as well as part of the drug abuse culture. Many middle-aged patients begin taking benzodiazepines for insomnia or anxiety, become dependent, and then seek multiple physicians to prescribe them. Sedative-hypnotics are used illicitly for their euphoriant effects, to augment the effects of other CNS depressant drugs such as opioids or alcohol, and to temper the excitatory and anxiogenic effects of stimulants, e.g., cocaine. Barbiturates have been replaced largely by benzodiazepines for two reasons: (1) benzodiazepines have a much larger therapeutic index (the lethal dose is much greater than the effective dose), and (2) barbiturates rapidly induce hepatic microsomal enzymes, causing physiological tolerance, whereas the benzodiazepines do not.

### A. Drugs

1. **Benzodiazepines.**  Diazepam (Valium), chlordiazepoxide (Librium), flurazepam (Dalmane), lorazepam (Ativan), alprazolam (Xanax), triazolam (Halcion), oxazepam (Serax), temazepam (Restoril), and others.

2. **Barbiturates.**  Secobarbital (Seconal), pentobarbital (Nembutal), and others.

3. **Similarly acting drugs.**  Meprobamate (Equanil, Meprospan, Miltown), methaqualone, glutethimide, ethchlorvynol (Placidyl), chloral hydrate (Noctec).

### B. Intoxication.  See Table 5–3. Intoxication also can cause disinhibition and amnesia.

### C. Withdrawal.  See Table 5–3. A potentially life-threatening condition, which often requires hospitalization. Interindividual differences in tolerance are large, and the dosages taken by some patients can be very large. All

sedatives, hypnotics, and anxiolytics have cross-tolerance with each other and with alcohol. The degree of tolerance can be measured with the pentobarbital challenge test (Table 5–5), which identifies the dose of pentobarbital needed to prevent withdrawal.

## IV. Stimulants (amphetamines and amphetaminelike substances)

Extremely addicting and dangerous. Powerful anorectic effects. Amphetamines are usually taken orally, but also can be injected or nasally inhaled. The clinical syndromes associated with amphetamines are similar to those associated with cocaine, although the oral route of amphetamine administration produces a less rapid euphoria and consequently is less addictive. IV amphetamine abuse is highly addictive. Commonly abused by students, long-distance truck drivers, and other groups who desire prolonged wakefulness and attentiveness. Amphetamines cause release of dopamine and may cause hallucinations and delusions, which are symptomatically identical to an acute schizophrenic episode (dopamine model of schizophrenia).

### A. Drugs

1. **Major amphetamines.** Amphetamines, dextroamphetamine (Dexedrine), methamphetamine (Desoxyn, speed), methylphenidate (Ritalin), pemoline (Cylert).

2. **Related substances.** Ephedrine, phenylpropanolamine (PPA), khat, methcathinone (crank).

3. **Substituted (designer) amphetamines.** (Also classified as hallucinogens.) Have neurochemical effects on both serotonergic and dopaminergic systems; with both amphetaminelike and hallucinogenlike behavioral effects, e.g., 3,4-methylenedioxymethamphetamine (MDMA, ecstasy), N-ethyl-3,4-methylenedioxyamphetamine (MDEA), 5-methoxy-3,4-methylenedioxyamphetamine (MMDA).

4. **Ice.** Pure form of methamphetamine (inhaled, smoked, injected).

### B. Intoxication and withdrawal.  See Table 5–3.

## V. Cocaine

Referred to as coke, blow, cane, freebase. The effects of cocaine are pharmacologically similar to those of other stimulants, but its widespread use warrants a separate discussion.

A natural product of the coca plant, cocaine has been used for its psychoactive effects in many cultures for centuries. Before its high addictiveness was well known, it was widely used as a stimulant and euphoriant. Cocaine is usually

TABLE 5–5
**PENTOBARBITAL[a] CHALLENGE TEST**

1. Give pentobarbital 200 mg orally.
2. Observe patient for intoxication after 1 hour, e.g., sleepiness, slurred speech, or nystagmus.
3. If patient is not intoxicated, give another 100 mg of pentobarbital every 2 hours (maximum 500 mg over 6 hours).
4. Total dose given to produce mild intoxication is equivalent to daily abuse level of barbiturates.
5. Substitute phenobarbital 30 mg (longer half-life) for each 100 mg of pentobarbital.
6. Decrease dose by about 10% a day.
7. Adjust rate if signs of intoxication or withdrawal are present.

[a]Other drugs can also be used.

inhaled, but can be smoked or injected. To be smoked, cocaine hydrochloride must be purified into a freebase form. The availability of a crystallized form of freebase cocaine (crack, rock) in small, inexpensive amounts (about $10 for a dose of 65–100 mg) in recent years has led to an epidemic of crack use, which has had devastating effects on society. Low socioeconomic groups have been particularly susceptible, leading to the further decay of many urban neighborhoods because of cocaine use and associated crime. Crack is smoked, has a rapid onset of action, and is highly addictive. The typical addict image previously associated with the heroin abuser now also applies to the crack abuser.

Smoking cocaine produces an onset of action comparable to that of an IV injection and is equally addictive. The euphoria is intense, and there is a risk of dependence after only one dose. Like amphetamines, cocaine can be taken in binges lasting up to several days. This phenomenon is partly the result of greater euphoric effects from subsequent doses (sensitization). During binges, the abuser will take the cocaine repeatedly until exhausted or out of drug. This is followed by a crash of lethargy, hunger, and prolonged sleep, followed by another binge. With repeated use, tolerance develops to the euphoriant, anorectic, hyperthermic, and cardiovascular effects.

IV cocaine use is associated with the same risks of other forms of IV drug abuse, including AIDS, septicemia, and venous thrombus. Long-term snorting can lead to a rebound rhinitis, which is often self-treated with nasal decongestants; it also causes nosebleeds and eventually may lead to a perforated nasal septum.

**A. Cocaine intoxication.**  See Table 5–3. Can cause restlessness, agitation, anxiety, talkativeness, pressured speech, paranoid ideation, aggressiveness, increased sexual interest, heightened sense of awareness, grandiosity, hyperactivity, and other manic symptoms. Physical signs include tachycardia, hypertension, pupillary dilation, chills, anorexia, insomnia, and stereotyped movements. Cocaine has also been associated with sudden death through cardiac complications and delirium. Delusional disorders are typically paranoid. Delirium may involve tactile or olfactory hallucinations. Delirium may lead to seizures and death. Treatment is largely symptomatic. Agitation can be treated with restraints, benzodiazepines, or, if severe (delirium or psychosis), low doses of high-potency antipsychotics (only as a last resort because the medications lower the seizure threshold). Somatic symptoms, e.g., tachycardia, hypertension, can be treated with β-adrenergic receptor antagonists (β-blockers). Evaluate for possible medical complications.

**B. Withdrawal.**  The most prominent sign of cocaine withdrawal is craving for cocaine. The tendency to develop dependence is related to the route of administration (lower with snorting, higher with IV injection or smoking freebase cocaine). Withdrawal symptoms include fatigue, lethargy, guilt, anxiety, and feelings of helplessness, hopelessness, and worthlessness. Long-term use can lead to depression, which may require antidepressant treatment. Observe for possible suicidal ideation. Withdrawal symptoms usually peak in several days, but the syndrome (especially depressive symptoms) may last for weeks.

## VI. Cannabis (marijuana)

About one third of Americans have tried marijuana. Marijuana and hashish contain Δ-9-tetrahydrocannabinol (THC), which is the main active euphoriant (many other active cannabinoids are probably responsible for the other varied effects). Sometimes, purified THC also is abused. Cannabinoids usually are smoked, but also can be eaten (delays onset, but one can eat very large doses).

A. **Cannabis intoxication.** Symptoms include euphoria or dysphoria, anxiety, suspiciousness, inappropriate laughter, time distortion, social withdrawal, impaired judgment, and the following objective signs: conjunctival injection, increased appetite, dry mouth, and tachycardia. It also causes a dose-dependent hypothermia and mild sedation. Often used with alcohol, cocaine, and other drugs. Treatment of intoxication usually is not required. Can cause depersonalization and, rarely, hallucinations. More commonly causes mild persecutory delusions, which seldom require medication. In very high doses, can cause mild delirium with panic symptoms or a prolonged cannabis psychosis (may last up to 6 weeks). Long-term use can lead to anxiety or depression and an apathetic amotivational syndrome. Urine THC testing is positive for many days after intoxication.

B. **Cannabis dependence.** Dependence and withdrawal are controversial diagnoses—there are certainly many psychologically dependent abusers, but forced abstinence even in heavy users does not consistently cause a characteristic withdrawal syndrome. (Marijuana is often considered a gateway drug, leading to abuse of so-called hard drugs.)

## VII. Hallucinogens

About 10% of Americans have used hallucinogens—1–2% in the last 12 months.

A. **Drugs**
   1. Lysergic acid diethylamide (LSD)
   2. Psilocybin (from some mushrooms)
   3. Mescaline (peyote cactus)
   4. Harmine and harmaline
   5. Ibogaine
   6. Substituted amphetamines, e.g., MDMA, MDEA, 2,5-dimethoxy-4-methylamphetamine (DOM, STP), dimethyltryptamine (DMT), MMDA, trimethoxyamphetamine (TMA), which are also commonly classified with amphetamines

B. **General considerations.** Hallucinogens usually are eaten, sucked out of paper (bucally ingested), or smoked. This category includes many different drugs with different effects. Hallucinogens act as sympathomimetics and cause hypertension, tachycardia, hyperthermia, and dilated pupils. Psychological effects range from mild perceptual changes to frank hallucinations; most users only experience mild effects. Usually used sporadically because of tolerance. Hallucinogens often are contaminated with anticholinergic drugs.

C. **Hallucinogen intoxication (hallucinosis)**
   1. **Diagnosis, signs, and symptoms.** In a state of full wakefulness and alertness, maladaptive behavioral changes (anxiety, depression, ideas of reference, paranoid ideation); changes in perception (hallucinations, illusions, depersonalization); and pupillary dilation, tachycardia or palpitations, sweating, blurring of vision, tremors, and incoordination. Panic reactions (bad trips) can occur, even in experienced users. The user

typically develops the conviction that the disturbed perceptions are real. In the typical bad trip, the user feels as if he or she is going mad, has damaged his or her brain, and will never recover. Treatment involves reassurance and keeping the patient with trusted supportive people (friends, nurses). In general, avoid using medications, but if the patient is severely anxious, benzodiazepines may be used. If the patient is psychotic and agitated, high-potency antipsychotics, such as haloperidol (Haldol), fluphenazine (Prolixin), or thiothixene (Navane) may be used (avoid low-potency antipsychotics because of anticholinergic effects). A controlled environment is necessary to prevent possible dangerous actions due to grossly impaired judgment. Physical restraints may be required. Prolonged psychosis resembling schizophreniform disorder occasionally develops in vulnerable patients. Delusional syndromes and mood (usually depressive) disorders may also develop.

**D. Posthallucinogen perception disorder.** A distressing reexperience of impaired perception after cessation of hallucinogen use, i.e., a **flashback.** The patient may require low doses of benzodiazepine (for an acute episode) or antipsychotic drug (if persistent).

## VIII. PCP

PCP is a dissociative anesthetic with hallucinogenic effects. Similarly acting drugs include ketamine (Ketalar), also referred to as Special K, and 1-(1-2-thienylcyclohenxyl) piperidine (TCP). PCP commonly causes paranoia and unpredictable violence, which often brings abusers to medical attention.

### A. PCP intoxication

**1. Diagnosis, signs, and symptoms.** Belligerence, assaultiveness, agitation, impulsiveness, unpredictability, and the following signs: nystagmus, increased blood pressure or heart rate, numbness or diminished response to pain, ataxia, dysarthria, muscle rigidity, seizures, and hyperacusis.

Typically, PCP is smoked with marijuana (a laced joint) or tobacco but can be eaten, injected, or inhaled nasally. PCP should be considered in patients who describe unusual experiences with marijuana or LSD.

Effects are dose-related. At low doses, PCP acts as a CNS depressant, producing nystagmus, blurred vision, numbness, and incoordination. At moderate doses, PCP produces hypertension, dysarthria, ataxia, increased muscle tone (especially in face and neck), hyperactive reflexes, and sweating. At higher doses, PCP produces agitation, fever, abnormal movements, rhabdomyolysis, myoglobinuria, and renal failure. Overdose can cause seizures, severe hypertension, diaphoresis, hypersalivation, respiratory depression, stupor (with eyes open), coma, and death. Violent actions are common with intoxication. Because of the analgesic effects, patients may have no regard for their own bodies and may severely injure themselves while agitated and combative. Psychosis, sometimes persistent (may resemble schizophreniform disorder), may develop. This is especially likely in patients with underlying schizophrenia. Other possible complications include delirium, mood disorder, and delusional disorder.

**2. Treatment.** Isolate the patient in a nonstimulating environment. Do not try to talk down the intoxicated patient as you might with an anxiety disorder patient; wait for the PCP to clear first. Urine acidification may increase drug clearance (ascorbic acid or ammonium chloride). Screen for other drugs. If acutely agitated, use benzodiazepines. If agitated and psychotic, a high-potency antipsychotic may be used. If physical restraint is required, immobilize the body completely to avoid self-injury. Recovery is usually rapid. Protect the patient and staff. Always evaluate for concomitant medical conditions.

## IX. Inhalants

A wide variety of glues, solvents, and cleaners are volatile and can be inhaled for psychotropic effects. Most are aromatic hydrocarbons; they include gasoline, kerosene, plastic and rubber cements, airplane and household glues, paints, lacquers, enamels, paint thinners, aerosols, polishes, fingernail polish remover, nitrous oxide, amyl nitrate, butyl nitrate, and cleaning fluids.

Inhalants typically are abused by adolescents in lower socioeconomic groups. Some homosexual men use poppers (amyl nitrate, butyl nitrate) during sex to intensify orgasm from the vasodilation, which produces lightheadedness, giddiness, and euphoria.

Symptoms of mild intoxication are similar to intoxication with alcohol or sedative-hypnotics. The diagnosis requires a high level of suspicion. Psychological effects include mild euphoria, belligerence, assaultiveness, impaired judgment, and impulsiveness. Physical effects include ataxia, confusion, disorientation, slurred speech, dizziness, depressed reflexes, and nystagmus. These can progress to delirium and seizures. Possible toxic effects include reports of brain damage, liver damage, bone marrow depression, peripheral neuropathies, and immunosuppression. Withdrawal is unknown. Short-term treatment is supportive medical care, e.g., fluids and blood pressure monitoring.

## X. Caffeine

Caffeine is present in coffee, tea, chocolate, cola and other carbonated beverages, cocoa, cold medications, and over-the-counter stimulants. The average cup of coffee contains 100–150 mg of caffeine, whereas tea and cola are about one half as strong. Stimulants usually contain 100 mg per pill. Intoxication is characterized by restlessness, nervousness, excitement, insomnia, flushed face, diuresis, gastrointestinal disturbance, muscle twitching, rambling flow of thought and speech, tachycardia or cardiac arrhythmia, periods of inexhaustibility, and psychomotor agitation. High doses can increase symptoms of psychiatric disorders, e.g., anxiety, psychosis. Tolerance develops. Withdrawal is usually characterized by headache and lasts 4–5 days. Inquire about all possible sources of caffeine.

## XI. Nicotine

Nicotine is taken through tobacco smoking and chewing.

**A. Nicotine dependence.** Develops rapidly and is strongly affected by environmental conditioning. Often coexists with dependence on other substances, e.g., alcohol, marijuana. Treatments for dependence include hypnosis, aversive therapy, acupuncture, nicotine nasal sprays and gums, and transdermal nicotine (nicotine patches). High relapse rates. Smoking is more habit-forming than chewing. Smoking is associated with chronic obstructive pulmonary disease, cancers, coronary heart disease, and peripheral vascular disease. Tobacco chewing is associated with peripheral vascular disease.

**B. Nicotine withdrawal.** Characterized by nicotine craving, irritability, frustration, anger, anxiety, difficulty concentrating, restlessness, bradycardia, and increased appetite. The withdrawal syndrome may last for up to several weeks and is often superimposed on withdrawal from other substances.

---

*For a more detailed discussion of this topic, see Jaffe JH: Introduction and Overview, Sec 11.1, p 755; Jaffe JH: Amphetamine (or Amphetaminelike)-Related Disorders, Sec 13.3, p 791; Greden JF, Pomerleau OF: Caffeine-Related Disorders and Nicotine-Related Disorders, Sec 13.4, p 799; Woody GE, Macfadden W: Cannabis-Related Disorders, Sec 13.5, p 810; Jaffe JH: Cocaine-Related Disorders, Sec 13.6, p 817; Crowley TJ: Hallucinogen-Related Disorders, Sec 13.7, p 831; Crowley TJ: Inhalant-Related Disorders, Sec 13.8, p 838; Jaffe JH: Opioid-Related Disorders, Sec 13.8, p 838; Jaffe JH: Opioid-Related Disorders, Sec 13.9, p 842; Crowley TJ: Pencyclidine (or Phencyclidinelike)-Related Disorders, Sec 13.10, p 864; Ciraulo DA, Greenblatt DJ: Sedative-, Hypnotic-, or Anxiolytic-Related Disorders, Sec 13.11, p 872; Wiseman EJ: Drug and Alcohol Abuse, Sec 49.6g, p 49.6g, in CTP/VI.*

---

# 6
# Disorders Associated with Alcohol

## I. General introduction

Alcohol, a central nervous system (CNS) depressant and intoxicant, is the most commonly used psychoactive substance in both the mentally healthy and the mentally ill. More than two thirds of all Americans consume alcohol, and the distinction between recreational or social drinking and alcohol abuse is often vague and unclear.

**Alcoholism** is the excessive use of ethanol-containing beverages. Although alcoholism does not describe a specific mental disorder, the disorders associated with alcoholism generally can be divided into two groups: (1) disorders related to the direct effects of alcohol on the brain (including alcohol intoxication, withdrawal, withdrawal delirium, and hallucinosis), (2) disorders related to behavior associated with alcohol (alcohol abuse and dependence), and (3) disorders with persisting effects (including alcohol-induced persisting amnestic disorder, dementia, Wernicke's encephalopathy, and Korsakoff's syndrome).

## II. Alcohol dependence and abuse

### A. Definition

1. **Alcohol dependence.** Excessive use of alcohol that is harmful to physical and mental health. It has three common forms: (1) continuous use of a large quantity of alcohol, (2) heavy use only on weekends or when job functioning is least likely to be impaired, and (3) binges of heavy drinking (lasting days to weeks) interspersed with long periods of sobriety.

2. **Alcohol abuse.** The continual use of alcohol that interferes with a person's overall functioning and that usually evolves into dependence. Generally, this category applies to a person whose drinking problem is not yet sufficient to warrant a diagnosis of alcohol dependence.

### B. Epidemiology

1. 14% lifetime prevalence for dependence.
2. More prevalent in men than in women (2–3:1), but rates for women may be increasing.
3. Many men and women over age 50 choose abstinence.
4. In the United States half the alcohol is consumed by 10% of alcohol drinkers.

### C. Etiology. Alcohol dependence runs in families, and children of alcohol-abusing parents are at high risk of developing alcohol abuse whether or not they are raised by their biological parents. The familial association is strongest for the male child of an alcohol-dependent father. There are ethnic and cultural differences in susceptibility to alcohol and its effects. For example,

many Asians show acute toxic effects, such as intoxication, flushing, dizziness, and headache after consuming only minimal amounts of alcohol. Some cultural groups, such as Jews, conservative Protestants, and Asians, have lower rates of alcohol dependence, whereas others, such as Native Americans, Eskimos, and some groups of Hispanic men, show high rates. These findings have led to a genetic theory about the etiology of alcoholism, but a definitive cause remains unknown.

1. **Comorbidity with other mental disorders.** Alcohol's sedative effect and its ready availability make it the most commonly used substance for the relief of anxiety, depression, and insomnia. However, long-term use may cause depression, and withdrawal in a dependent person may cause anxiety. Proper evaluation of depressed or anxious patients who drink heavily may require observation and reevaluation after a period of sobriety lasting up to several weeks. Many psychotic patients medicate themselves with alcohol when prescribed medications do not sufficiently reduce psychotic symptoms or when prescription medications are not available. In bipolar patients, heavy alcohol use often leads to a manic episode. Among patients with personality disorders, antisocial personalities are particularly likely to develop long-standing patterns of alcohol dependence. Alcohol abuse is prevalent in persons with other substance use disorders, and there is a particularly high correlation between alcohol dependence and nicotine dependence.

D. **Diagnosis, signs, and symptoms**

1. **Alcohol dependence.** See Table 6–1. Usually, the patient has some alcohol-related impairment in at least one of the following areas: work or school; health; family relationships; social functioning, such as seeing only drinking friends; or legal problems, such as arrests for driving while intoxicated or alcohol-related violence.

TABLE 6–1
**DSM-IV DIAGNOSTIC CRITERIA FOR ALCOHOL OR OTHER SUBSTANCE DEPENDENCE**

A. At least three of the following:
   (1) substance often taken in larger amounts or over a longer period than the person intended
   (2) persistent desire or one or more unsuccessful efforts to cut down or control substance use
   (3) a great deal of time spent in activities necessary to get the substance (e.g., theft), taking the substance (e.g., chain smoking), or recovering from its effects
   (4) frequent intoxication or withdrawal symptoms when expected to fulfill major role obligations at work, school, or home (e.g., does not go to work because hung over, goes to school or work "high," intoxicated while taking care of his or her children), or when substance use is physically hazardous (e.g., drives when intoxicated)
   (5) important social, occupational, or recreational activities given up or reduced because of substance use
   (6) continued substance use despite knowledge of having a persistent or recurrent social, psychological, or physical problem that is caused or exacerbated by the use of the substance (e.g., keeps using heroin despite family arguments about it, cocaine-induced depression, or having an ulcer made worse by drinking)
   (7) marked tolerance: need for markedly increased amounts of the substance (i.e., at least a 50% increase) in order to achieve intoxication or desired effect, or markedly diminished effect with continued use of the same amount
   (8) characteristic withdrawal symptoms
   (9) substance often taken to relieve or avoid withdrawal symptoms
B. Some symptoms of the disturbance have persisted for at least 1 month, or have occurred repeatedly over a longer period of time.

Used with permission, APA.

**Tolerance** is the phenomenon of the drinker needing, over time, greater amounts of alcohol to obtain the same effect. The development of tolerance, especially marked tolerance, usually indicates dependence. Mild tolerance for alcohol is common, but severe tolerance, such as that which is possible with opioids and barbiturates, is uncommon. Tolerance varies widely among persons. Dependence may only become apparent to the tolerant patient when he or she is forced to stop and develops withdrawal symptoms.

2. **Alcohol abuse.** See Table 6–2.

3. **Evaluation.** The proper evaluation of the alcohol user requires some suspiciousness on the part of the evaluator. In general, most people, when questioned, minimize the amount of alcohol they say they consume. When obtaining a history of degree of alcohol use, it might be helpful to phrase questions in a manner likely to elicit positive responses. For example, ask, "How much alcohol do you drink?" rather than, "Do you drink alcohol?" Other questions that may give important clues include how often the patient drinks in the morning, how often he or she has **blackouts** (amnesia while intoxicated), and how often friends or relatives have told the patient to cut down on drinking. Always look for subtle signs of alcohol abuse and always inquire about use of other substances. Does the patient seem to be accident prone (head injury, rib fracture, motor vehicle accidents)? Is he or she often in fights? Often absent from work? Are there social or family problems?

E. **Treatment.** The goal is the prolonged maintenance of total sobriety. Relapses are common. Initial treatment requires detoxification, inpatient if necessary, and treatment of any withdrawal symptoms. Coexisting mental disorders should be treated when the patient is sober.

1. **Insight.** Critically necessary but often difficult to achieve. The patient must acknowledge that he or she has a drinking problem. Severe denial may have to be overcome before the patient will cooperate in seeking treatment. Often, this requires the collaboration of family, friends, employers, and others. The patient may need to be confronted with the potential loss of career, family, and health if he or she continues to drink. Individual psychotherapy has been used, but group therapy may be more effective. Group therapy may also be more acceptable to many patients who perceive alcohol dependence as a social problem rather than a personal psychiatric problem.

TABLE 6–2
**DSM-IV DIAGNOSTIC CRITERIA FOR ALCOHOL OR OTHER SUBSTANCE ABUSE**

A. A maladaptive pattern of psychoactive substance use indicated by at least one of the following:
    (1) continued use despite knowledge of having a persistent or recurrent social, occupational, psychological, or physical problem that is caused or exacerbated by use of the psychoactive substance
    (2) recurrent use in situations in which use is physically hazardous (e.g., driving while intoxicated)
B. Some symptoms of the disturbance have persisted for at least 1 month, or have occurred repeatedly over a longer period of time.
C. Never met the criteria for psychoactive substance dependence for this substance.

Used with permission, APA.

2. **Alcoholics Anonymous (AA) and Al-Anon.** Supportive organizations, such as AA (for patients) and Al-Anon (for families of patients), can be effective in maintaining sobriety and helping the family to cope. AA emphasizes the inability of the member to cope alone with addiction to alcohol and encourages dependence on the group for support; AA also utilizes many techniques of group therapy.

3. **Psychosocial interventions.** Often necessary and very effective. **Family therapy** should focus on describing the effects of alcohol use on other family members. Patients must be forced to relinquish the perception of their right to be able to drink and recognize the detrimental effects on the family.

4. **Psychopharmacotherapy**
   a. **Disulfiram (Antabuse)**—125–500 mg a day of disulfiram may be used if the patient desires enforced sobriety. Patients taking disulfiram develop an extremely unpleasant reaction when they ingest even small amounts of alcohol. The reaction, caused by an accumulation of acetaldehyde, includes flushing, headache, throbbing in head and neck, dyspnea, hyperventilation, tachycardia, hypotension, sweating, anxiety, weakness, and confusion. Life-threatening complications, although uncommon, can occur. Disulfiram is useful only temporarily to help establish a long-term pattern of sobriety and to change long-standing alcohol-related coping mechanisms.
   b. **Naltrexone (ReVia)**—decreases alcohol craving, probably by blocking the release of endogenous opioids. This aids in achieving the goal of abstinence by preventing relapse and decreasing alcohol consumption. A dosage of 50 mg once daily is recommended for most patients.
   c. **Lithium**—probably ineffective in maintaining abstinence in patients with alcohol abuse or dependence or in treating depression in alcoholics.

5. **After recovery.** Most experts recommend that a recovered alcohol-dependent patient maintain lifelong sobriety and discourage attempts by recovered patients to learn to drink normally. (A dogma of AA is, "It's the first drink that gets you drunk.")

F. **Medical complications.** Alcohol is toxic to numerous organ systems. Complications of chronic alcohol abuse and dependence (or associated nutritional deficiencies) include cerebral atrophy, cerebellar degeneration, epilepsy, peripheral neuropathy, cardiomyopathy, myopathy, alcoholic hepatitis, cirrhosis, gastritis, pancreatitis, peptic ulcer, and many other gastrointestinal (GI) tract problems. In addition, nutritional deficiencies—e.g., thiamine, vitamin $B_{12}$, nicotinic acid, folate—often accompany chronic alcoholism. Alcohol use during pregnancy is toxic to the developing fetus and can cause congenital defects, as well as fetal alcohol syndrome.

## III. Alcohol intoxication

A. **Definition.** Recent ingestion of a sufficient amount of alcohol to produce maladaptive behavioral changes.

**B. Diagnosis, signs, and symptoms.** Whereas mild intoxication may produce a relaxed, talkative, euphoric, or disinhibited person, severe intoxication often leads to more maladaptive changes, such as aggressiveness, irritability, labile mood, impaired judgment, and impaired social or work functioning, among others.

Persons exhibit at least one of the following: slurred speech, incoordination, unsteady gait, nystagmus, memory impairment, stupor, and flushed face. Severe intoxication can lead to withdrawn behavior, psychomotor retardation, blackouts, and eventually obtundation, coma, and death. Common complications of alcohol intoxication include motor vehicle accidents, head injury, rib fracture, criminal acts, homicide, and suicide.

**1. Evaluation.** A thorough medical evaluation should be conducted; consider a possible subdural hematoma or a concurrent infection. Always evaluate for possible intoxication with other substances. Alcohol is frequently used in combination with other CNS depressants, such as benzodiazepines and barbiturates. The CNS depressant effects of such combinations can be synergistic and potentially fatal.

Appropriate examination of mental status and diagnosis of other concurrent mental disorders usually require reevaluation after the patient is no longer intoxicated, because almost any psychiatric symptom may acutely be due to alcohol intoxication. Blood alcohol levels are seldom important in the clinical evaluation (except to determine legal intoxication) because there may be differences in tolerance.

**2. Alcohol idiosyncratic intoxication.** Maladaptive behavior (often aggressive or assaultive) after ingesting a small amount of alcohol that would not cause intoxication in most people, i.e., pathological intoxication. Uncommon and controversial. The behavior must be atypical for the person when he or she is not drinking. Brain-damaged persons may also be more susceptible to alcohol idiosyncratic intoxication.

**C. Treatment**

1. Usually only supportive.
2. May give nutrients (especially thiamine, vitamin $B_{12}$, folate).
3. May require observation for complications, e.g., combativeness, coma, head injury, falling.

**D. Blackouts.** Periods of intoxication for which there is complete anterograde amnesia and during which the patient appears awake and alert. They occasionally can last for days with the intoxicated person performing complex tasks, such as long-distance travel, with no subsequent recollection. Brain-damaged persons may be more susceptible to blackouts.

## IV. Alcohol-induced psychotic disorder, with hallucinations

(Previously known as alcohol hallucinosis.) Vivid, persistent hallucinations (often visual and auditory), without delirium, following (usually within 2 days) a decrease in alcohol consumption in an alcohol-dependent person. May persist and progress to a more chronic form that is clinically similar to schizophrenia. Rare. The male-to-female ratio is 4:1. The condition usually requires at least 10 years of alcohol dependence. If the patient is agitated, possible treatments include benzodiazepines, e.g., lorazepam (Ativan) 1–2 mg orally or intramuscularly (IM), diazepam (Valium) 5–10 mg orally, or low doses of a high-potency antipsychotic, such as haloperidol (Haldol) 2–5 mg orally or IM as needed every 4–6 hours.

## V. Alcohol withdrawal

Begins within several hours after cessation of, or reduction in, prolonged (at least days) heavy alcohol consumption. At least two of the following must be present: autonomic hyperactivity, hand tremor, insomnia, nausea or vomiting, transient illusions or hallucinations, anxiety, grand mal seizures, and psychomotor agitation. May occur with perceptual disturbances, e.g., hallucinations, with intact reality testing.

## VI. Alcohol withdrawal delirium

(Also known as delirium tremens [DTs]). Usually only occurs after recent cessation of or reduction in severe, heavy alcohol use in medically compromised patients with a long history of dependence. Less common than uncomplicated alcohol withdrawal.

### A. Diagnosis, signs, and symptoms

1. Delirium.
2. Marked autonomic hyperactivity. Tachycardia, sweating, fever, anxiety, or insomnia.
3. Associated features. Vivid hallucinations that may be visual, tactile, or olfactory; delusions; agitation; tremor; fever; and seizures or so-called rum fits (if seizures develop, they always occur before delirium).
4. Typical features. Paranoid delusions, visual hallucinations of insects or small animals, and tactile hallucinations.

### B. Medical workup

1. Complete history and physical.
2. Lab tests—complete blood count (CBC) with differential, electrolytes, calcium, magnesium, blood chemistry panel, liver function tests, bilirubin, blood urea nitrogen (BUN), creatinine, fasting glucose, prothrombin time, albumin, total protein, hepatitis type B surface antigen, vitamin $B_{12}$ levels, folate levels, serum amylase, stool guaiac, urinalysis, urine drug screen, electrocardiogram (EKG), and chest x-ray. Other possible tests: electroencephalogram (EEG), lumbar puncture (LP), computed tomography (CT) of head, and GI series.

### C. Treatment

1. Take vital signs every 6 hours.
2. Observe the patient constantly.
3. Decrease stimulation.
4. Correct electrolyte imbalances and treat other coexisting medical problems, e.g., infection, head trauma.
5. If the patient is dehydrated, hydrate.
6. Chlordiazepoxide (Librium) 25–100 mg orally every 6 hours (other sedative-hypnotics could be substituted, but this is the convention). Use as needed for agitation, tremor, or increased vital signs (temperature, pulse, blood pressure).
7. Thiamine 100 mg orally 1–3 times a day.

8. Folic acid 1 mg orally daily.
9. One multivitamin daily.
10. Magnesium sulfate 1 g IM every 6 hours for 2 days (in patients who have had postwithdrawal seizures).
11. After patient is stabilized, taper chlordiazepoxide by 20% every 5–7 days.
12. Provide medication for adequate sleep.
13. Treat malnutrition if present.
14. This regimen allows for a very flexible dosage range of chlordiazepoxide. If prescribing a sedative on a standing regimen, be sure that the medication will be held if the patient is asleep or not easily arousable. The necessary total dose of benzodiazepine will vary greatly among patients owing to inherent individual differences, differing levels of alcohol intake, and concomitant use of other substances. Because many of these patients have liver function impairment, it also may be difficult to accurately estimate the sedative's elimination half-life.
15. Generally avoid antipsychotics because they can precipitate seizures. If the patient is agitated, psychotic, and shows signs of benzodiazepine toxicity (ataxia, slurred speech) in spite of being agitated, then consider using a high-potency antipsychotic, such as haloperidol or fluphenazine (Prolixin, Permitil), which is less likely to precipitate seizures than low-potency antipsychotics are.

## VII. Alcohol-induced persisting amnestic disorder

Disturbance in short-term memory due to prolonged heavy use of alcohol; rare in persons under the age of 35. The classic names for the disorder are Wernicke's encephalopathy (an acute set of neurological symptoms) and Korsakoff's syndrome (a chronic condition).

**A. Wernicke's encephalopathy.** (Also known as alcoholic encephalopathy.) An acute syndrome caused by thiamine deficiency. Characterized by nystagmus, abducens and conjugate gaze palsies, ataxia, and global confusion. Other symptoms may include confabulation, lethargy, indifference, mild delirium, anxious insomnia, or fear of the dark. Thiamine deficiency usually is due to chronic alcohol dependence. Treat with thiamine until ophthalmoplegia resolves. May also require magnesium (a cofactor for thiamine metabolism). With treatment, most symptoms resolve except ataxia, nystagmus, and sometimes peripheral neuropathy. The syndrome may clear in a few days or weeks or progress to Korsakoff's syndrome.

**B. Korsakoff's syndrome.** (Also known as Korsakoff's psychosis.) A chronic condition usually related to alcohol dependence, wherein alcohol represents a large portion of caloric intake for years. Caused by thiamine deficiency. Rare. Characterized by retrograde and anterograde amnesia. The patient also often will show confabulation, disorientation, and polyneuritis. In addition to thiamine replacement, clonidine (Catapres) and propranolol (Inderal) may be of some limited use. Often coexists with alcohol-related dementia.

## VIII. Substance-induced persisting dementia

This diagnosis should be made when other etiologies of dementia have been excluded and a history of chronic heavy alcohol abuse is evident. The symptoms persist past intoxication or withdrawal states. The dementia is usually mild. Management is similar to that of dementia from other etiologies.

For a more detailed discussion of this topic, see Schuckit MA: Alcohol-Related Disorders, Sec 13.2, p 775; Wiseman EJ: Drug and Alcohol Abuse, Sec 49.6g, p 2580, in **CTP/VI**.

# 7
# Schizophrenia

## I. Definition

Schizophrenia is a disorder of unknown causes; it is characterized by psychotic symptoms that significantly impair functioning and that involve disturbances in feeling, thinking, and behavior. The disorder is chronic and generally has (1) a prodromal phase, (2) an active phase with delusions, hallucinations, or both, and (3) a residual phase in which the disorder may be in remission.

## II. History

**1852**—Schizophrenia was first formally described by Belgian psychiatrist Benedict Morel, who called it "démence précoce."

**1896**—Emil Kraepelin, a German psychiatrist, applied the term "dementia precox" to a group of illnesses that began in adolescence and ended in dementia.

**1911**—Swiss psychiatrist Eugen Bleuler introduced the term "schizophrenia." There are no pathognomonic signs or symptoms; instead, a cluster of characteristic findings make the diagnosis. The diagnostic criteria in current use are from DSM-IV (Table 7-1). The criteria formulated by Kraepelin, Bleuler (the four As), and Kurt Schneider (first rank symptoms) are useful criteria (Tables 7-2, 7-3, 7-4); however, DSM-IV criteria are the most widely used and accepted.

## III. Diagnosis, signs, and symptoms

See Table 7-1. Schizophrenia is a phenomenological diagnosis based on observation and description of the patient.

**A. Impaired overall functioning.** The patient's level of functioning declines or fails to achieve the expected level.

**B. Abnormal content of thought.** For example, delusions, ideas of reference, poverty of content.

**C. Illogical form of thought.** For example, derailment, loosening of associations, incoherence, circumstantiality, tangentiality, overinclusiveness, neologisms, blocking, echolalia (all incorporated as a thought disorder).

**D. Distorted perception.** For example, hallucinations: visual, olfactory, tactile, and most frequently, auditory.

**E. Changed affect.** For example, flat, blunted, silly, labile, inappropriate.

**F. Impaired sense of self.** For example, loss of ego boundaries, gender confusion, inability to distinguish internal from external reality.

**G. Altered volition.** For example, inadequate drive or motivation and marked ambivalence.

**H. Impaired interpersonal functioning.** For example, social withdrawal and emotional detachment, aggressiveness, sexual inappropriateness.

TABLE 7–1
**DSM-IV DIAGNOSTIC CRITERIA FOR SCHIZOPHRENIA**

A. *Characteristic symptoms:* Two (or more) of the following, each present for a significant portion of time during a 1-month period (or less if successfully treated):
   (1) delusions
   (2) hallucinations
   (3) disorganized speech (e.g., frequent derailment or incoherence)
   (4) grossly disorganized or catatonic behavior
   (5) negative symptoms, i.e., affective flattening, alogia, or avolition
   **Note:** Only one criterion A symptom is required if delusions are bizarre or hallucinations consist of a voice keeping up a running commentary on the person's behavior or thoughts, or two or more voices conversing with each other.

B. *Social/occupational dysfunction:* For a significant portion of the time since the onset of the disturbance, one or more major areas of functioning such as work, interpersonal relations, or self-care are markedly below the level achieved prior to the onset (or when the onset is in childhood or adolescence, failure to achieve expected level of interpersonal, academic, or occupational achievement).

C. *Duration:* Continuous signs of the disturbance persist for at least 6 months. This 6-month period must include at least 1 month of symptoms (or less if successfully treated) that meet criterion A (i.e., active-phase symptoms) and may include periods of prodromal or residual symptoms. During these prodromal or residual periods, the signs of the disturbance may be manifested by only negative symptoms or two or more symptoms listed in criterion A present in an attenuated form (e.g., odd beliefs, unusual perceptual experiences).

D. *Schizoaffective and mood disorder exclusion:* Schizoaffective disorder and mood disorder with psychotic features have been ruled out because either (1) no major depressive, manic, or mixed episodes have occurred concurrently with the active-phase symptoms; or (2) if mood episodes have occurred during active-phase symptoms, their total duration has been brief relative to the duration of the active and residual periods.

E. *Substance/general medical condition exclusion:* The disturbance is not due to the direct physiological effects of a substance (e.g., a drug of abuse, a medication) or a general medical condition.

F. *Relationship to a pervasive developmental disorder:* If there is a history of Autistic Disorder or another Pervasive Developmental Disorder, the additional diagnosis of Schizophrenia is made only if prominent delusions or hallucinations are also present for at least a month (or less if successfully treated).

*Classification of longitudinal course* (can be applied only after at least 1 year has elapsed since the initial onset of active-phase symptoms):
   **Episodic with interepisode residual symptoms** (episodes are defined by the reemergence of prominent psychotic symptoms); *also specify if:* **with prominent negative symptoms**
   **Episodic with no interepisode residual symptoms**
   **Continuous** (prominent psychotic symptoms are present throughout the period of observation); *also specify if:* **with prominent negative symptoms**
   **Single episode in partial remission;** *also specify if:* **with prominent negative symptoms**
   **Single episode in full remission**
   **Other or unspecified pattern**

Used with permission, APA.

I. **Change in psychomotor behavior.** For example, agitation versus withdrawal, grimacing, posturing, rituals, catatonia.

J. **Sensorium.** For example, intact orientation to time, place, and person, intact memory, concreteness.

## IV. Types

### A. Paranoid

1. Preoccupation with systematized delusions or with frequent auditory hallucinations related to a single theme.
2. None of the following: incoherence, loosening of associations, flat or grossly inappropriate affect, catatonic behavior, grossly disorganized behavior.

TABLE 7–2
**EMIL KRAEPELIN'S CRITERIA**

- Disturbances of attention and comprehension
- Hallucinations, especially auditory (voices)
- Gedankenlautwerden (audible thoughts)
- Experiences of influenced thought
- Disturbances in the flow of thought, above all a loosening of associations
- Impairment of cognitive function and judgment
- Affective flattening
- Appearance of morbid behavior
  Reduced drive
  Automatic obedience
  Echolalia, echopraxia
  Acting out
  Catatonic frenzy
  Stereotypy
  Negativism
  Autism
  Disturbance of verbal expression

Table from World Psychiatric Association.

TABLE 7–3
**EUGEN BLEULER'S SYMPTOM CRITERIA**

*Basic or fundamental disturbances*
- Formal thought disorders[a]
- Disturbances of affect[a]
- Disturbances of the subjective experience of self
- Disturbances of volition and behavior
- Ambivalence[a]
- Autism[a]

*Accessory symptoms*
- Disorders of perception (hallucinations)
- Delusions
- Certain memory disturbances
- Modification of personality
- Changes in speech and writing
- Somatic symptoms
- Catatonic symptoms
- Acute syndrome (such as melancholic, manic, catatonic, and other states)

[a]Bleuler's four As: association, affect, ambivalence, and autism.
Table from the World Psychiatric Association.

## B. Disorganized
1. Incoherence, marked loosening of associations, or grossly disorganized behavior.
2. Flat or grossly inappropriate affect.
3. Does not meet criteria for catatonic type.

## C. Catatonic
1. Stupor or mutism.
2. Negativism.
3. Rigidity.
4. Purposeless excitement.
5. Posturing.
6. Echolalia or echopraxia.

TABLE 7–4
**KURT SCHNEIDER'S CRITERIA, FIRST AND SECOND RANK SYMPTOMS**

*First rank symptoms*
- Audible thoughts
- Voices arguing and/or discussing
- Voices commenting
- Somatic passivity experiences
- Thought withdrawal and other experiences of influenced thought[a]
- Thought broadcasting
- Delusional perceptions
- All other experiences involving made volition, made affect, and made impulses

*Second rank symptoms*
- Other disorders of perception
- Sudden delusional ideas
- Perplexity
- Depressive and euphoric mood changes
- Feelings of emotional impoverishment
- "... and several others as well."

[a]The symptom "thought insertion" was originally included under "other experiences of influenced thought."
Table from the World Psychiatric Association.

### D. Undifferentiated type
1. Prominent delusions, hallucinations, incoherence, or grossly disorganized behavior.
2. Does not meet the criteria for paranoid, catatonic, or disorganized type.

### E. Residual type
1. Absence of prominent delusions, hallucinations, incoherence, or grossly disorganized behavior.
2. Continuing evidence of the disturbance through two or more of the residual symptoms.

### F. Type I and type II.
Another system proposes classification of schizophrenia into type I and type II. The system is based on the presence of positive or negative symptoms, sometimes referred to, respectively, as productive and negative symptoms. The negative symptoms include affective flattening or blunting, poverty of speech or speech content, blocking, poor grooming, lack of motivation, anhedonia, social withdrawal, cognitive defects, and attentional deficits. Positive symptoms include loose associations, hallucinations, bizarre behavior, and increased speech. Type I patients have mostly positive symptoms, and type II patients have mostly negative symptoms.

### G. Paraphrenia.
Sometimes used as a synonym for "paranoid schizophrenia." The term also is used for either a progressively deteriorating course of illness or the presence of a well systematized delusional system. These multiple meanings have reduced the term's usefulness.

### H. Simple schizophrenia.
The term "simple schizophrenia" was used when schizophrenia had a broad diagnostic conceptualization. Simple schizophrenia was characterized by a gradual, insidious loss of drive and ambition. Patients with the disorder were usually not overtly psychotic and did not experience persistent hallucinations or delusions. The primary symptom is the withdrawal of the patient from social and work-related situations.

## V. Epidemiology

**A. Incidence and prevalence.** Lifetime prevalence is approximately 1–1.5%. An estimated 2 million Americans suffer from schizophrenia; worldwide, 2 million new cases appear each year. Prevalence, morbidity, and severity of presentation are greater in urban than in rural areas. Furthermore, morbidity and severity of presentation are greater in industrialized than in nonindustrialized areas.

**B. Sex ratio.** The male-to-female ratio is 1:1.

**C. Socioeconomic status.** Increased prevalence in lower socioeconomic groups, but equal incidence across socioeconomic classes (reflects downward drift theory, which states that although those with the disorder originally may have been born into any socioeconomic class, they eventually will tend to drift downward into the lower socioeconomic classes owing to their significant impairments).

**D. Age of onset.** Most common between ages 15 and 35 (50% below age 25). Rare before age 10 or after age 40. Earlier onset for men than for women.

**E. Religion.** Jews are affected less than Protestants and Catholics.

**F. Race.** Prevalence is reported to be higher among blacks and Hispanics than among whites, but this assertion may reflect the bias of diagnosticians or a higher percentage of minority persons living in lower socioeconomic groups and in industrialized urban areas.

**G. Seasonality.** Higher incidences in both winter and early spring (January–April in the northern hemisphere, July–September in the southern hemisphere).

**H. Inpatient versus outpatient.** From 1965 to 1975, the number of schizophrenic patients in hospitals decreased by 40–50%. Currently, up to 80% of schizophrenic patients are treated as outpatients.

**I. Cost.** Direct and indirect cost to the United States is approximately $100 billion a year.

## VI. Etiology

Owing to the heterogeneity of symptomatic and prognostic presentations of schizophrenia, no single etiological factor is considered causative. The stress-diathesis model is most often used, which states that the person who develops schizophrenia has a specific biological vulnerability, or diathesis, that is triggered by stress and leads to schizophrenic symptoms. Stresses may be genetic, biological, and psychosocial or environmental.

**A. Genetic.** Both single gene and polygenic theories have been proposed (Table 7–5). Although neither theory has been definitively substantiated, the

TABLE 7–5
**FEATURES CONSISTENT WITH POLYGENIC INHERITANCE**[a]

1. Disorder can be transmitted with two normal parents
2. Presentation of disorder ranges from very severe to less severe
3. More severely affected persons have a greater number of ill relatives than mildly affected persons do
4. Risk decreases as the number of shared genes decreases
5. Disorder present in both mother's and father's side of family

[a]The number of affected genes determines a person's risk and symptomatic picture.

polygenic theory appears to be more consistent with the presentation of schizophrenia.

1. **Consanguinity.** Incidence in families is higher than in the general population, and monozygotic (MZ) twin concordance is greater than dizygotic (DZ) (Table 7–6).

2. **Adoption studies.** Risk is secondary to biological parent, not adoptive parent.

   a. Risk to an adopted child (approximately 10–12%) is the same as if the child had been reared by his or her biological parents.

   b. The prevalence of schizophrenia is increased in biological parents of schizophrenic adoptees over adoptive parents.

   c. MZ twins reared apart have same concordance rate as twins reared together.

   d. Children who are born to nonaffected parents but raised by a schizophrenic parent do not have increased rates of schizophrenia.

B. **Biological**

1. **Dopamine hypothesis.** Schizophrenic symptoms are in part a result of hypersensitive dopamine receptors or increased dopamine activity. Antipsychotic medications bind to dopamine type 2 ($D_2$) receptors and cause functional decreases in dopamine activity. The mesocortical and mesolimbic central nervous system (CNS) dopaminergic tracts are those most implicated in schizophrenia. Drugs that increase dopamine (e.g., amphetamine, cocaine) worsen or trigger psychosis. Dopamine is important in the symptomatic manifestations of schizophrenia, but in a complex way that is not yet fully understood.

2. **Norepinephrine hypothesis.** Increased activity in schizophrenia leads to increased sensitization to sensory input.

3. **g-Aminobutyric acid (GABA) hypothesis.** Decreased GABA activity results in increased dopamine activity.

4. **Serotonin hypothesis.** Serotonin metabolism apparently is abnormal in some chronically schizophrenic patients, with both hyperserotonemia and hyposerotonemia being reported. Specifically, antagonism at the serotonin (5-hydroxytryptamine) type 2 ($5\text{-}HT_2$) receptor has been emphasized as important in reducing psychotic symptoms and in mitigating against the development of movement disorders related to $D_2$ antagonism. Research on mood disorders has implicated serotonin

TABLE 7–6
**PREVALENCE OF SCHIZOPHRENIA IN SPECIFIC POPULATIONS**

| Population | Prevalence |
|---|---|
| General population | 1–1.5% |
| First-degree relative[a] | 10–12% |
| Second-degree relative | 5–6% |
| Child of two schizophrenic parents | 40% |
| DZ twin | 12–15% |
| MZ twin | 45–50% |

[a]Schizophrenia is not a sex-linked disorder; it does not matter which parent has the disorder in terms of risk.

activity in suicidal and impulsive behavior, which schizophrenic patients also can exhibit.

**5. Hallucinogens.** It has been suggested that some endogenous amines act as substrates for abnormal methylation, resulting in endogenous hallucinogens. This hypothesis is not supported by reliable data.

**C. Psychosocial and environmental**

**1. Family factors.** Patients whose families have high expressed emotion (EE) have higher relapse rates than those whose families have low EE. EE has been defined as any overly involved, intrusive behavior, be it hostile and critical or controlling and infantilizing. Relapse rates are better when family behavior is modified to lower EE. Most observers believe that family dysfunction is a consequence, rather than a cause, of schizophrenia.

**2. Psychodynamic issues.** Understanding which psychosocial and environmental stressors may be specific to individual schizophrenic patients is crucial. Knowing what psychological and environmental stresses are most likely to trigger psychotic decompensation in a patient helps the clinician supportively address these issues and, in the process, helps the patient to feel and remain more in control.

**D. Infectious theory.** Evidence for slow virus etiology includes neuropathological changes consistent with past infections: gliosis, glial scarring, and presence of antiviral antibodies in the serum and cerebrospinal fluid of some schizophrenic patients. Increased frequency of perinatal complications and seasonality of birth data also can support an infectious theory.

**VII. Lab and psychological tests**

**A. Brain imaging**

**1. Computed tomography (CT).** Cortical atrophy in 10–35% of patients; enlargement of the lateral and third ventricle in 10–50% of patients; atrophy of the cerebellar vermis and decreased radiodensity of brain parenchyma. Abnormal CT scan findings may correlate with the presence of negative symptoms, e.g., flattened affect, social withdrawal, psychomotor retardation, lack of motivation, neuropsychiatric impairment, increased frequency of extrapyramidal symptoms from antipsychotic medications, and poor premorbid history.

**2. Positron emission tomography (PET).** In some patients, decreased frontal and parietal lobe metabolism, relatively high posterior metabolism, and abnormal laterality.

**3. Cerebral blood flow (CBF).** In some patients, decreased resting levels of frontal blood flow, increased parietal blood flow, and decreased whole brain blood flow. When PET scan and CBF studies are placed together with CT scan findings, dysfunction of the frontal lobe is most clearly implicated. Frontal lobe dysfunction may be secondary, however, to pathology elsewhere in the brain.

**B. Electroencephalogram (EEG).** Most schizophrenic patients have normal EEGs, but some have decreased alpha and increased theta and delta activity, paroxysmal abnormalities, and increased sensitivity to activation procedures, e.g., sleep deprivation.

C. **Evoked potential (EP) studies.** Initial hypersensitivity to sensory stimulation, with later compensatory blunting of information processing at higher
cortical levels.

D. **Immunological studies.** In some patients, atypical lymphocytes and
decreased numbers of natural killer cells.

E. **Endocrinological studies.** In some patients, decreased levels of luteinizing hormone (LH) and follicle-stimulating hormone (FSH); diminished
release of prolactin and growth hormone when stimulated by gonadotropin-
releasing hormone or thyrotropin-releasing hormone (TRH).

F. **Neuropsychological testing.** Thematic Apperception Test (TAT) and
Rorschach test usually reveal bizarre responses. When compared with parents
of normal controls, parents of schizophrenic patients show more deviation
from normals in projective tests (may be a consequence of living with
schizophrenic family member). Halstead-Reitan Battery reveals impaired
attention and intelligence, decreased retention time, and disturbed problem-
solving ability in approximately 20–35% of patients. Schizophrenic patients
have decreased intelligence quotients (I.Q.s) when compared with nonschizo-
phrenic patients, although the range of I.Q. scores is wide. Decline in I.Q.
occurs with progression of the illness.

## VIII. Pathophysiology

No consistent structural defects; changes noted include decreased number of
neurons, increased gliosis, and disorganization of neuronal architecture. Degeneration in limbic system, especially the amygdala, hippocampus, and cingulate
cortex, as well as in the basal ganglia, especially substantia nigra and dorsolateral
prefrontal cortex.

Minor (soft) neurological findings occur in 50–100% of patients: increased
prevalence of primitive reflexes, such as grasp reflex, abnormal stereognosis
and two-point discrimination, and dysdiadochokinesia (impairment in ability to
perform rapidly alternating movements). Paroxysmal saccadic eye movements
(inability to follow object through space with smooth eye movements) occur in
50–80% of schizophrenic patients and in 40–45% of first-degree relatives of
schizophrenic patients (compared with an 8–10% prevalence in nonschizo-
phrenic persons). This may be a neurophysiological marker of a vulnerability
for schizophrenia. Resting heart rate levels have been found to be higher in
schizophrenic patients than in controls and may reflect a hyperaroused state.

## IX. Psychodynamic factors

Understanding a patient's dynamics (or psychological conflicts and issues)
is critical for complete understanding of the symbolic meaning of symptoms.
A patient's internal experience is usually one of confusion and overwhelming
sensory input, and defense mechanisms are the ego's attempt to deal with
powerful affects. Three major primitive defenses interfere with reality testing:
(1) Psychotic projection—attributing inner sensations of aggression, sexuality,
chaos, and confusion to the outside world as opposed to recognizing them as
emanating from within; boundaries between inner and outer experience are
confused. Projection is the major defense underlying paranoia. (2) Reaction
formation—turning a disturbing idea or impulse into its opposite. (3) Psychotic
denial—transforming confusing stimuli into delusions and hallucinations.

## X. Differential diagnosis

**A. Medical and neurological disorders.** Present with impaired memory, orientation, and cognition; visual hallucinations; signs of CNS damage. Many neurological and medical disorders can present with symptoms identical to those of schizophrenia, including substance intoxication (e.g., cocaine, phencyclidine [PCP]) and substance-induced psychotic disorder, CNS infections (e.g., herpes encephalitis), vascular disorders (e.g., systemic lupus erythematosus), complex partial seizures (e.g., temporal lobe epilepsy), and degenerative disease (e.g., Huntington's disease).

**B. Schizophreniform disorder.** Symptoms may be identical to schizophrenia, but last for less than 6 months. There is also less deterioration and a better prognosis.

**C. Brief psychotic disorder.** Symptoms last less than 1 month and procede a clearly identifiable psychosocial stress.

**D. Mood disorders.** Both manic episodes and major depressive episodes of bipolar I disorder and major depressive disorder may present with psychotic symptoms. The differential diagnosis is particularly important because of the availability of specific and effective treatments for the mood disorders. DSM-IV states that mood symptoms in schizophrenia must be brief relative to the essential criteria. Also, if hallucinations and delusions are present in a mood disorder, they develop after the mood disturbance and do not persist. Other factors that help differentiate mood disorders from schizophrenia include family history, premorbid history, course, e.g., age of onset, prognosis, e.g., absence of residual deterioration following the psychotic episode, and response to treatment. Patients may experience postpsychotic depressive disorder of schizophrenia, i.e., a major depressive episode occurring after the residual phase of schizophrenia. True depression in these patients must be differentiated from medication-induced adverse effects, such as sedation, akinesia, and flattening of affect.

**E. Schizoaffective disorder.** Mood symptoms develop concurrently with symptoms of schizophrenia, but delusions or hallucinations must be present for 2 weeks in the absence of prominent mood symptoms during some phase of the illness. The prognosis of this disorder is better than that expected for schizophrenia and worse than that for mood disorders.

**F. Psychotic disorder not otherwise specified.** An atypical psychosis in which there is a confusing clinical feature, e.g., persistent auditory hallucinations as the only symptom, many culture-bound psychoses.

**G. Delusional disorders.** Nonbizarre, systematized delusions that last at least 6 months in the context of an intact, relatively high-functioning personality in the absence of prominent hallucinations or other schizophrenic symptoms. Onset is in middle to late adult life.

**H. Personality disorders.** Generally no psychotic symptoms, but, if present, they tend to be transient and not prominent. The most important personality disorders in this differential diagnosis are schizotypal, schizoid, borderline, and paranoid.

**I. Factitious disorder with predominantly psychological signs and symptoms and malingering.** No lab test or biological marker can objectively confirm the diagnosis of schizophrenia. Schizophrenic symptoms are therefore possible to feign for either clear secondary gain (malingering) or deep psychological motivations (factitious disorder).

J. **Pervasive developmental disorders.** Pervasive developmental disorders, e.g., autistic disorder, are usually recognized before 3 years of age. Although behavior may be bizarre and deteriorated, there are no delusions, hallucinations, or clear formal thought disorder, e.g., loosening of associations.

K. **Mental retardation.** Intellectual, behavioral, and mood disturbances that suggest schizophrenia. However, mental retardation involves no overt psychotic symptoms and involves a constant low level of functioning rather than a deterioration. If psychotic symptoms are present, a diagnosis of schizophrenia may be made concurrently.

L. **Shared cultural beliefs.** Seemingly odd beliefs shared and accepted by a cultural group and thus not considered psychotic.

## XI. Course and prognosis

A. **Course.** Prodromal symptoms of anxiety, perplexity, terror, or depression generally precede the onset of schizophrenia, which may be acute or insidious. Prodromal symptoms may be present for months before definitive diagnosis is made. Onset is generally in the late teens and early 20s. Precipitating events, such as emotional trauma, drugs, and separations, may trigger episodes of illness in predisposed persons. Classically, the course of schizophrenia is one of deterioration over time, with acute exacerbations superimposed on a chronic picture. Vulnerability to stress is lifelong. Postpsychotic depressive episodes may occur in the residual phase. Over the course of the illness, the more florid positive psychotic symptoms, such as bizarre delusions and hallucinations, tend to diminish in intensity, while the more residual negative symptoms, such as poor hygiene, flattened emotional response, and various oddities of behavior, may actually increase.

Relapse rates are approximately 40% in 2 years on medication and 80% in 2 years off medication. Suicide is attempted in 50% of patients; 10% are successful. Violence is not greater than in the general population. There is increased risk of sudden death, medical illness, and shortened life expectancy.

B. **Prognosis.** See Table 7–7. In terms of overall prognosis, some investigators have described a loose rule of thirds: approximately one third of patients lead somewhat normal lives, one third continue to experience significant symptoms but can function within society, and the remaining one third are markedly impaired and require frequent hospitalizations. Approximately 10% of this final third of patients require long-term institutionalization.

## XII. Treatment

Clinical management of the schizophrenic patient may include hospitalization and antipsychotic medication, as well as psychosocial treatments, such as behavioral, family, group, individual, and social skills and rehabilitation therapies.

A. **Pharmacological.** The antipsychotics include dopamine receptor antagonists, serotonin-dopamine antagonists (SDAs), e.g., risperidone (Risperdal), and clozapine (Clozaril).

TABLE 7-7
**FEATURES WEIGHTING TOWARD GOOD OR POOR PROGNOSIS IN SCHIZOPHRENIA**

| Good Prognosis | Poor Prognosis |
|---|---|
| Late onset | Young onset |
| Obvious precipitating factors | No precipitating factors |
| Acute onset | Insidious onset |
| Good premorbid social, sexual, and work histories | Poor premorbid social, sexual, and work histories |
| Mood disorder symptoms (especially depressive disorders) | Withdrawn, autistic behavior |
| Married | Single, divorced, or widowed |
| Family history of mood disorders | Family history of schizophrenia |
| Good support systems | Poor support systems |
| Positive symptoms | Negative symptoms |
| | Neurological signs and symptoms |
| | History of perinatal trauma |
| | No remissions in three years |
| | Many relapses |
| | History of assaultiveness |

1. **Choice of drug**
   a. **Dopamine receptor antagonists**—the classic antipsychotic drugs, which are effective in the treatment of schizophrenia. However, only a small percentage of patients (perhaps 25%) are helped sufficiently to recover a reasonable amount of normal mental functioning. The most common annoying effects are akathisia and parkinsonian symptoms of rigidity and tremor. The potential serious adverse effects include tardive dyskinesia and neuroleptic malignant syndrome.
   b. **Risperidone**—a dopamine receptor antagonist with significant antagonist activity at the 5-HT$_2$ receptor and at the D$_2$ receptor. Risperidone may be more effective than currently available dopamine receptor antagonists at treating both the positive and the negative symptoms of schizophrenia. Risperidone is also associated with significantly fewer and less severe neurological adverse effects than are typical dopamine receptor antagonists.

2. **Dosage.** Use chlorpromazine as a reference for relative potency (Table 7-8). Start with 25 mg orally or intramuscularly (IM) and raise to 300-1,800 mg daily for acute attacks. Titrate dose upward until therapeutic effect is achieved. Haloperidol (Haldol) may be used for rapid tranquilization (1-10 mg orally or IM over 30-60 minutes); daily dosage may go as high as 100 mg. Long-acting depot fluphenazine (Prolixin, Permitil) concentrate or decanoate (25 mg IM) or haloperidol can be effective for 14-21 days and is helpful in increasing compliance.

3. **Maintenance.** After signs and symptoms abate and the patient is stabilized (usually after 4 weeks), dosage can be reduced to the lowest level to maintain freedom from symptoms. After 6 months in remission, the drug can be withdrawn for a trial period to see if relapse occurs, at which point therapy is reinstituted. Some patients may need lifelong maintenance therapy to prevent relapse.

4. **Other drugs.** If standard antipsychotic medication alone is ineffective, several other drugs have been reported to cause varying degrees of improvement. The addition of lithium may be helpful in a significant percentage of patients; propranolol (Inderal), benzodiazepines, val-

TABLE 7–8
**DOPAMINE RECEPTOR ANTAGONIST DRUGS**

| Generic Name | Trade Name | Potency[a] (mg of drug equivalent to 100 mg chlorpromazine) |
|---|---|---|
| Phenothiazines | | |
| Aliphatic | | |
| Chlorpromazine | Thorazine | 100—low |
| Triflupromazine | Vesprin | 25–50—low |
| Promazine | Sparine | 40—low |
| Piperazine | | |
| Prochlorperazine | Compazine | 15—medium |
| Perphenazine | Trilafon | 10—medium |
| Trifluoperazine | Stelazine | 3–5—high |
| Fluphenazine | Prolixin, Permitil | 1.5–3—high |
| Piperidine | | |
| Thioridazine | Mellaril | 100—low |
| Mesoridazine | Serentil | 50—low |
| Thioxanthene | | |
| Thiothixene | Navane | 2–5—high |
| Dibenzoxazepine | | |
| Loxapine | Loxitane | 10–15—medium |
| Dihydroindole | | |
| Molindone | Moban, Lidone | 6–10—medium |
| Butyrophenones | | |
| Haloperidol | Haldol | 2–5—high |
| Droperidol | Inapsine | 10—medium |
| Diphenylbutylpiperidine | | |
| Pimozide | Orap | 1—high |
| Benzisoxazole | | |
| Risperidone | Risperdal | 2–3—low |

[a]Recommended adult dosages are 200–400 mg a day of chlorpromazine or an equivalent amount of another drug.

proate, and carbamazepine (Tegretol) have been reported to lead to improvement in some cases.

**B. Electroconvulsive therapy.**   Used effectively in small percentage of schizophrenic patients, particularly those with the catatonic subtype. Patients in whom the illness has lasted less than 1 year are most responsive.

**C. Psychosocial.**   Antipsychotic medication alone is not as effective in treating schizophrenic patients as when the drugs are coupled with psychosocial interventions.

    **1. Behavior therapy.**   Token economy—desired behaviors are positively reinforced by rewarding targeted behaviors with specific tokens, such as trips or privileges. The intent is to generalize reinforced behavior to the world outside of the hospital ward.

    **2. Group therapy.**   Focus is on support and social skills development (activities of daily living). Groups are especially helpful in decreasing social isolation and increasing reality testing.

    **3. Family therapy.**   Family therapy techniques can significantly decrease relapse rates for the schizophrenic family member. High-EE family interaction can be diminished through family therapy. Multiple family groups, in which family members of schizophrenic patients discuss and share issues, have been particularly helpful.

4. **Supportive psychotherapy.** Traditional insight-oriented psychotherapy is not recommended in treating schizophrenic patient, because their egos are too fragile. Supportive therapy, which may include advice, reassurance, education, modeling, limit setting, and reality testing, is generally the therapy of choice. The rule is that as much insight as a patient desires and can tolerate is an acceptable goal.

5. **Interview techniques.**    One must first understand as much as possible what schizophrenic patients may be feeling and thinking. Schizophrenic patients are described as having extremely fragile ego structures, which leave them open to an unstable sense of self and others, primitive defenses, and severely impaired ability to modulate external stress.

   The critical task for the interviewer is to establish contact with the patient in a manner that allows for a tolerable balance of autonomy and interaction.

   a. There is both a deep wish for and a terrible fear of interpersonal contact, called the need-fear dilemma.

   b. The fear of contact may represent the fear of a fundamental intrusion, resulting in delusional fears of personal and world annihilation as well as loss of control, identity, and self.

   c. The wish for contact may represent fears that, without human interaction, the person is dead, nonhuman, mechanical, or permanently trapped.

   d. Schizophrenic patients may project their own negative, bizarre, and frightening self-images onto others, leading the interviewer to feel as uncomfortable, scared, or angry as the patient. Aggressive or hostile impulses are particularly frightening to these patients and may lead them to disorganization in thought and behavior.

   e. Offers of help may be experienced as coercion, attempts to force the person into helplessness, or a sense of being devoured.

6. **Dos and don'ts for the psychiatric and psychotherapeutic interview.**    There is no one right thing to say to a schizophrenic patient. The most important job of the interviewer is to help to diminish the inner chaos, loneliness, and terror that the schizophrenic patient is feeling. The challenge is to convey empathy without being regarded as being dangerously intrusive.

   a. *Don't* try to argue or rationally persuade the patient out of a delusion. Efforts to convince the patient that a delusion is not real will generally lead to more tenacious assertions of delusional ideas.

   b. *Do* listen. How patients experience the world, e.g., dangerous, bizarre, overwhelming, invasive, is conveyed through their thought content and process. Listen for the feelings behind the delusional ideas— are they afraid, sad, angry, hopeless? Do they feel as though they have no privacy, no control? What is their image of themselves?

   c. *Do* acknowledge these feelings to the patient, simply and clearly. For example, when the patient says, "When I walk into a room, people can see inside my head and read my thoughts," the clinician might respond with, "What is that like for you?"

d. *Don't* feel that anything must be said. Careful listening can convey that the clinician believes the person is human with something important to say.

e. *Do* be flexible about interview times, both the number of visits and how long each visit lasts. If a patient can only tolerate 10 minutes, tell him or her that the interview will resume later, and be clear and reliable about when; it can be an indicator of the clinician's trustworthiness.

f. *Do* be straightforward with a patient—don't pretend that a delusion is actually true, but convey that the delusion is true for the patient. Represent reality to the patient—the challenge is to be a consistent source of reality-testing without making the patient feel humiliated or rejected. For example, if a patient says, ''This song on the radio was written just for me, can't you hear the message?'' one might respond, ''I can hear that the song is about feeling sad after losing someone, and that you must be feeling like that yourself.''

g. *Do* pay attention to how the patient makes you feel, because this often reflects the patient's characteristic style of interaction. Be careful to sort out whether feelings are in direct response to the patient as opposed to something unrelated, e.g., being annoyed because of a fight with a supervisor that morning or because the patient is making subtle, insulting remarks about doctors.

h. *Don't* automatically laugh at a patient when something is said that seems funny. Actively psychotic people will describe delusions that can sound absurd or humorous, but clearly the patient does not experience them as funny. Laughing at a patient can convey disrespect and a lack of understanding of the underlying terror and despair that many patients feel. Keeping this in mind can help to decrease the urge to laugh. Laughter can be appropriate, such as when a patient purposefully tells a joke. Humor can be an indication of health, unless it is used excessively or inappropriately.

i. *Do* respect a paranoid patient's need for distance and control. Many paranoid patients feel more comfortable with a certain formality and respectful aloofness, as opposed to expressions of warmth and empathy.

j. *Do* answer certain personal questions. Try to turn the interview back to the patient. Answering some personal questions may help patients talk more freely about themselves. For example, if the patient asks ''Are you married?'' the clinician might respond, ''Can you tell me why that is important to you?'' *Patient:* ''I just want to know; are you married?'' *Interviewer:* ''I will tell you, but let's talk a bit first about why that information is so important to you.''

---

*For a more detailed discussion of this topic, see Schizophrenia, Chap 14, p 889; Szatmari P: Schizophrenia with Childhood Onset, Chap 45, p 2393; Harris MJ, Jeste DV: Schizophrenia and Delusional Disorders, Sec 49.6c, p 2569, in* CTP/VI.

# 8

# Delusional and Other Psychotic Disorders

## I. Delusional disorder

**A. Definition.** Disorder in which the primary or sole manifestation is a delusion that is fixed and unshakable.

**B. Diagnosis, signs, and symptoms.** See Table 8–1. Delusions last at least 1 month and are well systematized as opposed to bizarre or fragmented. The patient's emotional response to the delusional system is congruent with and appropriate to the content of the delusion. The personality remains intact or deteriorates minimally. Patients often are hypersensitive and hypervigilant, which may lead to social isolation despite their high-level functioning capacities. Under nonstressful circumstances, the patient may be judged to be without evidence of mental illness.

**C. Epidemiology.** Incidence is approximately 1–3 cases per 100,000 persons a year. Prevalence reported to be 0.025–0.03%, but may be higher because many patients do not seek help. Women outnumber men by a slight margin. Age of onset ranges from the mid-20s into the 90s, with average age of 40 years.

**D. Etiology**

**1. Genetic.** Genetic studies indicate that delusional disorder is neither a subtype nor an early or prodromal stage of schizophrenia or mood disorder. The risk of schizophrenia or mood disorder is not increased in first-degree relatives.

**2. Biological.** Patients may have discrete defects in the limbic system and basal ganglia.

**3. Psychosocial.** Delusional disorder is primarily psychosocial in origin. Common background characteristics include histories of physical or emotional abuse; cruel, erratic, and unreliable parenting; and overly demanding and perfectionistic upbringings. Basic trust (Erik Erikson) does not develop, with the child believing that the environment is consistently hostile and potentially dangerous. Other psychosocial factors include a history of deafness, blindness, social isolation and loneliness, recent immigration or other abrupt environmental changes, and advanced age.

**E. Lab and psychological tests.** No lab test can confirm the diagnosis. Projective psychological tests reveal a preoccupation with paranoid or grandiose themes and issues of inferiority, inadequacy, and anxiety.

**F. Pathophysiology.** No known pathophysiology except when patients have discrete anatomical defects of the limbic system or basal ganglia.

**G. Psychodynamic factors.** Defenses used: (1) denial, (2) reaction forma-

TABLE 8–1
**DSM-IV DIAGNOSTIC CRITERIA FOR DELUSIONAL DISORDER**

A. Nonbizarre delusions (i.e., involving situations that occur in real life, such as being followed, poisoned, infected, loved at a distance, or deceived by spouse or lover, or having a disease) of at least 1 month's duration.
B. Criterion A for schizophrenia has never been met. **Note:** Tactile and olfactory hallucinations may be present in Delusional Disorder if they are related to the delusional theme.
C. Apart from the impact of the delusion(s) or its ramifications, functioning is not markedly impaired and behavior is not obviously odd or bizarre.
D. If mood episodes have occurred concurrently with delusions, their total duration has been brief relative to the duration of the delusional periods.
E. The disturbance is not due to the direct physiological effects of a substance (e.g., a drug of abuse, a medication) or a general medical condition.

*Specify* type (the following types are assigned based on the predominant delusional theme):
   **Erotomanic type:** delusions that another person, usually of higher status, is in love with the individual
   **Grandiose type:** delusions of inflated worth, power, knowledge, identity, or special relationship to a deity or famous person
   **Jealous type:** delusions that the individual's sexual partner is unfaithful
   **Persecutory type:** delusions that the person (or someone to whom the person is close) is being malevolently treated in some way
   **Somatic type:** delusions that the person has some physical defect or general medical condition
   **Mixed type:** delusions characteristics of more than one of the above types, but no one theme predominates
   **Unspecified type**

Used with permission, APA


TABLE 8–2
**NEUROLOGICAL AND MEDICAL CONDITIONS THAT CAN PRESENT WITH DELUSIONS**

Basal ganglia disorders—Parkinson's disease, Huntington's disease

Deficiency states—$B_{12}$ folate, thiamine, niacin

Delirium

Dementia—Alzheimer's disease, Pick's disease

Endocrinopathies—adrenal, thyroid, parathyroid

Limbic system pathology—epilepsy, cerebrovascular diseases, tumors

Substance-induced—amphetamines, anticholinergics, antidepressants, antihypertensives, antituberculosis drugs, antiparkinson agents, cimetidine, cocaine, disulfiram (Antabuse), hallucinogens

Systemic—hepatic encephalopathy, hypercalcemia, hypoglycemia, porphyria, uremia


tion, (3) projection. Major defense is projection—symptoms are a defense against unacceptable ideas and feelings. Patients deny feelings of shame, humiliation, and inferiority; turn any unacceptable feelings into their opposites through reaction formation (inferiority into grandiosity); and project any unacceptable feelings outward onto others.

## H. Differential diagnosis

1. **Psychotic disorder due to general medical condition with delusions.** Conditions that may mimic delusional disorder include hypothyroidism and hyperthyroidism, Parkinson's disease, multiple sclerosis, Alzheimer's disease, tumors, and trauma to the basal ganglia. Many medical and neurological illnesses can present with delusions (Table 8–2). The most common sites for lesions are the basal ganglia and the limbic system.

2. **Substance-induced psychotic disorder with delusions.** Intoxication with sympathomimetics, e.g., amphetamines, marijuana, or L-dopa (Larodopa), is likely to result in delusional symptoms.

3. **Paranoid personality disorder.** No true delusions are present, although overvalued ideas that verge on being delusional may be present. Patients are predisposed to delusional disorders.

4. **Paranoid schizophrenia.** More likely to present with prominent auditory hallucinations, personality deterioration, and more marked disturbance in role functioning. Age of onset tends to be younger in schizophrenia than in delusional disorder.

5. **Major depressive disorder.** Depressed patients may have paranoid delusions secondary to major depressive disorder, but the mood symptoms and associated characteristics, such as vegetative symptoms, positive family history, and response to antidepressants, are prominent.

6. **Bipolar I disorder.** Manic patients may have grandiose or paranoid delusions, which are clearly secondary to the primary and prominent mood disorder; associated with such characteristics as euphoric and labile mood, positive family history, and response to lithium.

I. **Course and prognosis.** Disorder tends to be chronic and unremitting in 30–50% of patients. Less satisfactory response to pharmacotherapy than patients with delusional symptoms associated with schizophrenia or mood disorder. Psychotherapy is difficult because of lack of trust.

J. **Treatment.** Patients rarely enter therapy voluntarily; rather, they are brought by concerned friends and relatives. Establishing rapport is difficult; patient's hostility is fear-motivated. Successful psychotherapy may enable the patient to improve social adaption in spite of persistent delusion.

1. **Hospitalization.** Hospitalization is necessary if patient is unable to control suicidal or homicidal impulses; if there is extreme impairment, e.g., refusing to eat because of a delusion about food poisoning; or if there is a need for a thorough organic workup.

2. **Psychopharmacotherapy.** Patients tend to refuse medications because of suspiciousness. Severely agitated patients may require intramuscular antipsychotic medication. Otherwise, low-dose antipsychotics, e.g., 2 mg haloperidol (Haldol), may be tried. Delusional patients are more likely to react to adverse effects with delusional ideas; thus, a very gradual increase in dose is recommended to diminish the likelihood of disturbing adverse effects. Antidepressants may be of use with severe depression.

3. **Psychotherapy: Dos and Don'ts**

   a. *Don't* argue with or challenge the patient's delusions. A delusion may become even more entrenched if the patient feels that it must be defended.

   b. *Don't* pretend that the delusion is true, since the clinician must represent reality to the patient. However, do listen to the patient's concerns about the delusion and try to understand what the delusion may mean, specifically in terms of the patient's self-esteem.

   c. *Do* respond sympathetically to the fact that the delusion is disturbing and intrusive in the patient's life and offer to help the patient to develop ways to live more comfortably with the delusion.

   d. *Do* understand that the delusional system may be a means of grappling with profound feelings of shame and inadequacy and that the patient

TABLE 8–3
**DSM-IV DIAGNOSTIC CRITERIA FOR SCHIZOPHRENIFORM DISORDER**

A. Criteria A, D, and E of schizophrenia are met.
B. An episode of the disorder (including prodromal, active, and residual phases) lasts at least 1 month but less than 6 months. (When the diagnosis must be made without waiting for recovery, it should be qualified as "provisional.")

*Specify* if:
   **Without good prognostic features**
   **With good prognostic features:** as evidenced by two (or more) of the following:
      (1) onset of prominent psychotic symptoms within 4 weeks of the first noticeable change in usual behavior or functioning
      (2) confusion or perplexity at the height of the psychotic episode
      (3) good premorbid social and occupational functioning
      (4) absence of blunted or flat affect

Used with permission, APA.

may be hypersensitive to any imagined slights or condescensions, even when unintended.

   e. *Do* be straightforward, honest, and up-front in all dealings with the patient, since these patients are hypervigilant to being tricked or deceived. Explain side effects of medications and why you are giving medications, e.g., to help with anxiety, irritability, insomnia, anorexia; be reliable and on time for appointments; schedule regular appointments.

   f. *Do* examine what particular stresses or experiences triggered the first appearance of the delusion and try to understand why they led to the patient's feelings of shame or inadequacy. Understand that other similar stresses or experiences in the patient's life may exacerbate delusional symptoms. Help the patient develop alternative means of responding to stressful situations.

## II. Schizophreniform disorder

**A. Definition.** Symptoms identical to those of schizophrenia except that they resolve within 6 months and normal functioning returns.

**B. Diagnosis, signs, and symptoms.** See Table 8–3.

**C. Epidemiology.** Data are unavailable; however, the disorder may be less than half as common as schizophrenia.

**D. Etiology.** Related more to mood disorders than to schizophrenia. In general, schizophreniform patients have more mood symptoms and a better prognosis than schizophrenic patients. Schizophrenia occurs more often in families of mood disorder patients than in families of schizophreniform disorder.

**E. Differential diagnosis.** Identical to that of schizophrenia. See Chapter 7.

**F. Course and prognosis.** Good prognostic features include absence of blunted or flat affect, good premorbid functioning, confusion and disorientation at the height of the psychotic episode, shorter duration, acute onset, and onset of prominent psychotic symptoms within 4 weeks of any first noticeable change in behavior.

**G. Treatment.** Antipsychotic medications should be used to treat psychotic symptoms, but should be withdrawn after 3–6 months. Recurrent episodes

TABLE 8–4
**DSM-IV DIAGNOSTIC CRITERIA FOR SCHIZOAFFECTIVE DISORDER**

A.  An uninterrupted period of illness during which, at some time, there is either a major depressive episode, a manic episode, or a mixed episode concurrent with symptoms that meet criterion A for schizophrenia. **Note:** The major depressive episode must include criterion A1: depressed mood.
B.  During the same period of illness, there have been delusions or hallucinations for at least 2 weeks in the absence of prominent mood symptoms.
C.  Symptoms that meet criteria for a mood episode are present for a substantial portion of the total duration of the active and residual periods of the illness.
D.  The disturbance is not due to the direct physiological effects of a substance (e.g., a drug of abuse, a medication) or a general medical condition.

*Specify* type:
  **Bipolar type:** if the disturbance includes a maniac or a mixed episode (or a manic or a mixed episode and major depressive episodes)
  **Depressive type:** if the disturbance only includes major depressive episodes

Used with permission, APA.

warrant a trial with lithium. Psychotherapy is critical in helping patients to understand and deal with their psychotic experiences.

## III. Schizoaffective disorder

   **A. Definition.**    A disorder with concurrent features of both schizophrenia and a mood disorder that cannot be diagnosed as either one separately.

   **B. Diagnosis, signs, and symptoms.**    See Table 8–4.

   **C. Epidemiology.**    Lifetime prevalence is less than 1%; and occurs equally in men and women.

   **D. Etiology.**    Some patients may be misdiagnosed; they are actually schizophrenic with prominent mood symptoms or have a mood disorder with prominent psychotic symptoms. Prevalence of schizophrenia is not increased in schizoaffective families, but prevalence of mood disorders is. See etiology of schizophrenia (Chapter 7) and mood disorders (Chapter 9) for additional data and theories.

   **E. Differential diagnosis.**    Any medical, psychiatric, or drug-related condition that causes psychotic or mood symptoms must be considered.

   **F. Course and prognosis.**    Poor prognosis is associated with positive family history of schizophrenia, early and insidious onset without precipitating factors, predominance of psychotic symptoms, and poor premorbid history. Schizoaffective patients have a better prognosis than schizophrenic patients and a worse prognosis than mood disorder patients. Schizoaffective patients respond more often to lithium and are less likely to have a deteriorating course than schizophrenic patients are.

   **G. Treatment.**    Antidepressant or antimanic treatments should be attempted, and antipsychotic medications should be used to control acute psychoses.

## IV. Brief psychotic disorder

   **A. Definition.**    Symptoms last for less than 1 month and follow an obvious stress in the patient's life.

TABLE 8–5
**DSM-IV DIAGNOSTIC CRITERIA FOR BRIEF PSYCHOTIC DISORDER**

A. Presence of one (or more) of the following symptoms:
   (1) delusions
   (2) hallucinations
   (3) disorganized speech (e.g., frequent derailment or incoherence)
   **Note:** Do not include a symptom if it is a culturally sanctioned response pattern.
B. Duration of an episode of the disturbance is at least 1 day but less than 1 month, with eventual full return to premorbid level of functioning.
C. The disturbance is not better accounted for by a mood disorder with psychotic features, schizoaffective disorder, or schizophrenia and is not due to the direct physiological effects of a substance (e.g., a drug of abuse, a medication) or a general medical condition.

*Specify if:*
**With marked stressor(s)** (brief reactive psychosis): if symptoms occur shortly after and apparently in response to events that, singly or together, would be markedly stressful to almost anyone in similar circumsances in the person's culture
**Without marked stressor(s):** if psychotic symptoms do not occur shortly after, or are not apparently in response to events that, singly or together, would be markedly stressful to almost anyone in similar circumstances in the person's culture
**With postpartum onset:** if onset within 4 weeks postpartum

Used with permission, APA.

B. **Diagnosis, signs, and symptoms.**   See Table 8–5. Similar to those of other psychotic disorders, but with an increase in volatility and lability, confusion, disorientation, and affective symptoms.

C. **Epidemiology.**   No definitive data are available. More highly associated with persons with preexisting personality disorders and with those who have previously experienced major stressors, such as disasters or dramatic cultural changes.

D. **Etiology.**   Mood disorders are more common in the families of these patients. Psychosocial stress triggers psychotic episode. Psychosis is understood as a defensive response in a person with inadequate coping mechanisms.

E. **Differential diagnosis.**   Organic causes must be ruled out—in particular, drug intoxication and withdrawal. Seizure disorders must also be considered. Schizophrenia, mood disorders, and transient psychotic episodes associated with borderline and schizotypal personality disorders must be ruled out.

F. **Course and prognosis.**   Good prognostic indicators include a severe precipitating stressor (usually followed within hours by the psychosis), confusion and lability during the episode, good premorbid history, negative family history for schizophrenia, and short duration of symptoms (may last a few hours to days).

H. **Treatment.**   Short-term hospitalization may be required; antipsychotic medications may not be necessary, because often the symptoms can resolve very quickly on their own. If medication is required, use as low a dose as possible and discontinue as soon as possible. Psychotherapy is extremely important to address the nature and significance of the specific social stress that triggered the psychotic episode. Patients must build more adaptive and less devastating means of coping with future stress.

## V. Shared psychotic disorder

A. **Definition.**   Delusional system shared by two or more persons; previously called induced paranoid disorder and *folie à deux*.

B. **Diagnosis, signs, and symptoms.**   Persecutory delusions are most common, and the key presentation is the sharing and blind acceptance of these delusions between two people. Suicide or homicide pacts may be present.

**C. Epidemiology.** The disorder is rare; more common in women and in persons with physical disabilities that make them dependent on another person. Family members, usually two sisters, are involved in 95% of cases.

**D. Etiology.** The cause is primarily psychological; however, there may be a genetic influence because it most often affects members of the same family. There is a risk of schizophrenia in the families of people with this disorder. Psychological or psychosocial factors include a socially isolated relationship in which one person is submissive and dependent and the other is dominant with an established psychotic system.

**E. Psychodynamic factors.** The dominant psychotic personality maintains some contact with reality through the submissive person, while the submissive personality is desperately anxious to be cared for and accepted by the dominant person. The two often have a strongly ambivalent relationship.

**F. Differential diagnosis.** Rule out personality disorders, malingering, and factitious disorders in the submissive patient. Organic causes must always be considered.

**G. Course and prognosis.** Recovery rates vary; some are as low as 10–40%. Traditionally, the submissive partner is separated from the dominant, psychotic partner with the ideal outcome of a rapid diminution in the psychotic symptoms. If symptoms do not remit, the submissive person may meet the criteria for another psychotic disorder, such as schizophrenia or delusional disorder.

**H. Treatment.** Separate the persons and help the more submissive, dependent partner develop other means of support to compensate for the loss of the relationship. Antipsychotic medications are beneficial.

## VI. Postpartum psychosis

**A. Definition.** Syndrome occurring after childbirth and characterized by severe depression and delusions. Sometimes occurs as a part of a mood disorder, brief psychotic disorder, or secondary psychotic disorder.

**B. Diagnosis, signs, and symptoms.** Most cases occur 2–3 days postpartum. Initial complaints of insomnia, restlessness, and emotional lability progress to confusion, irrationality, delusions, and obsessive concerns about the infant. Thoughts of wanting to harm the baby or self are characteristic.

**C. Epidemiology.** Occurs in 1–2 per 1,000 deliveries. Most episodes occur in primiparas.

**D. Etiology.** Usually secondary to underlying mental illness, such as schizophrenia and bipolar disorders.

1. Sudden change in hormonal levels after parturition may contribute.
2. Psychodynamic conflicts about motherhood—unwanted pregnancy, trapped in unhappy marriage, fears of mothering.

TABLE 8–6
**DSM-IV DIAGNOSTIC CRITERIA FOR PSYCHOTIC DISORDER NOT OTHERWISE SPECIFIED**

This category includes psychotic symptomatology (i.e., delusions, hallucinations, disorganized speech, grossly disorganized or catatonic behavior) about which there is inadequate information to make a specific diagnosis or about which there is contradictory information, or disorders with psychotic symptoms that do not meet the criteria for any specific psychotic disorder.

Examples include:
1. Postpartum psychosis that does not meet criteria for mood disorder with psychotic features, brief psychotic disorder, psychotic disorder due to a general medical condition, or substance-induced psychotic disorder
2. Psychotic symptoms that have lasted for less than 1 month but that have not yet remitted, so that the criteria for brief psychotic disorder are not met
3. Persistent auditory hallucinations in the absence of any other features
4. Persistent nonbizarre delusions with periods of overlapping mood episodes that have been present for a substantial portion of the delusional disturbance
5. Situations in which the clinician has concluded that a psychotic disorder is present, but is unable to determine whether it is primary, due to a general medical condition, or substance-induced

Used with permission, APA.

### E. Differential diagnosis

1. **Postpartum blues.** Most women experience postpartum emotional lability. Clears spontaneously. No evidence of psychotic thinking.

2. **Substance-induced mood disorder.** Depression associated with postanesthetic states, such as that after cesarean section or scopolamine-meperidine (Demerol) analgesia (twilight sleep).

3. **Psychotic disorder due to a general medical condition.** Rule out infection, hormonal imbalance (e.g., hypothyroidism), encephalopathy associated with toxemia of pregnancy, preeclampsia.

### F. Course and prognosis.
Risk of infanticide, suicide, or both is high in untreated cases. Supportive family network, good premorbid personality, and appropriate treatment are associated with good to excellent prognosis.

### G. Treatment.
Suicidal precautions in presence of suicidal ideation. Do not leave the infant alone with the mother if delusions are present or if there are ruminations about the infant's health.

1. **Pharmacological.** Medication for primary symptoms: antidepressants for suicidal ideation and depression; antianxiety agents for agitation, insomnia, e.g., lorazepam [Ativan] 0.5 mg every 4–6 hours; lithium for manic behavior; antipsychotic agents for delusions, e.g., haloperidol 0.5 mg every 6 hours.

2. **Psychological.** Psychotherapy, both individual and marital therapy, to deal with intrapsychic or interpersonal conflicts. Consider discharging mother and infant to home only after arrangements for temporary homemaker are in place to reduce environmental stresses associated with care of the newborn.

## VII. Psychotic disorder not otherwise specified (NOS)

### A. Definition.
Patients whose psychotic presentation does not meet the diagnostic criteria for any established psychotic disorder; also known as atypical psychoses.

### B. Diagnosis, signs, and symptoms.
See Table 8–6. This diagnostic category includes disorders that present with various psychotic features (e.g., delusions, hallucinations, loosening of associations, catatonic behaviors) but

that cannot be delineated as any specific disorder. The disorders may include postpartum psychoses and rare or exotic syndromes, such as specific culture-bound syndromes.

1. **Autoscopic psychosis.**  Rare hallucinatory psychosis during which patient sees a phantom or specter of his or her own body. Usually psychogenic in origin, but consider irritable lesion of temporoparietal lobe. Responds to reassurance and antipsychotic medications.

2. **Capgras's syndrome.**  Delusion that persons in the environment are not their real selves but are doubles imitating the patient or impostors imitating someone else. May be part of schizophrenia and related disorders. Treat with antipsychotic medication. Psychotherapy is useful in understanding dynamics of the delusional belief, e.g., distrust of certain real persons in the environment.

3. **Cotard's syndrome.**  Delusions of nihilism, e.g., nothing exists, the body has disintegrated, the world is coming to an end. Usually seen as part of schizophrenia or severe bipolar disorder. May be early sign of Alzheimer's disease. May respond to antipsychotic or antidepressant medication.

---

*For a more detailed discussion of this topic, see Other Psychotic Disorders, Chap 15, p 1019; Harris MJ, Jeste DV: Schizophrenia and Delusional Disorders, Sec 49.6c, p 2569, in CTP/VI.*

# 9

# Mood Disorders

## I. General introduction

Mood is a sustained emotional tone perceived along a normal continuum of sad to happy. Mood disorders are characterized by abnormal feelings of depression or euphoria with associated psychotic features in some severe cases. Mood disorders are divided into bipolar and depressive disorders.

## II. Diagnosis, signs, and symptoms

### A. Depression (major depressive episode). See Table 9–1.

#### 1. Data obtained from history

a. Anhedonia—inability to experience pleasure.

b. Withdrawal from friends or family.

c. No motivation, low frustration tolerance.

d. Vegetative signs:

    i.   Loss of libido.

    ii.  Weight loss and anorexia.

    iii. Weight gain and hyperphagia.

    iv. Low energy level; fatigability.

    v.  Abnormal menses.

    vi. Early morning awakening (terminal insomnia); approximately 75% of depressed patients have sleep difficulties, either insomnia or hypersomnia.

    vii. Diurnal variation (symptoms worse in morning).

e. Constipation.

f. Dry mouth.

g. Headache.

#### 2. Data obtained from mental status examination (MSE)

a. **General appearance and behavior**—psychomotor retardation or agitation, poor eye contact, tearful, downcast, inattentive to personal appearance.

b. **Affect**—constricted, intense.

c. **Mood**—depressed, irritable, frustrated, sad.

d. **Speech**—little or no spontaneity, monosyllabic, long pauses, soft, low, monotone.

e. **Thought content**—60% of depressed patients have suicidal ideation, and 15% of depressed patients commit suicide; obsessive rumination; pervasive feelings of hopelessness, worthlessness, and guilt; somatic preoccupations; indecisiveness; poverty of content; hallucinations and delusions (mood-congruent themes of guilt, poverty, nihilism, deserved persecution, somatic preoccupation); little spontaneity.

TABLE 9–1
**DSM-IV CRITERIA FOR MAJOR DEPRESSIVE EPISODE**

A. Five (or more) of the following symptoms have been present during the same 2-week period and represent a change from previous functioning; at least one of the symptoms is either (1) depressed mood or (2) loss of interest or pleasure.
  **Note:** Do not include symptoms that are clearly due to a general medical condition, or mood-incongruent delusions or hallucinations.
  (1) depressed mood most of the day, nearly every day, as indicated by either subjective report (e.g., feels sad or empty) or observation made by others (e.g., appears tearful). **Note:** In children and adolescents, can be irritable mood.
  (2) markedly diminished interest or pleasure in all, or almost all, activities most of the day, nearly every day (as indicated by either subjective account or observation made by others)
  (3) significant weight loss when not dieting or weight gain (e.g., a change of more than 5% of body weight in a month), or decrease or increase in appetite nearly every day. **Note:** In children, consider failure to make expected weight gains.
  (4) insomnia or hypersomnia nearly every day
  (5) psychomotor agitation or retardation nearly every day (observable by others, not merely subjective feelings of restlessness or being slowed down)
  (6) fatigue or loss of energy nearly every day
  (7) feelings of worthlessness or excessive or inappropriate guilt (which may be delusional) nearly every day (not merely self-reproach or guilt about being sick)
  (8) diminished ability to think or concentrate, or indecisiveness, nearly every day (either by subjective account or as observed by others)
  (9) recurrent thoughts of death (not just fear of dying), recurrent suicidal ideation without a specific plan, or a suicide attempt or a specific plan for committing suicide
B. The symptoms do not meet criteria for a mixed episode.
C. The symptoms cause clinically significant distress or impairment in social, occupational, or other important areas of functioning.
D. The symptoms are not due to the direct physiological effects of a substance (e.g., a drug of abuse, a medication) or a general medical condition (e.g., hypothyroidism).
E. The symptoms are not better accounted for by bereavement, i.e., after the loss of a loved one, the symptoms persist for longer than 2 months or are characterized by marked functional impairment, morbid preoccupation with worthlessness, suicidal ideation, psychotic symptoms, or psychomotor retardation.

Used with permission, APA.

   **f. Sensorium**—distractable, difficulty concentrating, complaints of poor memory, apparent disorientation; abstract thought may be impaired.

   **g. Insight and judgment**—impaired because of cognitive distortions of personal worthlessness.

**3. Associated features**

   **a. Somatic complaints may mask depression**—in particular, cardiac, gastrointestinal (GI), genitourinary (GU), low back pain, or orthopedic complaints.

   **b.** Content of delusions and hallucinations, when present, tend to be congruent with depressed mood; most common are delusions of guilt, poverty, and deserved persecution, as well as somatic and nihilistic (end of the world) delusions. Mood-incongruent delusions are those with content not apparently related to the predominant mood, such as delusions of thought insertion, broadcasting, and control or persecutory delusions unrelated to depressive themes.

**4. Age-specific features.** Depression can present differently at different ages.

   **a. Prepubertal**—somatic complaints, agitation, single-voice auditory hallucinations, anxiety disorders, and phobias.

   **b. Adolescence**—substance abuse, antisocial behavior, restlessness, truancy, school difficulties, promiscuity, increased sensitivity to rejection, poor hygiene.

TABLE 9–2
**DSM-IV CRITERIA FOR MANIC EPISODE**

A. A distinct period of abnormally and persistently elevated, expansive, or irritable mood, lasting at least 1 week (or any duration if hospitalization is necessary).
B. During the period of mood disturbance, three (or more) of the following symptoms have persisted (four if the mood is only irritable) and have been present to a significant degree:
   (1) inflated self-esteem or grandiosity
   (2) decreased need for sleep (e.g., feels rested after only 3 hours of sleep)
   (3) more talkative than usual or pressure to keep talking
   (4) flight of ideas or subjective experience that thoughts are racing
   (5) distractibility (i.e., attention too easily drawn to unimportant or irrelevant external stimuli)
   (6) increase in goal-directed activity (either socially, at work or school, or sexually) or psychomotor agitation
   (7) excessive involvement in pleasurable activities that have a high potential for painful consequences (e.g., engaging in unrestrained buying sprees, sexual indiscretions, or foolish business investments)
C. The symptoms do not meet criteria for a mixed episode.
D. The mood disturbance is sufficiently severe to cause marked impairment in occupational functioning or in usual social activities or relationships with others, or to necessitate hospitalization to prevent harm to self or others, or there are psychotic features.
E. The symptoms are not due to the direct physiological effects of a substance (e.g., a drug of abuse, a medication, or other treatment) or a general medical condition (e.g., hyperthyroidism).
**Note:** Maniclike episodes that are clearly caused by somatic antidepressant treatment (e.g., medication, electroconvulsive therapy, light therapy) should not count toward a diagnosis of bipolar I disorder.

Used with permission, APA.

      c. **Elderly**—cognitive deficits (memory loss, disorientation, and confusion), pseudodementia or the dementia syndrome of depression, apathy, distractibility.

B. **Mania (manic episode).**   See Table 9–2.
   1. **Data obtained from history**
     a. Erratic and disinhibited behavior:
       i.  Excessive spending of money.
       ii.  Excessive gambling.
       iii.  Hypersexuality, promiscuity.
     b. Overextended in activities and responsibilities.
     c. Low frustration tolerance.
     d. Vegetative signs:
       i.  Increased libido.
       ii.  Weight loss, anorexia.
       iii.  Insomnia (expressed as no need to sleep).
       iv.  Excessive energy.
   2. **Data obtained from MSE**
     a. **General appearance and behavior**—psychomotor agitation, seductive, colorful clothes, excessive makeup, inattention to personal appearance or bizarre combinations of clothes, intrusive, entertaining, threatening, hyperexcited.
     b. **Affect**—labile, intense (may have rapid depressive shifts).
     c. **Mood**—euphoric, expansive, irritable, demanding, flirtatious.
     d. **Speech**—pressured, loud, dramatic, exaggerated, may become incoherent.
     e. **Thought content**—highly elevated self-esteem, grandiosity, highly egocentric, delusions and less frequently hallucinations (mood-congruent themes of inflated self-worth and power; most often grandiose and paranoid).

TABLE 9–3
**DSM-IV DIAGNOSTIC CRITERIA FOR MELANCHOLIC FEATURES SPECIFIER**

*Specify* if:
   **With melancholic features** (can be applied to the current or most recent major depressive episode
   in major depressive disorder and to a major depressive episode in bipolar I or bipolar II disorder
   only if it is the most recent type of mood episode)
A.  Either of the following, occurring during the most severe period of the current episode:
    (1) loss of pleasure in all, or almost all, activities
    (2) lack of reactivity to usually pleasurable stimuli (does not feel much better, even temporarily,
        when something good happens)
B.  Three (or more) of the following:
    (1) distinct quality of depressed mood (i.e., the depressed mood is experienced as distinctly
        different from the kind of feeling experienced after the death of a loved one)
    (2) depression regularly worse in the morning
    (3) early morning awakening (at least 2 hours before usual time of awakening)
    (4) marked psychomotor retardation or agitation
    (5) significant anorexia or weight loss
    (6) excessive or inappropriate guilt

Used with permission, APA.

   **f. Thought process**—flight of ideas (if severe, can lead to incoherence),
   racing thoughts, neologisms, clang associations, circumstantiality,
   tangentiality.

   **g. Sensorium**—highly distractible, difficulty concentrating; memory,
   if not too distracted, generally is intact; abstract thinking generally
   is intact.

   **h. Insight and judgment**—extremely impaired; often total denial of
   illness and inability to make any organized or rational decisions.

## C. Depressive disorders

   **1. Major depressive disorder (MDD).** (Also known as unipolar
   depression and unipolar disorder.) Severe episodic depressive disorder.
   Symptoms must be present for at least 2 weeks and represent a change
   from previous functioning. More common in women than in men by
   2:1. Precipitating event occurs in at least 25% of patients. Diurnal
   variation with symptoms worse early in morning. Psychomotor retardation or agitation is present. Associated with vegetative signs and mood-
   congruent delusions; hallucinations may be present. Median age of onset
   is 40 years, but can occur at any time. Genetic factor is present.

   **a. With melancholic features**—See Table 9–3. Severe and responsive
   to biological intervention.

   **b. Chronic major depressive episode**—present for at least 2 years;
   more common in elderly men, especially alcohol and substance abusers; and responds poorly to medications. Accounts for the condition
   of 10–15% of those with MDD. Can also occur as part of bipolar I
   and II disorders.

   **c. With seasonal pattern**—depression that comes with shortened day-
   light in winter and fall and disappears during spring and summer;
   also known as seasonal affective disorder (SAD). Characterized by
   hypersomnia, hyperphagia, and psychomotor slowing. Related to
   abnormal melatonin metabolism. Treated with exposure to bright,
   artificial light for 2–6 hours a day. May also occur as part of bipolar
   I and II disorders.

   **d. With postpartum onset**—severe depression beginning within 4
   weeks of birth. Most often occurs in women with underlying or

preexisting mood or other psychiatric disorder. Symptoms range from marked insomnia, lability, and fatigue to suicide. Homicidal and delusional beliefs can occur about the baby. Can be psychiatric emergency with both mother and baby at risk. Also applies to manic or mixed episodes or to brief psychotic disorder. See Chapter 8.

 **e. With atypical features**—sometimes called hysterical dysphoria. Major depressive episode characterized by weight gain and hypersomnia rather than weight loss and insomnia. More common in women than in men by 2–3:1. Common in MDD with seasonal pattern. May also occur as part of bipolar I or II disorder and dysthymic disorder.

 **f. Pseudodementia**—MDD presenting as cognitive dysfunction resembling dementia. Occurs in elderly persons. Occurs more often in patients with previous history of mood disorder. Depression is primary and preeminent, antedating cognitive deficits. Responsive to electroconvulsive therapy (ECT) or antidepressant medication.

 **g. Depression in children**—not uncommon. Same signs and symptoms as for adults. Masked depression seen in running away from home, school phobia, substance abuse. Suicide may occur.

 **h. Double depression**—dysthymic patients who develop superimposed MDD (about 10–15%).

 **i. Atypical depression**—known as depressive disorder not otherwise specified (NOS) in DSM-IV. Depressive features that do not meet criteria for specific mood disorder, e.g., minor depressive disorder, recurrent brief depressive disorder, and premenstrual dysphoric disorder.

 **2. Dysthymic disorder.** (Previously known as depressive neurosis.) Less severe than MDD, dysthymic disorder is more common and chronic in women than in men. Insidious onset. Occurs more often in persons with history of long-term stress or sudden losses; often coexists with other psychiatric disorders, such as substance abuse, personality disorders, and obsessive-compulsive disorder. Symptoms tend to be worse later in the day. Onset generally is in a person's 20s or 30s, although there is an early-onset type, which begins before age 21. More common among first-degree relatives with MDD. Symptoms should include at least two of the following: poor appetite, overeating, sleep problems, fatigue, low self-esteem, poor concentration or difficulty making decisions, and feelings of hopelessness.

**D. Bipolar disorders**

 **1. Bipolar I disorder.** Patient has met the criteria for a full manic or mixed episode, usually sufficiently severe to require hospitalization. May occur with major depressive or hypomanic episodes.

 **2. Bipolar II disorder.** Patient has had at least one major depressive episode and at least one hypomanic episode, but no manic episode.

 **3. Rapid-cycling bipolar disorder.** Alternating manic and depressive episodes separated by intervals of 48–72 hours. Bipolar disorder with mixed or rapid cycling episodes appears to be more chronic than bipolar disorder without alternating episodes.

 **4. Adolescent mania.** Signs of mania masked by substance abuse, alcoholism, antisocial behavior.

TABLE 9-4
**EPIDEMIOLOGY OF MAJOR DEPRESSIVE DISORDER AND BIPOLAR I DISORDER**

| | Major Depressive Disorder | Bipolar I Disorder |
|---|---|---|
| Incidence (new cases per year) | 1/100 men 3/100 women | 1.2/100 men 1.8/100 women |
| Prevalence (existing cases) | 2–3/100 men 5–10/100 women | 1/100 men and women |
| Lifetime expectancy | 10% men 20% women | 1% men and women |
| Sex | 2:1 women/men | Men or women (may be slightly higher in women) |
| Age | 40—mean age men/women 10% occur after age 60 Small peak in adolescence 50% occur before age 40 | 30—mean age men/women |
| Race | No difference | No difference |
| Sociocultural | ↑ risk with family history of alcohol/depression/parental loss before age 13 Slightly ↑ risk in lower socioeconomic groups | ↑ risk with family history of mania/ bipolar illness No difference urban/rural Slightly increased in higher socioeconomic groups |
| Family history | (Evidence for heritability stronger for bipolar disorder than for depression) Approximately 10–13% risk for first-degree relatives MZ concordance rate higher than DZ, but ratio not as high as seen in bipolar | 20–25% risk for first-degree relatives 50% of bipolar patients have parent with mood disorder Child with one bipolar parent = 25% risk of developing disorder Child with two bipolar parents = 50–75% risk Bipolar MZ concordance rate = 40–70% Bipolar DZ concordance rate = 20% |

Used with permission, APA.

5. **Cyclothymic disorder.**    Less severe bipolar disorder with alternating periods of hypomania and moderate depression. The condition is chronic and nonpsychotic. Symptoms must be present for at least 2 years. Equally common in men and women. Onset usually is insidious and occurs in late adolescence or early adulthood. Substance abuse is common. MDD and bipolar disorder are more common among first-degree relatives than among the general population. Recurrent mood swings may lead to social and professional difficulties. May respond to lithium.

## III. Epidemiology

See Table 9–4.

## IV. Etiology

### A. Biological

1. **Neurochemical.**    Decreased biogenic amine (serotonin, norepinephrine, dopamine) activity in depression—increased activity in mania. Biogenic amine metabolites 5-hydroxyindoleacetic acid

(5-HIAA) (from serotonin), homovanillic acid (HVA) (from dopamine), 3-methoxy-4-hydroxyphenylglycol (MHPG) (from norepinephrine)—altered in blood, urine, and cerebrospinal fluid (CSF). Some assaultive, violent, depressed suicidal patients show decreased 5-HIAA in CSF. Dysregulation of adrenergic-cholinergic system with cholinergic dominance.

2. **Hormonal.** In general, neuroendocrine abnormalities probably reflect disruptions in biogenic amine input to the hypothalamus. The hypothalamic-pituitary-adrenal axis is hyperactive in depression, leading to increased cortisol secretion. Also in depression—blunted release of thyroid-stimulating hormone (TSH), decreased growth hormone (GH), decreased follicle-stimulating hormone (FSH), decreased luteinizing hormone (LH), and decreased testosterone. Immune functions are decreased in both mania and depression.

3. **Sleep.** Abnormalities in 60–65% of mood disorder patients. In depression, increased rapid eye movement (REM) density in first half of sleep, increased REM time overall, decreased REM latency (beginning of first REM period after falling asleep), decreased stage 4 sleep. Multiple awakenings common in mania, with overall decrease in sleep time.

4. **Genetic.** Both bipolar disorders and depressive disorders run in families, but evidence for heritability is higher for bipolar disorder.

One parent with bipolar I disorder—25% chance of mood disorder in child. Two parents with bipolar I disorder—50–75% chance of mood disorder in child. One parent with MDD—10–13% chance of mood disorder in child. One monozygotic (MZ) twin bipolar I—33–90% chance of bipolar I in other twin (dizygotic [DZ] twins—5–25%). One MZ twin with MDD—about 50% chance of MDD in other twin (DZ twins—10–25%).

No genetic association has been consistently replicated. Associations between the mood disorders, particular bipolar I disorder, and genetic markers have been reported for chromosomes 5, 11, and X.

B. **Psychosocial**
   1. **Psychoanalytic.** Symbolic or real loss of loved person (love object) perceived as rejection. Mania and elation viewed as defense against underlying depression. Rigid superego serves to punish person for guilt feelings about unconscious sexual or aggressive impulses. Freud described internalized ambivalence toward love object, which can produce a pathological form of mourning if the object is lost or perceived as lost. This mourning takes the form of severe depression with feelings of guilt, worthlessness, and suicidal ideation.
   2. **Cognitive.** Cognitive triad of Aaron Beck: (1) negative self-view ("things are bad because I'm bad"); (2) negative interpretation of experience ("everything has always been bad"); (3) negative view of future (anticipation of failure). Learned helplessness is a theory that attributes depression to a person's inability to control events. Theory is derived from observed behavior of animals experimentally given unexpected random shocks from which they could not escape.

## V. Lab and psychological tests

**A. Dexamethasone suppression test (DST).**  Nonsuppression (a positive DST) due to hypersecretion of cortisol secondary to hyperactivity of hypothalamic-pituitary-adrenal axis. Abnormal in 50% of major depressives. Of limited clinical usefulness owing to frequency of false-positives and -negatives. **TSH**—diminished release in response to thyrotropin-releasing hormone (TRH); reported in both depression and mania. **Prolactin release**—decreased in response to tryptophan. Tests are not definitive.

**B. Psychological tests**

1. **Zung Self-Rating Scale.**  Scored by patients; index of depressive intensity.
2. **Hamilton Depression Scale.**  Scored by examiner.
3. **Rorschach test.**  Standardized set of 10 inkblots scored by examiner—few associations, slow response time in depression.
4. **Thematic Apperception Test (TAT).**  Series of 30 pictures depicting ambiguous situations and interpersonal events. Patient creates a story about each scene—depressives will create depressed stories, manics more grandiose and dramatic ones.

**C. Brain imaging.**  No gross brain changes Enlarged cerebral ventricles on computed tomography (CT) scan in some patients with mania or psychotic depression; diminished basal ganglia blood flow in some depressive patients. Magnetic resonance imaging (MRI) studies have also indicated that patients with MDD have smaller caudate nuclei and smaller frontal lobes than do control subjects. Magnetic resonance spectroscopy (MRS) studies of patients with bipolar I disorder have produced data consistent with the hypothesis that the pathophysiology of the disorder may involve an abnormal regulation of membrane phospholipid metabolism.

## VI. Psychodynamics

In depression, introjection of ambivalently viewed lost object leading to an inner sense of conflict, guilt, rage, pain, and loathing; a pathological mourning, which becomes depression as ambivalent feelings meant for the introjected object are directed at the self. In mania, feelings of inadequacy and worthlessness are converted by means of denial, reaction formation, and projection to grandiose delusions.

## VII. Differential diagnosis

Table 9–5 lists the clinical differences between depression and mania.

**A. Mood disorder due to general medical condition.**  Depressive, manic, or mixed features or major depressivelike episode secondary to medical illness, e.g., brain tumor, metabolic illness, human immunodeficiency virus (HIV) disease, Cushing's syndrome (Table 9–6). Cognitive deficits are common.

1. **Myxedema madness.**  Hypothyroidism associated with fatigability, depression, and suicidal impulses. May mimic schizophrenia with thought disorder, delusions, hallucinations, paranoia, and agitation. More common in women.

TABLE 9–5
**CLINICAL DIFFERENCES BETWEEN DEPRESSION AND MANIA**

|  | Depressive Syndrome | Manic Syndrome |
|---|---|---|
| Mood | Depressed, irritable, or anxious (the patient may, however, smile or deny subjective mood change and instead complain of pain or other somatic distress) | Elated, irritable, or hostile |
|  | Crying spells (the patient may, however, complain of inability to cry or to experience emotions) | Momentary tearfulness (as part of mixed state) |
| Associated psychologic manifestations | Lack of self-confidence; low self-esteem; self-reproach | Inflated self-esteem; boasting; grandiosity |
|  | Poor concentration; indecisiveness | Racing thoughts; clang associations (new thoughts triggered by word sounds rather than meaning); distractibility |
|  | Reduction in gratification; loss of interest in usual activities; loss of attachments; social withdrawal | Heightened interest in new activities, people, creative pursuits; increased involvement with people (who are often alienated because of the patient's intrusive and meddlesome behavior); buying sprees; sexual indiscretions; foolish business investments |
|  | Negative expectations; hopelessness; helplessness; increased dependency |  |
|  | Recurrent thoughts of death and suicide |  |
| Somatic manifestations | Psychomotor retardation; fatigue Agitation | Psychomotor acceleration; eutonia (increased sense of physical well-being) |
|  | Anorexia and weight loss, or weight gain | Possible weight loss from increased activity and inattention to proper dietary habits |
|  | Insomnia, or hypersomnia | Decreased need for sleep |
|  | Menstrual irregularities; amenorrhea |  |
|  | Anhedonia; loss of sexual desire | Increased sexual desire |
| Psychotic symptoms | Delusions of worthlessness and sinfulness | Grandiose delusions of exceptional talent |
|  | Delusions of reference and persecution | Delusions of assistance; delusions of reference and persecution |
|  | Delusions of ill health (nihilistic, somatic, or hypochondriacal) | Delusions of exceptional mental and physical fitness |
|  | Delusions of poverty | Delusions of wealth, aristocratic ancestry, or other grandiose identity |
|  | Depressive hallucinations in the auditory, visual, and (rarely) olfactory spheres | Fleeting auditory or visual hallucinations |

Table from Berkow R., ed: *Merck Manual*, ed 15, p 1518. Merck Sharp & Dohme Research Laboratories, Rahway, NJ, 1987. Used with permission.

TABLE 9–6
**NEUROLOGICAL AND MEDICAL CAUSES OF DEPRESSIVE (AND MANIC) SYMPTOMS**

*Neurological*
Cerebrovascular diseases
Dementias (including dementia of the Alzheimer's
   type with depressed mood)
Epilepsy[a]
Fahr's disease[a]
Huntington's disease[a]
Hydrocephalus
Infections (including HIV and neurosyphilis)[a]
Migraines[a]
Multiple sclerosis[a]
Narcolepsy
Neoplasms[a]
Parkinson's disease
Progressive supranuclear palsy
Sleep apnea
Trauma[a]
Wilson's disease[a]

*Endocrine*
Adrenal (Cushing's, Addison's diseases)
Hyperaldosteronism
Menses-related[a]

Parathyroid disorders (hyper- and hypo-)
Postpartum[a]
Thyroid disorders (hypothyroidism and apathetic
   hyperthyroidism)[a]

*Infectious and Inflammatory*
Acquired immune deficiency syndrome (AIDS)[a]
Chronic fatigue syndrome
Mononucleosis
Pneumonia—viral and bacterial
Rheumatoid arthritis
Sjögren's arteritis
Systemic lupus erythematosus[a]
Temporal arteritis
Tuberculosis

*Miscellaneous Medical*
Cancer (especially pancreatic and other GI)
Cardiopulmonary disease
Porphyria
Uremia (and other renal diseases)[a]
Vitamin deficiencies ($B_{12}$, folate, niacin, thiamine)[a]

[a]These conditions are also associated with manic symptoms.

2. **Mad hatter's syndrome.**   Chronic mercury intoxication (poisoning) producing manic (and sometimes depressive) symptoms.

B. **Schizophrenia.**   Schizophrenia can look like a manic, major depressive, or mixed episode with psychotic features. To differentiate, rely on such factors as family history, course, premorbid history, and response to medication. Depressive or manic episode with presence of mood-incongruent psychotic features (delusions or hallucinations, such as thought insertion and broadcasting, loose associations or flight of ideas, poor reality testing, inattention to personal hygiene, or bizarre behavior) can be mistaken for schizophrenia and may have a poorer prognosis than depression or mania with mood-congruent psychotic features.

C. **Grief.**   Not a true disorder. Known as bereavement in DSM-IV. Profound sadness secondary to major loss. Presentation may be similar to that of MDD with anhedonia, withdrawal, and vegetative signs. Remits with time. Differentiated from MDD by absence of suicidal ideation or profound feelings of hopelessness and worthlessness. Usually resolves within a year. May develop into major depressive episode in predisposed persons.

D. **Substance-induced mood disorder.**   Mood disorders caused by a drug or toxin, e.g., cocaine, amphetamine, propranolol (Inderal), steroids. Must always rule out when patient presents with depressive or manic symptoms. Mood disorders are often comorbid with substance abuse and dependence.

E. **Personality disorders.**   Lifelong behavioral pattern associated with rigid defensive style; depression may occur more readily after stressful life event because of inflexibility of coping mechanisms. Manic episode may also occur more readily in predisposed people with preexisting personality disorder. A mood disorder may be diagnosed on Axis I simultaneously with a personality disorder on Axis II.

**F. Schizoaffective disorder.** Signs and symptoms of schizophrenia accompany prominent mood symptoms. Course and prognosis are between those of schizophrenia and mood disorders.

**G. Adjustment disorder with depressed mood.** Moderate depression in response to clearly identifiable stress, which resolves as stress diminishes. Considered a maladaptive response due to either impairment in functioning or excessive and disproportionate intensity of symptoms. Persons with personality disorders or organic deficits may be more vulnerable.

## VIII. Course and prognosis

15% of depressed patients eventually commit suicide. An untreated, average depressed episode lasts about 10 months. At least 75% of affected patients have a second episode of depression, usually in the first 6 months after the initial episode. Average number of depressive episodes in a lifetime is five. Prognosis generally is good: 50% recover, 30% partially recover, 20% have a chronic course. About 20–30% of dysthymic patients develop, in descending order of frequency, MDD (called "double depression"), bipolar II disorder, or bipolar I disorder. About one-third of cyclothymic disorder patients develop major mood disorder, usually bipolar II disorder. 45% of manic episodes recur. Untreated, manic episodes last 3–6 months with a high rate of recurrence (average of 10 recurrences). Some 80–90% of manic patients eventually experience a full depressive episode. Prognosis is fair: 15% recover; 50–60% partially recover (multiple relapses with good interepisodic functioning), and one-third have some evidence of chronic symptoms and social deterioration.

## IX. Treatment

**A. Depressive disorders.** Major depressive episodes are treatable in 70–80% of patients. The physician must integrate pharmacotherapy with psychotherapeutic interventions. If physicians view mood disorders as fundamentally evolving from psychodynamic issues, their ambivalence about the use of drugs may result in a poor response, noncompliance, and probably inadequate dosages for too short a treatment period. Conversely, if physicians ignore the psychosocial needs of the patient, the outcome of pharmacotherapy may be compromised.

  1. **Pharmacological.** Almost always indicated in MDD and may be used in some cases of dysthymic disorder. See Table 9–7.

  a. If there is family history of positive response to a particular drug, that drug should be tried first.

  b. Begin with a tricyclic or tetracyclic antidepressant or a serotonin-specific reuptake inhibitor (SSRI), depending on clinician's preference, and monitor for 2–3 weeks. Response usually is seen within 4 weeks. About 75% of patients respond positively. If symptoms are still present at 4–6 weeks, serum drug levels should be measured. Consider switching to a different class, e.g., tricyclic to SSRI, if response is poor or adverse side effects occur. SSRIs should be considered when anticholinergic side effects need to be avoided. SSRIs may be the drugs of choice for dysthymic disorder.

TABLE 9–7
**CRITERIA FOR ADEQUACY OF ANTIDEPRESSANT TRIALS**

| | Criteria | |
|---|---|---|
| | Definite Trials with Durations ≥6 wk | Probable Trials with Duration ≥4 and <6 wk |
| Antidepressant | Daily Dose | Daily Dose |
| **Tricyclics** | | |
| Imipramine, desipramine | ≥250 mg or plasma levels of desipramine ≥125 mg/mL and of imipramine ≥200 ng/mL | 200–249 mg |
| Nortriptyline | ≥100 mg of plasma levels between 50 and 150 ng/mL | 75–99 mg |
| Amitriptyline, doxepin | ≥250 mg | 200–249 mg |
| Maprotiline | ≥200 mg | 150–199 mg |
| Protriptyline | >60 mg | 40–59 mg |
| **Monoamine oxidase inhibitors** | | |
| Phenelzine | ≥60 mg | 45–59 mg |
| Isocarboxazid or tranylcypromine | >40 mg | 30–39 mg |
| **Serotonin-specific reuptake inhibitors** | | |
| Fluoxetine | ≥20 mg | 5–19 mg |
| **Other agents** | | |
| Bupropion | >400 mg | 300–399 mg |
| Trazodone | ≥300 mg | 200–299 mg |
| Amoxapine | >300 mg | 200–299 mg |
| Lithium | plasma levels, 0.7–1.1 mEq/L | plasma levels, 0.4–0.69 mEq/L |
| **Electroconvulsive therapy** | ≥12 total, with at least six bilateral | ≥9–11 unilateral |

Table adapted from Nirenberg AA. A systematic approach to treatment-resistant depression, J Clin Psychiatry Monogr 10: 7, 1992.

   c. L-Triiodothyronine ($T_3$) (Cytomel), lithium, or amphetamine may be added to supplement the antidepressant.
   d. If symptoms still do not improve, try a monoamine oxidase inhibitor (MAOI). An MAOI is safe with reasonable dietary restrictions of tyramine-containing substances. Major depressive episodes with atypical features, with psychotic features, or related to bipolar I disorder may preferentially respond to MAOIs. MAOIs must not be administered for 2–5 weeks after discontinuation of an SSRI, e.g., 5 weeks for fluoxetine, 2 weeks for paroxetine (Paxil). SSRI or other serotonergic drug, e.g., clomipramine (Anafranil), must not be administered for 2 weeks after discontinuation of an MAOI (Table 9–8).
   e. Bupropion (Wellbutrin) is a safe and effective antidepressant drug. Sympathomimetics are rarely used as first-line drugs because of their high potential for abuse. Alprazolam (Xanax) is not a common first-line drug because of its potential for sedation, motor impairment, and abuse. As a first-line drug, trazodone (Desyrel) is limited by its significant sedative properties and its association with priapism in men.
   f. Maintenance treatment for at least 6 months with antidepressants helps to prevent relapse. Long-term treatment may be indicated in patients with recurrent MDDs. Lithium appears to be effective as an adjunct in treating recurrent MDD.

TABLE 9-8
**DRUGS TO BE AVOIDED DURING MAOI TREATMENT**

**Never use:**
Anesthetic—never spinal anesthetic or local anesthetic containing epinephrine (lidocaine and procaine are safe)
Antiasthmatic medications
Antihypertensives α-methyldopa, guanethidine, reserpine, pargyline)
Diuretics
L-Dopa, L-tryptophan
SSRIs, clomipramine, trazodone, venlafaxine
Narcotics (especially meperidine (Demerol); morphine or codeine may be less dangerous)
Over-the-counter cold, hay fever, and sinus medications, especially those containing dextromethorphan (aspirin, acetaminophen, and menthol lozenges are safe)
Sympathomimetics amphetamine, cocaine, methylphenidate, dopamine, metaruminol, epinephrine, norepinephrine, isoproterenol)

**Use carefully:**
Antihistamines
Disulfiram
Hydralazine (Apresoline)
Propranolol (Inderal)
Terpin hydrate with codeine
Tricyclic and tetracyclic drugs

---

g. ECT is useful in refractory MDD and major depressive episodes with psychotic features; ECT also is indicated when rapid therapeutic response is desired or when side effects of antidepressant medications must be avoided. (ECT is underused as first-line antidepressant treatment.)

h. Lithium should be a first-line antidepressant in treatment of the depression of bipolar disorder. A heterocyclic antidepressant, T₃, or MAOI may be added as necessary, but monitor the patient carefully for emergence of manic symptoms.

2. **Psychological.** Psychotherapy in conjunction with antidepressants is more effective than either treatment alone in treatment of MDD.

a. **Cognitive therapy**—short-term treatment with interactive therapist and assigned homework aimed at testing and correcting negative cognitions and the unconscious assumptions that underlie them; based on correcting chronic distortions in thinking, which lead to depression, in particular the cognitive triad; feelings of helplessness and hopelessness about oneself, one's future, and one's past.

b. **Behavior therapy**—based on learning theory (classical and operant conditioning)—generally short-term and highly structured; aimed at specific, circumscribed undesired behaviors. The operant conditioning technique of positive reinforcement may be an effective adjunct in the treatment of depression.

c. **Interpersonal therapy (IPT)**—developed as specific short-term treatment for nonbipolar, nonpsychotic, outpatient depression. Emphasis on ongoing, current interpersonal issues as opposed to unconscious, intrapsychic dynamics.

d. **Psychoanalytically oriented psychotherapy**— insight-oriented therapy of indeterminate length aimed at achieving understanding of unconscious conflicts and motivations that may be fueling and sustaining depression.

    **e. Supportive psychotherapy**—therapy of indeterminate length with the primary aim of providing emotional support. Indicated particularly in acute crisis, such as grief, or when the patient is beginning to recover from a major depressive episode but cannot yet engage in more demanding, interactive therapy.

    **f. Group therapy**—not indicated for acutely suicidal patients. Other depressed patients may benefit from support, ventilation, and positive reinforcement of groups, as well as from interpersonal interaction and immediate correction of cognitive and transference distortions by other group members.

    **g. Family therapy**—particularly indicated when patient's depression is disrupting family stability, when depression is related to family events, or when depression is supported or maintained by family patterns.

## B. Bipolar disorders

### 1. Pharmacological

    a. Lithium is the treatment of choice for bipolar I and cyclothymic disorders; it is effective in 80% of bipolar I patients. With acute manic symptoms, lithium plus an antipsychotic (generally haloperidol [Haldol]) is necessary because the clinical response to lithium generally takes 7–10 days. A complete lithium trial should last at least 4 weeks before deciding to discontinue.

    b. A lithium blood level of 0.8–1.2 mEq per L is generally necessary for control of acute symptoms. A lower blood level, e.g., 0.4–0.8 mEq per L, is often sufficient as a maintenance level. For most adult patients, a reasonable starting dose is 300 mg three times a day. Eventually, the maintenance dosage usually ranges between 900 and 2,100 mg a day. Toxicity can occur quickly at blood levels close to therapeutic levels, e.g., 2.0 mEq per L and above.

    c. The need for maintenance lithium is determined by the patient's history of previous severe manic episodes. Maintenance dose should be the lowest possible amount that controls symptoms and produces minimal side effects. If manic symptoms occur while the patient is on lithium, an antipsychotic may be added or the dose of lithium increased.

    d. Lithium is the drug of choice for the treatment (including prevention) of the depressed phase of bipolar I or cyclothymic disorder. (40–50% of cyclothymic patients treated with antidepressants experience antidepressant-induced manic or hypomanic episodes.) If major depressive episodes occur while a patient is on lithium, an antidepressant may be added or the dosage of lithium increased.

    e. Pretreatment workup for lithium includes a serum creatinine level, electrolyte screen, thyroid function tests, complete blood count (CBC), electrocardiogram (EKG), and a pregnancy test as indicated. Lithium toxicity is potentially fatal and may consist of vomiting, severe diarrhea, severe tremor, ataxia, seizures, mental confusion, focal neurological signs, hyperreflexia, dysarthria, and coma. Generally, less serious adverse effects include gastric distress, weight gain, tremor, fatigue, and mild cognitive deficits. Other adverse effects involve the kidneys, thyroid, heart, and skin. Lithium is teratogenic and has been associated with birth defects affecting the heart.

   f. After 4 weeks, if lithium is ineffective by itself in controlling manic symptoms, other drugs may be tried, in particular, carbamazepine (Tegretol) or valproate (Depakene, Depakote), either alone or in conjunction with lithium. Other drugs used in treatment of mania include verapamil (Isoptin, Calan), nimodipine (Nimotop), clonidine (Catapres), clonazepam (Klonopin), and L-thyroxine (Levoxyl, Levothroid, Synthroid). See Chapter 24.

**2. Psychological.** Psychotherapy in conjunction with antimanic drugs, e.g., lithium, is more effective than either treatment alone. Psychotherapy is not indicated when a patient is experiencing a manic episode. In this situation, the safety of the patient and others must be paramount, and pharmacological and physical steps must be taken to protect and calm the patient.

   **a. Cognitive therapy**—has been studied in relation to increasing compliance with lithium therapy among bipolar patients.

   **b. Behavior therapy**—can be most effective during inpatient treatment of manic patients in helping to set limits on impulsive or inappropriate behavior through such techniques as positive and negative reinforcement and token economies.

   **c. Psychoanalytically oriented psychotherapy**—can be beneficial in the recovery and stabilization of manic patients, if patient is capable of and desires insight into underlying conflicts that may trigger and fuel manic episodes. Can also help patients understand resistances to medication and thus increase compliance.

   **d. Supportive psychotherapy**—indicated particularly during acute phases and in early recompensation. Some patients can only tolerate supportive therapy, whereas others can tolerate insight-oriented therapy. Supportive therapy more often is indicated with chronic bipolar disorder patients who may have significant interepisodic residual symptoms and social deterioration.

   **e. Group therapy**—can be helpful in challenging denial and defensive grandiosity of manic patients. Useful in addressing such common issues among manic people as loneliness, shame, inadequacy, fear of mental illness, and loss of control. Helpful in reintegrating patients socially.

   **f. Family therapy**—particularly important with bipolar patients, because their disorder is strongly familial (20–25% of first-degree relatives) and because manic episodes are so disruptive to patients' interpersonal relationships and jobs. During manic episodes, patient may spend huge amounts of family money or act with sexual inappropriateness; residual feelings of anger, guilt, and shame among family members must be addressed. Ways to help with compliance and recognizing triggering events can be explored.

---

*For a more detailed discussion of this topic, see Mood Disorders, Chap 16, p 1067; Parry BL, Rausch JL: Premenstrual Dysphoric Disorder, Sec 29.5, p 1707; Carlson GA, Abbott SF: Mood Disorders and Suicide, Chap 44, p 2367; Alexopoulous GS: Mood Disorders, Sec 49.6b, p 2566, in* CTP/VI.

---

# 10

# Anxiety Disorders

## I. Definition

Anxiety is a pathological state characterized by a feeling of dread accompanied by somatic signs that indicate a hyperactive autonomic nervous system. It is differentiated from fear, which is a response to a known cause.

## II. Diagnosis, signs, and symptoms

See Table 10–1.

A. **Panic disorder and agoraphobia.** See Table 10–2. Characterized by spontaneous panic attacks (Table 10–3) and may be associated with agoraphobia (fear of being in open spaces, outside the home alone, or in a crowd). Agoraphobia can occur alone, although patients usually have associated panic attacks. Anticipatory anxiety is characterized by the feeling that panic and helplessness or humiliation will occur. Agoraphobics may become housebound and never leave the home or only go outside with a companion.

B. **Generalized anxiety disorder.** See Table 10–4. Characterized by chronic, generalized anxiety for at least 1 month. Includes overanxious disorder of childhood.

C. **Specific phobia.** See Table 10–5. Irrational fear of an object, e.g., horses, or isolated situation, e.g., heights, and need to avoid it.

D. **Social phobia.** See Table 10–6. Irrational fear of public situations, e.g., public speaking.

E. **Obsessive-compulsive disorder.** See Table 10–7. Recurrent intrusive ideas, impulses, thoughts (obsessions), or patterns of behavior (compulsions) that are ego-alien and produce anxiety if resisted.

F. **Posttraumatic and acute stress disorders.** See Table 10–8. Anxiety produced by extraordinary major life stress. Event is relived in dreams and waking thoughts. The symptoms of reexperiencing, avoidance, and hyperarousal last more than 1 month. For patients in whom symptoms have been present less than 1 month, the appropriate diagnosis may be acute stress disorder.

## III. Epidemiology

See Table 10–9.

## IV. Etiology

### A. Biological

1. Excessive autonomic reaction with increased sympathetic tone.
2. Increased release of catecholamines.

**TABLE 10–1**
**SIGNS AND SYMPTOMS OF ANXIETY DISORDERS**

| Physical Signs | Psychological Symptoms |
|---|---|
| Trembling, twitching, feeling shaky | Feeling of dread |
| Backache, headache | Difficulty concentrating |
| Muscle tension | Hypervigilance |
| Shortness of breath, hyperventilation | Insomnia |
| Fatigability | Decreased libido |
| Startle response | "Lump in the throat" |
| Autonomic hyperactivity | Upset stomach ("butterflies") |
|   Flushing and pallor | |
|   Tachycardia, palpitations | |
|   Sweating | |
|   Cold hands | |
|   Diarrhea | |
|   Dry mouth (xerostomia) | |
|   Urinary frequency | |
| Paresthesia | |
| Difficulty swallowing | |

**TABLE 10–2**
**DSM-IV DIAGNOSTIC CRITERIA FOR PANIC DISORDER WITHOUT AGORAPHOBIA**

A. Both (1) and (2):
  (1) recurrent unexpected panic attacks
  (2) at least one of the attacks has been followed by 1 month (or more) of one (or more) of the following:
    (a) persistent concern about having additional attacks
    (b) worry about the implications of the attack or its consequences (e.g., losing control, having a heart attack, "going crazy")
    (c) a significant change in behavior related to the attacks
B. Absence of agoraphobia
C. The panic attacks are not due to the direct physiological effects of a substance (e.g., a drug of abuse, a medication) or a general medical condition (e.g., hyperthyroidism).
D. The panic attacks are not better accounted for by another mental disorder, such as social phobia (e.g., occurring on exposure to feared social situations), specific phobia (e.g., on exposure to a specific phobic situation), obsessive-compulsive disorder (e.g., on exposure to dirt in someone with an obsession about contamination), posttraumatic stress disorder (e.g., in response to stimuli associated with a severe stressor), or separation anxiety disorder (e.g., in response to being away from home or close relatives).

Used with permission, APA.

3. Increased norepinephrine metabolites, e.g., 3-methoxy-4-hydroxyphenylglycol (MHPG). Experimental lactate infusion increases norepinephrine, producing anxiety.
4. Decreased rapid eye movement (REM) latency and stage 4 sleep (similar to depression).
5. Decreased γ-aminobutyric acid (GABA) causes central nervous system (CNS) hyperactivity (GABA inhibits CNS ability).
6. Serotonin increase causes anxiety; increased dopaminergic activity associated with anxiety.
7. Hyperactive center in temporal cerebral cortex.
8. Locus ceruleus, center of noradrenergic neurons, hyperactive in anxiety states.

## B. Psychoanalytic

1. Unconscious impulses, e.g., sex, aggression, threaten to burst into consciousness and produce anxiety.

Table 10-3
**DSM-IV DIAGNOSTIC CRITERIA FOR PANIC ATTACK**

**Note:** A panic attack is not a codable disorder. Code the specific diagnosis in which the panic attack occurs (e.g., panic disorder with agoraphobia).

A discrete period of intense fear or discomfort, in which four (or more) of the following symptoms developed abruptly and reached a peak within 10 minutes:
 (1) palpitations, pounding heart, or accelerated heart rate
 (2) sweating
 (3) trembling or shaking
 (4) sensations of shortness of breath or smothering
 (5) feeling of choking
 (6) chest pain or discomfort
 (7) nausea or abdominal distress
 (8) feeling dizzy, unsteady, lightheaded, or faint
 (9) derealization (feelings of unreality) or depersonalization (being detached from oneself)
 (10) fear of losing control or going crazy
 (11) fear of dying
 (12) paresthesias (numbness or tingling sensations)
 (13) chills or hot flushes

Used with permission, APA.

TABLE 10-4
**DSM-IV DIAGNOSTIC CRITERIA FOR GENERALIZED ANXIETY DISORDER**

A. Excessive anxiety and worry (apprehensive expectation), occurring more days than not for at least 6 months, about a number of events or activities (such as work or school performance).
B. The person finds it difficult to control the worry.
C. The anxiety and worry are associated with three (or more) of the following six symptoms (with at least some symptoms present for more days than not for the past 6 months). **Note:** Only one item is required in children.
 (1) restlessness or feeling keyed up or on edge
 (2) being easily fatigued
 (3) difficulty concentrating or mind going blank
 (4) irritability
 (5) muscle tension
 (6) sleep disturbance (difficulty falling or staying asleep, or restless, unsatisfying sleep)
D. The focus of the anxiety and worry is not confined to features of an Axis I disorder, e.g., the anxiety or worry is not about having a panic attack (as in panic disorder), being embarrassed in public (as in social phobia), being contaminated (as in obsessive-compulsive disorder), being away from home or close relatives (as in separation anxiety disorder), gaining weight (as in anorexia nervosa), having multiple physical complaints (as in somatization disorder), or having a serious illness (as in hypochondriasis), and the anxiety and worry do not occur exclusively during posttraumatic stress disorder.
E. The anxiety, worry, or physical symptoms cause clinically significant distress or impairment in social, occupational, or other important areas of functioning.
F. The disturbance is not due to the direct physiological effects of a substance (e.g., a drug of abuse, a medication) or a general medical condition (e.g., hyperthyroidism) and does not occur exclusively during a mood disorder, a psychotic disorder, or a pervasive development disorder.

Used with permission, APA

 2. Defense mechanisms are used to ward off anxiety.
 3. Displacement produces phobias.
 4. Reaction formation, undoing, and displacement produce obsessive-compulsive disorder.
 5. Breakdown of repression produces panic or generalized anxiety disorder.
 6. Agoraphobia related to:
     i. Hostile-dependent relationship with companion.
     ii. Fear of aggressive or sexual impulses from self to others or vice versa.

TABLE 10-5
**DSM-IV DIAGNOSTIC CRITERIA FOR SPECIFIC PHOBIA**

A. Marked and persistent fear that is excessive or unreasonable, cued by the presence or anticipation of a specific object or situation (e.g., flying, heights, animals, receiving an injection, seeing blood).
B. Exposure to the phobic stimulus almost invariably provokes an immediate anxiety response, which may take the form of a situationally bound or situationally predisposed panic attack. **Note:** In children, the anxiety may be expressed by crying, tantrums, freezing, or clinging.
C. The person recognizes that the fear is excessive or unreasonable. **Note:** In children, this feature may be absent.
D. The phobic situation(s) is avoided or else is endured with intense anxiety or distress.
E. The avoidance, anxious anticipation, or distress in the feared situation(s) interferes significantly with the person's normal routine, occupational (or academic) functioning, or social activities or relationships, or there is marked distress about having the phobia.
F. In individuals under age 18 years, the duration is at least 6 months.
G. The anxiety, panic attacks, or phobic avoidance associated with the specific object or situation are not better accounted for by another mental disorder, such as obsessive-compulsive disorder (e.g., fear of dirt in someone with an obsession about contamination), posttraumatic stress disorder (e.g., avoidance of stimuli associated with a severe stressor), separation anxiety disorder (e.g., avoidance of school), social phobia (e.g., avoidance of social situations because of fear of embarrassment), panic disorder with agoraphobia, or agoraphobia without history of panic disorder.

*Specify* type:
**Animal type**
**Natural environment type** (e.g., heights, storms, water)
**Blood-injection-injury type**
**Situational type** (e.g., airplanes, elevators, enclosed places)
**Other type** (e.g., phobic avoidance of situations that may lead to choking, vomiting, or contracting an illness; in children, avoidance of loud sounds or costumed characters)

Used with permission, APA.


TABLE 10-6
**DSM-IV DIAGNOSTIC CRITERIA FOR SOCIAL PHOBIA**

A. A marked and persistent fear of one or more social or performance situations in which the person is exposed to unfamiliar people or to possible scrutiny by others. The individual fears that he or she will act in a way (or show anxiety symptoms) that will be humiliating or embarrassing. **Note:** In children, there must be evidence of the capacity for age-appropriate social relationships with familiar people and the anxiety must occur in peer settings, not just in interactions with adults.
B. Exposure to the feared social situation almost invariably provokes anxiety, which may take the form of a situationally bound or situationally predisposed panic attack. **Note:** In children, the anxiety may be expressed by crying, tantrums, freezing, or shrinking from social situations with unfamiliar people.
C. The person recognizes that the fear is excessive or unreasonable. **Note:** In children, this feature may be absent.
D. The feared social or performance situations are avoided or else are endured with intense anxiety or distress.
E. The avoidance, anxious anticipation, or distress in the feared social or performance situation(s) interferes significantly with the person's normal routine, occupational (academic) functioning, or social activities or relationships, or there is marked distress about having the phobia.
F. In individuals under age 18 years, the duration is at least 6 months.
G. The fear or avoidance is not due to the direct physiological effects of a substance (e.g., a drug of abuse, a medication) or a general medical condition and is not better accounted for by another mental disorder (e.g., panic disorder with or without agoraphobia, separation anxiety disorder, body dysmorphic disorder, a pervasive developmental disorder, or schizoid personality disorder).
H. If a general medical condition or another mental disorder is present, the fear in criterion A is unrelated to it, e.g., the fear is not of stuttering, trembling in Parkinson's disease, or exhibiting abnormal eating behavior in anorexia nervosa or bulimia nervosa.

*Specify* if:
**Generalized:** if the fears include most social situations (also consider the additional diagnosis of avoidant personality disorder)

Used with permission, APA.

TABLE 10-7
**DSM-IV DIAGNOSTIC CRITERIA FOR OBSESSIVE-COMPULSIVE DISORDER**

A.  Either obsessions or compulsions:
    *Obsessions as defined by (1), (2), (3), and (4):*
    (1) recurrent and persistent thoughts, impulses, or images that are experienced, at some time during the disturbance, as intrusive and inappropriate and that cause marked anxiety or distress
    (2) the thoughts, impulses, or images are not simply excessive worries about real-life problems
    (3) the person attempts to ignore or suppress such thoughts, impulses, or images, or to neutralize them with some other thought or action
    (4) the person recognizes that the obsessional thoughts, impulses, or images are a product of his or her own mind (not imposed from without as in thought insertion)
    *Compulsions as defined by (1) and (2):*
    (1) repetitive behaviors (e.g., hand washing, ordering, checking) or mental acts (e.g., praying, counting, repeating words silently) that the person feels driven to perform in response to an obsession, or according to rules that must be applied rigidly
    (2) the behaviors or mental acts are aimed at preventing or reducing distress or preventing some dreaded event or situation; however, these behaviors or mental acts either are not connected in a realistic way with what they are designed to neutralize or prevent or are clearly excessive
B.  At some point during the course of the disorder, the person has recognized that the obsessions or compulsions are excessive or unreasonable. **Note:** This does not apply to children.
C.  The obsessions or compulsions cause marked distress, are time consuming (take more than 1 hour a day), or significantly interfere with the person's normal routine, occupational (or academic) functioning, or usual social activities or relationships.
D.  If another Axis I disorder is present, the content of the obsessions or compulsions is not restricted to it (e.g., preoccupation with food in the presence of an eating disorder; hair pulling in the presence of trichotillomania; concern with appearance in the presence of body dysmorphic disorder; preoccupation with drugs in the presence of a substance use disorder; preoccupation with having a serious illness in the presence of hypochondriasis; preoccupation with sexual urges or fantasies in the presence of a paraphilia; or guilty ruminations in the presence of major depressive disorder).
E.  The disturbance is not due to the direct physiological effects of a substance (e.g., a drug of abuse, a medication) or a general medical condition.

*Specify* if:
    **With poor insight:** if, for most of the time during the current episode, the person does not recognize that the obsessions and compulsions are excessive or unreasonable

Used with permission, APA.

## C. Learning theory

1.  Anxiety is produced by frustration or stress. Once experienced, anxiety becomes a conditioned response to other, less severe, frustrating or stressful situations.
2.  May be learned through identification and imitation of anxiety patterns in parents (social learning theory).
3.  Anxiety is associated with naturally frightening stimulus, e.g., accident, transferred to another stimulus through conditioning, producing phobia.

# V. Psychological tests

## A. Rorschach test

1.  Anxiety responses. For example, animal movements, unstructured forms, heightened color.
2.  Phobic responses. For example, anatomy forms, bodily harm.
3.  Obsessive-compulsive responses. For example, overattention to detail.

## B. Thematic Apperception Test (TAT)

1.  Increased fantasy productions.
2.  Themes of aggression, sexuality.
3.  Feelings of tension.

TABLE 10–8
**DSM-IV DIAGNOSTIC CRITERIA FOR POSTTRAUMATIC STRESS DISORDER**

A.  The person has been exposed to a traumatic event in which both of the following were present:
    (1) the person experienced, witnessed, or was confronted with an event or events that involved actual or threatened death or serious injury, or a threat to the physical integrity of self or others
    (2) the person's response involved intense fear, helplessness, or horror. **Note:** In children, this may be expressed instead by disorganized or agitated behavior
B.  The traumatic event is persistently reexperienced in one (or more) of the following ways:
    (1) recurrent and intrusive distressing recollections of the event, including images, thoughts, or perceptions. **Note:** In young children, repetitive play may occur in which themes or aspects of the trauma are expressed.
    (2) recurrent distressing dreams of the event. **Note:** In children, there may be frightening dreams without recognizable content.
    (3) acting or feeling as if the traumatic event were recurring (includes a sense of reliving the experience, illusions, hallucinations, and dissociative flashback episodes, including those that occur on awakening or when intoxicated). **Note:** In young children, trauma-specific reenactment may occur.
    (4) intense psychological distress at exposure to internal or external cues that symbolize or resemble an aspect of the traumatic event
    (5) physiological reactivity on exposure to internal or external cues that symbolize or resemble an aspect of the traumatic event
C.  Persistent avoidance of stimuli associated with the trauma and numbing of general responsiveness (not present before the trauma), as indicated by three (or more) of the following:
    (1) efforts to avoid thoughts, feelings, or conversations associated with the trauma
    (2) efforts to avoid activities, places, or people that arouse recollections of the trauma
    (3) inability to recall an important aspect of the trauma
    (4) markedly diminished interest or participation in significant activities
    (5) feeling of detachment or estrangement from others
    (6) restricted range of affect (e.g., unable to have loving feelings)
    (7) sense of a foreshortened future (e.g., does not expect to have a career, marriage, children, or a normal life span)
D.  Persistent symptoms of increased arousal (not present before the trauma), as indicated by two (or more) of the following:
    (1) difficulty falling or staying asleep
    (2) irritability or outbursts of anger
    (3) difficulty concentrating
    (4) hypervigilance
    (5) exaggerated startle response
E.  Duration of the disturbance (symptoms in criteria B, C, and D) is more than 1 month.
F.  The disturbance causes clinically significant distress or impairment in social, occupational, or other important areas of functioning.

*Specify* if:
   **Acute:** if symptoms last less than 3 months
   **Chronic:** if symptoms last 3 months or more
*Specify* if:
   **With delayed onset:** if symptoms begin at least 6 months after the stressor

Used with permission, APA.

### C. Bender-Gestalt
1. No organic changes.
2. Use of small area in obsessive-compulsive disorder.
3. Spread out on page in anxiety states.

### D. Draw-A-Person
1. Attention to head and general detailing in obsessive-compulsive disorder.
2. Body image distortions in phobia.
3. Rapid drawing in anxiety disorders.

### E. Minnesota Multiphasic Personality Inventory (MMPI)
1. High hypochondriasis, psychasthenia, hysteria scales in anxiety.

TABLE 10–9
**EPIDEMIOLOGY OF ANXIETY DISORDERS**

| | Panic Disorder | Phobia | Obsessive-Compulsive Disorder | Generalized Anxiety Disorder | Posttraumatic Stress Disorder |
|---|---|---|---|---|---|
| Lifetime prevalence | 1.5–4% of population | Most common anxiety disorder: 3–5% of population | 2–3% of population | 3–8% of population | 1–3% of population; 30% of Vietnam veterans |
| Male:female ratio | 1:1 (without agoraphobia) 1:2 (with agoraphobia) | 1:2 | 1:1 | 1:2 | 1:2 |
| Age at onset | Late 20s | Late childhood | Adolescence or early adulthood | Variable; early adulthood | Any age, including childhood |
| Family history | 20% of first-degree (1) relatives of agoraphobic patients have agoraphobia | May run in families, especially blood, injection, injury type | 35% in 1 relatives | 25% of 1 relatives affected | — |
| Twin studies | Higher concordance in monozygotic (MZ) twins than in dizygotic (DZ) twins | — | Higher concordance in MZ twins than in DZ twins | 80–90% concordance in MZ twins; 10–15% in DZ twins | — |

TABLE 10-10
**PSYCHODYNAMICS OF ANXIETY DISORDERS**

| Disorder | Defense | Comment |
|---|---|---|
| Phobia | Displacement<br>Symbolization | Anxiety detached from idea or situation and displaced on some other symbolic object or situation |
| Agoraphobia | Projection<br>Displacement | Repressed hostility, rage, or sexuality projected on environment, which is seen as dangerous |
| Obsessive-compulsive disorder | Undoing<br>Isolation<br>Reaction formation | Severe superego acts against impulses about which patient feels guilty; anxiety controlled by repetitious act or thought |
| Anxiety | Regression | Repression of forbidden sexual, aggressive, or dependency strivings breaks down |
| Panic | Regression | Anxiety overwhelms personality and is discharged in panic state<br>Total breakdown of repressive defense and regression occurs |
| Posttraumatic stress disorder | Regression<br>Repression<br>Denial<br>Undoing | Trauma reactivates unconscious conflicts; ego relives anxiety and tries to master it |

## VI. Lab tests

No specific test for anxiety.

## VII. Pathophysiology

A. No pathognomonic changes.

B. In obsessive-compulsive disorder, decreased metabolism on positron emission tomography (PET) in orbital gyrus, caudate nuclei, cingulate gyrus.

C. Increased PET blood flow in right parahippocampus in panic, frontal lobe in anxiety.

D. Mitral valve prolapse in 50% of patients with panic disorder.

E. Nonspecific electroencephalogram (EEG) changes, nonsuppression of dexamethasone suppression test (DST) in some obsessive-compulsive patients.

## VIII. Psychodynamics

See Table 10-10.

## IX. Differential diagnosis

Anxiety is a major component of psychological, medical, and neurological disorders.

**A. Depressive disorders.** 50–70% of depressed patients have anxiety or obsessive brooding; 20–30% of primarily anxious patients also experience depression.

**B. Schizophrenia.** May be anxious and have severe obsessions in addition to hallucinations or delusions.

**C. Bipolar I disorder.** Characterized by massive anxiety during manic episode.

TABLE 10–11
**MEDICAL AND NEUROLOGICAL CAUSES OF ANXIETY**

**Neurological disorders**
  Cerebral neoplasms
  Cerebral trauma and postconcussive syndromes
  Cerebrovascular disease
  Subarachnoid hemorrhage
  Migraine
  Encephalitis
  Cerebral syphilis
  Multiple sclerosis
  Wilson's disease
  Huntington's disease
  Epilepsy

**Systemic conditions**
  Hypoxia
    Cardiovascular disease
    Pulmonary insufficiency
    Anemia

**Endocrine disturbances**
  Pituitary dysfunction
  Thyroid dysfunction
  Parathyroid dysfunction
  Adrenal dysfunction
  Pheochromocytoma
  Virilization disorders of females

**Inflammatory disorders**
  Lupus erythematosus
  Rheumatoid arthritis
  Polyarteritis nodosa
  Temporal arteritis

**Deficiency states**
  Vitamin $B_{12}$ deficiency
  Pellagra

**Miscellaneous conditions**
  Hypoglycemia
  Carcinoid syndrome
  Systemic malignancies
  Premenstrual syndrome
  Febrile illnesses and chronic infections
  Porphyria
  Infectious mononucleosis
  Posthepatitis syndrome
  Uremia

**Toxic conditions**
  Alcohol and drug withdrawal
  Amphetamines
  Sympathomimetic agents
  Vasopressor agents
  Caffeine and caffeine withdrawal
  Penicillin
  Sulfonamides
  Cannabis
  Mercury
  Arsenic
  Phosphorus
  Organophosphates
  Carbon disulfide
  Benzene
  Aspirin intolerance

Table from Cummings JL: *Clinical Neuropsychiatry.* Grune & Stratton, Orlando, 1985, p 214. Used with permission.

TABLE 10–12
**DIFFERENTIAL DIAGNOSIS OF COMMON MEDICAL CONDITIONS MIMICKING ANXIETY**

| | |
|---|---|
| Angina pectoris/ Myocardial Infarction (MI) | Electrocardiogram (EKG) with ST depression in angina; cardiac enzymes in MI. Crushing chest pain usually associated with angina/MI. Anxiety pains usually sharp and more superficial |
| Hyperventilation syndrome | History of rapid, deep respirations; circumoral pallor; carpopedal spasm; responds to rebreathing in paper bag |
| Hypoglycemia | Fasting blood sugar usually under 50 mg/dL; signs of diabetes mellitus— polyuria, polydypsia, polyphagia |
| Hyperthyroidism | Elevated triiodothyronine ($T_3$), thyroxine ($T_4$); exophthalmos in severe cases |
| Carcinoid syndrome | Hypertension accompanies anxiety; elevated urinary catecholamines (5-hydroxyindoleacetic acid (5-HIAA)) |

**D. Atypical psychosis.** (Called psychotic disorder not otherwise specified in DSM-IV.) Massive anxiety in addition to psychotic features.

**E. Adjustment disorder with anxiety.** History of psychosocial stressor within 3 months of onset.

**F. Medical and neurological conditions.** Secondary psychotic disorder caused by specific organic factor (Tables 10–11 and 10–12); cognitive impairment is present.

**G. Substance-related disorders.**    Panic or anxiety associated with intoxication (especially caffeine, amphetamines) and withdrawal states.

## X. Course and prognosis

### A. Panic disorder
1. Panic attacks tend to recur 2–3 times a week.
2. Chronic course with remissions and exacerbations.
3. Prognosis is excellent with therapy.

### B. Phobic disorder
1. Chronic course.
2. Phobias may worsen if untreated.
3. Good to excellent prognosis with therapy.
4. Agoraphobia is the most resistant of all phobias.

### C. Obsessive-compulsive disorder
1. Chronic course with waxing and waning of symptoms.
2. Fair prognosis with therapy, but some cases are intractable.

### D. Generalized anxiety disorder
1. Chronic course; symptoms may diminish as patient gets older.
2. Over time, patient may develop secondary depression—not uncommon if left untreated.

### E. Posttraumatic stress disorder
1. Chronic course.
2. Trauma periodically is reexperienced over several years.
3. Worse prognosis with preexisting psychopathological state.

## XI. Treatment

### A. Pharmacological
1. **Diazepam (Valium)**
   a. **Dosage**—2–10 mg orally 2–4 times a day; 2–10 mg intramuscularly or intravenously for acute agitation.
   b. **Indication**—generalized anxiety disorder, posttraumatic stress disorder.
   c. **Common adverse effects**—drowsiness, fatigue, hypotension, paradoxical excitement.
   d. **Cautions**—long-term use can cause physical dependence, i.e., withdrawal symptoms upon abrupt discontinuation; most often in patients with history of alcoholism or drug abuse.
2. **Alprazolam (Xanax)**
   a. **Dosage**—0.25–0.5 mg orally 3 times a day; may be increased to 6–8 mg every day.
   b. **Indications**—rapidly acting, good short-term treatment for panic disorder and agoraphobia.
   c. **Common adverse effects**—drowsiness, cognitive impairment, hypotension.
3. **Imipramine (Tofranil)**
   a. **Dosage**—75 mg a day orally to start; increase to 150–300 mg. **Note:** In elderly or adolescent patients, start with 25–50 mg a day and

increase to 75–100 mg a day. See Chapter 24 for other heterocyclic compounds useful in anxiety.

b. **Indications**—primarily for mood disorder but useful in panic disorder, social phobia.

c. **Common adverse effects**—drowsiness, confusion, anticholinergic effect (dry mouth, tachycardia, arrhythmias), constipation, delayed micturition. **Note:** Obtain electrocardiogram (EKG) in patients over age 40 to test cardiac function. Do not prescribe monoamine oxidase inhibitors (MAOIs) until 14 days after stopping imipramine therapy.

**4. Tranylcypromine (Parnate)**

a. **Dosage**—10 mg orally in morning and 10 mg in afternoon; increase to 30–50 mg a day in divided doses.

b. **Indications**—primarily for depression but useful in panic disorder. See Chapter 24 for other MAOIs useful in anxiety. **Note:** Do not use in elderly persons. Do not use with narcotics (especially meperidine [Demerol]); coadministration may be fatal.

c. **Major adverse effect**—hypertensive crisis caused by foods with tryptophan or tyramine, sympathomimetic agents, other MAOIs, tricyclics, and narcotics; all may produce fatal intracranial bleeding secondary to acute hypertensive episode.

**5. Buspirone (BuSpar)**

a. **Dosage**—5 mg twice daily; increase to 15–60 mg a day in divided doses.

b. **Indications**—generalized anxiety disorder.

c. **Common adverse effects**—headache, dizziness. **Note:** Not cross-tolerant with benzodiazepines.

**6. Propranolol (Inderal)**

a. **Dosage**—10 mg orally twice daily; increase to 80–160 mg a day in divided doses; administer dose of 20–40 mg 30 minutes before phobic situation, e.g., public speaking.

b. **Indications**—social phobia.

c. **Adverse effects**—bradycardia, hypotension, drowsiness. **Note:** Do not use with history of asthma. Not useful in chronic anxiety unless caused by hypersensitive β-adrenergic state.

**7. Clonazepam (Klonopin)**

a. **Dosage**—0.5 mg twice daily; increase to 2–10 mg a day.

b. **Indications**—generalized anxiety disorder, panic disorder, posttraumatic stress disorder.

c. **Adverse effects**—drowsiness, ataxia. **Note:** Food and Drug Administration (FDA) approved use is for petit mal, myoclonic, and akinetic seizures, but a medically approved use is for anxiety disorders.

**8. Clomipramine (Anafranil)**

a. **Dosage**—150–300 mg a day.

b. **Indication**—obsessive-compulsive disorder.

**9. Fluoxetine (Prozac)**

a. **Dosage**—20–80 mg a day.

b. **Indications**—used primarily in depression, also of use in obsessive-compulsive disorder.

**10. Fluvoxamine (Luvox)**

**a. Dosage**—50–30 mg a day.

**b. Indications**—major use is obsessive-compulsive disorder, also of use in depression.

**B. Psychological.** Some of the anxiety disorders, such as posttraumatic stress disorder, are treated primarily with psychotherapy; others, such as phobias, generalized anxiety, panic disorder, and obsessive-compulsive disorder, are treated with a combination of modalities. The following can be viewed as an introduction to the topic discussed in greater detail in Chapter 24.

**1. Insight-oriented psychotherapy.** Goal is to increase the patient's development of insight into psychological conflicts, which if unresolved can manifest as symptomatic behavior, such as anxiety, phobias, obsessions and compulsions, and posttraumatic stress. Particularly indicated if (1) anxiety symptoms are clearly secondary to underlying neurotic conflict, (2) anxiety continues after behavioral or pharmacological treatments are instituted, (3) new anxiety symptoms develop after the original symptoms resolve (symptom substitution), and (4) the anxieties are more generalized, less specific, and circumscribed.

**2. Behavior therapy.** Basic assumption is that change can occur without developing psychological insight into underlying causes. Techniques include positive and negative reinforcement, punishment, systematic desensitization, flooding, implosion, graded exposure, and self-monitoring.

a. Indicated for clearly delineated, circumscribed, maladaptive behaviors, such as phobias, compulsions, and obsessions. (Compulsive behavior generally is more responsive than obsessional thinking.)

b. Most current strategies for treatment of anxiety disorders include a combination of pharmacological and behavioral interventions.

c. Current thinking generally maintains that although drugs can reduce anxiety early, treatment with drugs alone leads to equally early relapse. Patients treated with cognitive and behavioral therapies appear to do significantly and consistently better than do those receiving drugs alone.

**3. Cognitive therapy.** Based on the premise that maladaptive behavior is secondary to distortions in how people perceive themselves and in how others perceive them. Treatment is short-term and interactive, with assigned homework and tasks to be performed between sessions that focus on correcting distorted assumptions and cognitions. Emphasis is on confronting and examining situations that elicit interpersonal anxiety and associated mild depression.

**4. Group therapy.** Groups range from those that solely provide support and an increase in social skills, to those focusing on relief of specific symptoms, to those that are primarily insight-oriented. Groups may be heterogeneous or homogeneous in terms of diagnosis; homogeneous groups are most commonly used in the treatment of such diagnoses as posttraumatic stress disorder, in which therapy is aimed at education about and exposure to social skills, with practice in a group setting.

---

*For a more detailed discussion of this topic, see Anxiety Disorders, Chap 17, p 1191; Mattison RE: Separation Anxiety Disorder and Anxiety in Children, Sec 43.1, p 2345; Lesser RM: Anxiety Disorders, Sec 29.6d, p 2572, in CTP/VI.*

---

# 11

## Somatoform Disorders, Factitious Disorders, and Malingering

### I. Somatoform disorders

The essential feature of these disorders is a physical or somatic complaint without any demonstrable organic findings to account for the complaint or without any known physiological mechanisms to explain the findings. There is also the presumption of associated psychological factors or unconscious conflicts to account for the presenting syndrome.

There are seven categories of somatoform disorders: (1) somatization disorder, (2) undifferentiated somatoform disorder, (3) conversion disorder, (4) pain disorder, (5) hypochondriasis, (6) body dysmorphic disorder, and (7) somatoform disorder not otherwise specified (NOS).

#### A. Somatization disorder

1. **Definition.** Somatic complaints not limited to one organ system and not caused by known medical disorder. (Previously known as Briquet's syndrome.)
2. **Diagnosis, signs, and symptoms.** See Table 11–1.
3. **Epidemiology**
   a. Lifetime prevalence in general population is 0.1–0.5%.
   b. Affects more women than men.
   c. Affects 1–2% of all women.
   d. More common in less well-educated persons and low socioeconomic groups.
   e. Usual onset is in adolescence and young adulthood.
4. **Etiology**
   a. **Psychosocial**—suppression or repression of anger toward others, with turning of anger toward self, can account for symptoms. Punitive personality organization with strong superego. Low self-esteem is common. Identification with parent who models sick role. Some dynamic similarity to depression.
   b. **Genetic**—positive family history; present in 10–20% of mothers and sisters of affected patients; twins—concordance rate of 29% in monozygotic (MZ) and 10% in dizygotic (DZ) twins.
5. **Lab and psychological tests.** Minor neuropsychological abnormality in some patients, e.g., faulty assessment of somatosensory input.
6. **Pathophysiology.** None. Prolonged use of medications may cause adverse side effects unrelated to somatization complaint.

TABLE 11–1
**DSM-IV DIAGNOSTIC CRITERIA FOR SOMATIZATION DISORDER**

A. A history of many physical complaints beginning before age 30 years that occur over a period of several years and result in treatment being sought or significant impairment in social, occupational, or other important areas of functioning.

B. Each of the following criteria must have been met, with individual symptoms occurring at any time during the course of the disturbance:
    (1) *four pain symptoms:* a history of pain related to at least four different sites or functions (e.g., head, abdomen, back, joints, extremities, chest, rectum, during menstruation, during sexual intercourse, or during urination)
    (2) *two gastrointestinal symptoms:* a history of at least two gastrointestinal symptoms other than pain (e.g., nausea, bloating, vomiting other than during pregnancy, diarrhea, or intolerance of several different foods)
    (3) *one sexual symptom:* a history of at least one sexual or reproductive symptom other than pain (e.g., sexual indifference, erectile or ejaculatory dysfunction, irregular menses, excessive menstrual bleeding, vomiting throughout pregnancy)
    (4) *one pseudoneurological symptom:* a history of at least one symptom or deficit suggesting a neurological condition not limited to pain (conversion symptoms such as impaired coordination or balance, paralysis or localized weakness, difficulty swallowing or lump in throat, aphonia, urinary retention, hallucinations, loss of touch or pain sensation, double vision, blindness, deafness, seizures; dissociative symptoms such as amnesia; or loss of consciousness other than fainting)

C. Either (1) or (2):
    (1) after appropriate investigation, each of the symptoms in criterion B cannot be fully explained by a known general medical condition or the direct effects of a substance (e.g., a drug of abuse, a medication)
    (2) when there is a related general medical condition, the physical complaints or resulting social or occupational impairment are in excess of what would be expected from the history, physical examination, or laboratory findings

D. The symptoms are not intentionally feigned or produced (as in factitious disorder or malingering).

Used with permission, APA.

**7. Psychodynamics.** Repression of wish or impulse expressed through body complaints. Superego conflicts, partially expressed by symptom. Anxiety converted into specific symptom.

**8. Differential diagnosis**

    a. Rule out organic cause for somatic symptom.

    b. Multiple sclerosis for weakness.

    c. Epstein-Barr virus for chronic fatigue syndrome.

    d. Porphyria for abdominal pain.

    e. Somatic delusion occurs in schizophrenia.

    f. Panic attacks have cardiovascular symptoms that are intermittent, episodic.

    g. Conversion disorder has fewer symptoms with clearer symbolic meaning.

    h. Factitious disorder—conscious faking of symptoms to achieve patient role; usually eager to be in hospital.

    i. Pain disorder—pain is usually only complaint.

**9. Course and prognosis**

    a. Chronic course with few remissions; however, severity of complaints can fluctuate. Complications include unnecessary surgery, repeated medical workups, substance dependence, and adverse effects of unnecessary prescribed drugs.

    b. Depression is frequent.

**10. Treatment**

    a. **Pharmacological**—avoid psychotropics, except under period of acute anxiety or depression, because patients tend to become psychologically dependent. Antidepressants are useful in secondary depressions.

TABLE 11–2
**DSM-IV DIAGNOSTIC CRITERIA FOR UNDIFFERENTIATED SOMATOFORM DISORDER**

A. One or more physical complaints (e.g., fatigue, loss of appetite, gastrointestinal or urinary complaints)
B. Either (1) or (2):
    (1) after appropriate investigation, the symptoms cannot be fully explained by a known general medical condition or the direct effects of a substance (e.g., a drug of abuse, a medication)
    (2) when there is a related general medical condition, the physical complaints or resulting social or occupational impairment is in excess of what would be expected from the history, physical examination, or laboratory findings
C. The symptoms cause clinically significant distress or impairment in social, occupational, or other important areas of functioning.
D. The duration of the disturbance is at least 6 months.
E. The disturbance is not better accounted for by another mental disorder (e.g., another somatoform disorder, sexual dysfunction, mood disorder, anxiety disorder, sleep disorder, or psychotic disorder).
F. The symptom is not intentionally produced or feigned (as in factitious disorder or malingering).

Used with permission, APA.


TABLE 11–3
**DIFFERENTIAL DIAGNOSIS FOR UNDIFFERENTIATED SOMATOFORM DISORDER**

**Somatoform disorder**—multiple symptoms, several years' duration, onset before 30 years of age

Somatoform disorder NOS—symptoms for less than 6 months.

Major depressive disorder, anxiety disorders, adjustment disorder—frequently include unexplained symptoms

**Factitious disorder and malingering**—symptoms intentionally produced or fabricated


    **b. Psychological**—Long-term insight or supportive psychotherapy is required to provide understanding of dynamics, support through distressing life events, or both; also to follow patient to prevent substance abuse, doctor-shopping, unnecessary procedures, or diagnostic tests.

**B. Undifferentiated somatoform disorder**

  **1. Definition.**  Residual category used to describe a partial picture of somatoform disorder.

  **2. Diagnosis, signs, and symptoms.**  See Table 11–2. The patient may have multiple somatic complaints that are not severe enough or too vague to warrant a diagnosis of full somatoform disorder. General fatigue is the most common syndrome.

  **3. Course and prognosis.**  Unpredictable. Frequently another mental disorder or medical condition is ultimately diagnosed.

  **4. Differential diagnosis.**  See Table 11–3.

**C. Conversion disorder**

  **1. Definition.**  Characterized by one or more neurological symptoms associated with psychological conflict or need, not physical, neurological or substance-related disorder.

  **2. Diagnosis, signs, and symptoms**

    a. Motor abnormalities—paralysis, ataxia, dysphagia, vomiting, aphonia.

    b. Disturbances of consciousness—pseudoseizures, unconsciousness.

    c. Sensory disturbances or alterations—blindness, deafness, anosmia, anesthesia, analgesia, diplopia; glove and stocking anesthesia (does not follow known sensory pathways).

d. Close temporal relationship between symptom and stress or intense emotion.

e. Left-sided symptoms more common than right-sided symptoms.

f. The person is not conscious of intentionally producing the symptom.

g. The symptom is not a culturally sanctioned response pattern and after appropriate investigation cannot be explained by a known physical disorder.

## 3. Epidemiology

a. Incidence and prevalence—10% of hospital inpatients and 5–15% of all psychiatric outpatients.

b. Age—early adulthood, but can occur in middle or old age.

c. The male-to-female ratio is 1:2.

d. Family history—higher in family members.

e. More common in low socioeconomic groups and less well-educated persons.

## 4. Etiology

### a. Biological

i. Symptom depends on activation of inhibitory brain mechanisms.

ii. Excessive cortical arousal triggers inhibitory central nervous system (CNS) mechanisms at synapses, brain stem, reticular activating system.

iii. Increased susceptibility in patients with frontal lobe trauma or other neurological deficits.

### b. Psychological

i. Expression of unconscious psychological conflict, which is repressed.

ii. Premorbid personality disorder—avoidant, histrionic.

iii. Impulse, e.g., sex or aggression, is unacceptable to ego and is disguised through symptom.

iv. Identification with family member with same symptoms from real disease.

## 5. Lab and psychological tests

a. Evoked potential shows disturbed somatosensory perception; diminished or absent on side of defect.

b. Mild cognitive impairment, attentional deficits, and visuoperceptive changes on Halstead-Reitan Battery.

c. Minnesota Multiphasic Personality Inventory (MMPI), Rorschach test show increased instinctual drives, sexual repression, inhibited aggression.

## 6. Pathophysiology.   No changes.

## 7. Psychodynamics

a. *La belle indifférence* is a lack of concern about illness present in some patients.

b. Primary gain refers to reduction of anxiety by repression of unacceptable impulse. Symbolization of impulse onto symptom, e.g., paralyzed arm prevents expression of aggressive impulse.

c. Other defense mechanisms—reaction formation, denial, displacement.

d. Secondary gain refers to benefits of illness, e.g., compensation from lawsuit (compensation neurosis), avoiding work, depending on family. Patient usually lacks insight about this dynamic.

8. **Differential diagnosis.**   Major task is to distinguish from organically based disorder. 25–50% of patients are eventually diagnosed with physical or medical disorder.

   **a. Paralysis**—in conversion, paralysis is inconsistent; it does not follow motor pathways. There are no pathological reflexes, e.g., Babinski's sign. Spastic paralysis, clonus, cogwheel rigidity absent in conversion disorder.

   **b. Ataxia**—bizarre character in conversion disorder—leg may be dragged and not circumducted as in organic lesion. Astasia-abasia is unsteady gait in which patient with conversion disorder does not fall or injure self.

   **c. Blindness**—no pupillary response is seen in neurological blindness (except that occipital lobe lesions produce cortical blindness with intact pupillary response). Tracking movements are absent in true blindness. Monocular diplopia, triplopia, and tunnel vision can be conversion complaint. Ophthalmologists use tests with distorting prisms and colored lenses to detect hysterical blindness.

   **d. Deafness**—loud noise will awaken sleeping conversion patient but not organic deaf patient. Audiometric tests reveal varying responses in conversion.

   **e. Sensory**—sensory loss does not follow dermatomes; hemisensory loss, which stops at midline, or glove and stocking anesthesia occur in conversion disorder.

   **f. Hysterical**—pain most often relates to head and face, back and abdomen. Look for organic findings—muscular spasm, osteoarthritis.

   **g. Pseudoseizures**—incontinence, loss of motor control, and tongue biting are rare in pseudoseizures; an aura usually is present in organic epilepsy. Look for abnormal electroencephalogram (EEG). (Note that 10–15% of the normal adult population have abnormal EEG results.) Babinski's sign occurs in organic seizure and postictal state but not in conversion seizures.

   **h. Differentiate conversion from:**
      **i. Schizophrenia**—thought disorder.
      **ii. Mood disorder**—depression or mania.
      **iii. Malingering and factitious disorder with physical symptoms**—difficult to distinguish, but malingerers are aware that they are faking symptoms and have insight into what they are doing; factitious patients also are aware that they are faking, but do so because they want to be patients and be in a hospital.

   **i. Drug-assisted interview**—intravenous amobarbital (Amytal) (100–500 mg) in slow infusion will often cause conversion symptoms to abate. For example, patient with hysterical aphonia will begin to talk. Test can be used to aid in diagnosis but is not always reliable.

9. **Course and prognosis.**   Tends to be recurrent, separated by asymptomatic periods. Major concern is to not miss early neurological symp-

TABLE 11–4
**FACTORS ASSOCIATED WITH GOOD AND POOR PROGNOSES**

**Good prognosis**
Sudden onset
Clearly identifiable stress at onset
Short time between onset and treatment
Above-average I.Q.
Symptoms of paralysis, aphonia, blindness

**Poor prognosis**
Comorbid mental disorders
Ongoing litigation
Symptoms of tremor, seizures

tom, which then progresses into full-blown syndrome, e.g., multiple sclerosis may begin with spontaneously remitting diplopia or hemiparesis. Table 11–4 lists factors associated with good and bad prognoses.

10. **Treatment**
   a. **Pharmacological**—benzodiazepines for anxiety and muscular tension; antidepressants or serotonergic agents for obsessive rumination about symptoms.
   b. **Psychological**
      i. Insight-oriented therapy is useful in understanding dynamic principles and conflicts behind symptoms. Patient learns to accept sexual or aggressive impulses and not to use conversion disorder as a defense.
      ii. Behavior therapy is used to induce relaxation and to reduce or eliminate the need for symptom reduction.
      iii. Hypnosis and reeducation are useful in uncomplicated situations.
      iv. Do not accuse patient of trying to get attention or of not wanting to get better.
      v. Narcoanalysis sometimes removes symptoms.

D. **Pain disorder**
   1. **Definition.**   Somatoform pain disorder is a preoccupation with pain in the absence of physical disease to account for its intensity. It does not follow a neuroanatomical distribution. Stress and conflict may closely correlate with the initiation or exacerbation of the pain.
   2. **Diagnosis, signs, and symptoms.**   See Table 11–5. Pain may be accompanied by localized sensorimotor symptoms, such as anesthesia, paresthesia. Symptoms of depression are common.
   3. **Epidemiology.**   Any age of onset, especially during 30s and 40s. More common in women than in men. Some evidence of first-degree biological relatives having a high incidence of pain, depression, and alcoholism.
   4. **Etiology.**
      a. **Behavioral**—Pain behaviors are reinforced when rewarded, e.g., pain symptoms may become intense when followed by attentive behavior from others or avoidance of unliked activity.
      b. **Interpersonal**—Pain is a way to manipulate and gain advantage in a relationship, e.g., to stabilize a fragile marriage.
      c. **Biological**—Some patients may have pain disorder, rather than another mental disorder, because of sensory and limbic structural or chemical abnormalities that predispose them to pain.

TABLE 11–5
**DSM-IV DIAGNOSTIC CRITERIA FOR PAIN DISORDER**

A. Pain in one or more anatomical sites is the predominant focus of the clinical presentation and is of sufficient severity to warrant clinical attention.
B. The pain causes clinically significant distress or impairment in social, occupational, or other important areas of functioning.
C. Psychological factors are judged to have an important role in the onset, severity, exacerbation, or maintenance of the pain.
D. The symptom or deficit is not intentionally produced or feigned (as in factitious disorder or malingering).
E. The pain is not better accounted for by a mood, anxiety, or psychotic disorder and does not meet criteria for dyspareunia.

*Code* as follows:
**Pain disorder associated with psychological factors:** psychological factors are judged to have the major role in the onset, severity, exacerbation, or maintenance of the pain. (If a general medical condition is present, it does not have a major role in the onset, severity, exacerbation, or maintenance of the pain.) This type of pain disorder is not diagnosed if criteria are also met for somatization disorder.

*Specify* if:
**Acute:** duration of less than 6 months
**Chronic:** duration of 6 months or longer

**Pain disorder associated with both psychological factors and a general medical condition:** both psychological factors and a general medical condition are judged to have important roles in the onset, severity, exacerbation, or maintenance of the pain. The associated general medical condition or anatomical site of the pain is coded on Axis III.

*Specify* if:
**Acute:** duration of less than 6 months
**Chronic:** duration of 6 months or longer

---

5. **Psychodynamics.** Patients may be symbolically expressing an intrapsychic conflict through the body. Persons may unconsciously regard emotional pain as weak and displace it to the body. Pain can be a method to obtain love or can be used as a punishment. Defense mechanisms involved in the disorder include displacement, substitution, and repression.

## E. Hypochondriasis

1. **Definition.** Morbid fear or belief that one has a serious disease even though none exists.

2. **Diagnosis, signs, and symptoms**
   a. Any organ or functional system can be affected. Gastrointestinal (GI) and cardiovascular (CV) systems are most commonly affected.
   b. Patient believes that disease or malfunction is present.
   c. Negative physical examination or lab test reassures patient but only briefly, then symptoms return (in somatic delusion, patient cannot be reassured).
   d. Disturbance lasts at least 6 months.
   e. The belief is not of delusional intensity.

3. **Epidemiology**
   a. Prevalence—10% of all medical patients.
   b. Men and women are affected equally.
   c. Occurs at all ages; peaks in 30s for men and 40s for women.
   d. Seen in MZ twins and in first-degree relatives.

4. **Etiology**
   a. Psychogenic, but patient may have congenital hypersensitivity to bodily functions and sensations and low threshold for pain or physical discomfort.

  b. Aggression toward others is turned against the self through a particular body part.

  c. Affected organ may have important symbolic meaning.

5. **Lab and psychological tests**

  a. Repeated physical examinations to rule out medical illness are negative.

  b. MMPI shows elevated hysterical scale.

  c. Many color responses on Rorschach test.

6. **Psychodynamics.** Repression of anger toward others; displacement of anger toward physical complaints; pain and suffering used as punishment for unacceptable guilty impulses; undoing.

7. **Differential diagnosis.** Diagnosis is made by inclusion, *not* by exclusion. Physical disorders must be ruled out; however, 15–30% of patients with hypochondriacal disorder have physical problems. Workup for organic disease may aggravate the condition by placing too much emphasis on the physical complaint.

  a. **Depression**—patient may have a somatic complaint or somatic complaint could be part of depressive syndrome. Look for signs of depression, e.g., apathy, anhedonia, feelings of worthlessness.

  b. **Anxiety disorder**—manifested by marked anxiety or obsessive-compulsive signs or symptoms; *la belle indifférence* is not present.

  c. **Somatization disorder**—multiple organ systems are involved; vague complaints.

  d. **Pain disorder**—pain is major and usually sole complaint.

  e. **Malingering and factitious disorders**—history is associated with frequent hospitalizations, marked secondary gain; symptoms lack symbolic value and are under conscious control. *La belle indifférence* is not present.

  f. **Sexual dysfunction**—if sex is complaint, diagnose as sexual disorder.

8. **Course and prognosis.** Chronic course with remissions. Exacerbations usually are associated with identifiable life stress. Good prognosis is associated with minimal premorbid personality, poor prognosis with antecedent or superimposed physical disorder.

9. **Treatment**

  a. **Pharmacological**—pharmacological targeting of symptoms: antianxiety drugs and antidepressant drugs for anxiety and depression. Serotonergic drugs useful for depression and obsessive-compulsive disorder. Drug-assisted interview can induce catharsis and potential removal of symptoms; however, such relief usually is only temporary.

  b. **Psychological**

    i. Insight-oriented dynamic psychotherapy uncovers symbolic meaning of symptom and is useful. Do not confront patient with such statements as, ''It's all in your head.'' Long-term relationship with physician or psychiatrist is valuable with reassurance that no physical disease is present.

    ii. Hypnosis and behavioral therapy are useful to induce relaxation. Prolonged conversion disorder can produce physical deterioration (e.g., muscle atrophy or contractures, osteoporosis), so attention to these issues is necessary.

## F. Body dysmorphic disorder

1. **Definition.**   Imagined belief (not of delusional proportions) that there is a defect in appearance of all or a part of the body.

2. **Diagnosis, signs, and symptoms.**   Patient complains of defect, e.g., wrinkles, hair loss, too small breasts or penis, age spots, stature. Complaint is out of proportion to any minor objective physical abnormality.

   If a slight physical anomaly is present, the person's concern is grossly excessive; however, the belief is not of delusional intensity, as in delusional disorder, somatic type, i.e., the person can acknowledge the possibility that he or she may be exaggerating the extent of the defect or that there may be no defect at all.

3. **Epidemiology.**   Onset from adolescence through early adulthood. Men and women are affected equally.

4. **Etiology.**   Unknown.

   a. **Biological**—responsiveness to serotonergic agents suggests involvement of serotonin or relation to another mental disorder.

   b. **Psychological**—look for unconscious conflict relating to a distorted body part.

5. **Lab and psychological tests.**   Draw-A-Person test shows exaggeration, diminution, or absence of affected body part.

6. **Pathophysiology.**   No known pathological abnormalities. Minor body deficits may actually exist upon which imagined belief develops.

7. **Psychodynamics.**   Defense mechanisms include repression (of unconscious conflict), distortion and symbolization (of body part), and projection (belief that other persons also see imagined deformity).

8. **Differential diagnosis.**   Distorted body image occurs in schizophrenia, mood disorders, medical disorders, anorexia nervosa, bulimia nervosa, obsessive-compulsive disorder, gender identity disorder, *koro* (worry that penis is shrinking into abdomen).

9. **Course and prognosis.**   Chronic course with repeated visits to doctors, plastic surgeons, or dermatologists. Secondary depression may occur. In some cases, imagined body distortion progresses to delusional belief.

10. **Treatment**

    a. **Pharmacological**—serotonergic drugs, e.g., fluoxetine (Prozac), clomipramine (Anafranil), effectively reduce symptoms in at least 50% of patients. Treatment with surgical, dermatological, and dental procedures is rarely never successful.

    b. **Psychological**—psychotherapy is useful; uncovers conflicts relating to symptoms, feelings of inadequacy.

## II. Factitious disorders

### A. Definition.   Symptoms are deliberately and consciously simulated by patient. May be psychological, e.g., hallucinations or physical, e.g., pain.

### B. Diagnosis, signs, and symptoms

1. **With predominantly physical signs and symptoms.** Also known as Munchausen's syndrome. Intentional production of physical symptoms—nausea, vomiting, pain, seizures. Patients may intentionally put blood in feces or urine, artificially raise body temperature, take insulin to lower blood sugar. Gridiron abdomen sign is the result of scars from multiple surgical operations.

2. **With predominantly psychological signs and symptoms.** Intentional production of psychiatric symptoms—hallucinations, delusions, depression, bizarre behavior. Patients may make up story that they suffered major life stress to account for symptoms. *Pseudologia fantastica* consists of making up extravagant lies that the patient believes. Substance abuse, especially of opioids, is common in both types.

3. **With combined physical and psychological signs and symptoms.** Intentional production of both physical and psychological symptoms.

4. **Factitious disorder NOS.** Includes disorders that do not meet criteria for factitious disorder, e.g., factitious disorder by proxy (intentionally feigning symptoms in another person who is under the person's care in order to indirectly assume the sick role).

C. **Epidemiology.** Unknown. More common in men than in women. Usually adult onset. 5–10% of all hospital admissions are for factitious illness, especially feigned fevers. More common in health care workers.

D. **Etiology.** Early real illness coupled with parental abuse or rejection is typical. Patient recreates illness as an adult to gain loving attention from doctors. Masochistic gratification for some patients who want to undergo surgical procedures. Others identify with important past figure who had psychological or physical illness.

E. **Psychodynamics.** Repression, identification with the aggressor, regression, symbolization.

F. **Differential diagnosis**

1. **Physical illness.** Physical examination and laboratory workup should be done; results will be negative. The nursing staff should observe carefully for deliberate elevation of temperature, alteration of body fluids.

2. **Somatoform disorder.** Symptoms are voluntary in factitious disorder and not caused by unconscious or symbolic factors. *La belle indifférence* is not present in factitious disorder. Hypochondriacs do not want to undergo extensive tests or surgery.

3. **Malingering.** Most difficult differential diagnosis. Malingerers have specific goals, e.g., insurance payments, avoidance of jail term.

4. **Ganser's syndrome.** Found in prisoners who give approximate answers to questions and talk past the point. Classified as a dissociative disorder NOS.

G. **Course and prognosis.** Usually chronic course, which begins in adulthood but may have earlier onset. Frequent consultation with doctors and history of hospitalizations as patient seeks repeated care. High risk of substance abuse over time. Prognosis improves if there is associated depression or anxiety that responds to pharmacotherapy. Risk of death if patient undergoes multiple life-threatening surgical procedures.

### H. Treatment

1. Avoid unnecessary laboratory tests or medical procedures. Confront patient with diagnosis of factitious disorder and feigned symptoms. Patients rarely enter psychotherapy because of poor motivation; however, working alliance with doctor is possible over time, and patient may gain insights into behavior. Good management, however, is more likely than a cure. A data bank of patients with repeated hospitalizations for factitious illness is available in some areas of the United States.

2. Psychopharmacological therapy is useful with associated anxiety or depression. Substance abuse should be treated if present.

3. Contact child welfare services if a child is at risk, e.g., with factitious disorder by proxy.

## III. Malingering

### A. Definition.
Voluntary production of physical or psychological symptoms in order to accomplish specific goal, e.g., to receive insurance payments, avoid jail term or punishment.

### B. Diagnosis, signs, and symptoms.
Patient has many vague or poorly localized complaints that are presented in great detail; patients are easily irritated if a doctor is skeptical of the history. Psychosocial history reveals a need to avoid some situation, to obtain money, presence of legal problems. Look for defined goal (secondary gain).

### C. Epidemiology.
Unknown. It occurs most frequently in settings with a preponderance of men—the military, prisons, factories, and other industrial settings—although the condition also occurs in women.

### D. Etiology.
Unknown. May be associated with antisocial personality disorder.

### E. Differential diagnosis

1. **Factitious disorders.** No obvious secondary gain.
2. **Somatoform disorder.** Symbolic or unconscious component to symptom. Symptoms are not voluntarily and willfully produced.

### F. Treatment.
Results of physical and laboratory workups often are negative. Patient should be monitored as if there were real disease, but no treatment should be offered. At some time, identify areas of secondary gain and encourage patient to ventilate and help provide ways of managing stress. Patient may then be willing to give up symptoms.

---

*For a more detailed discussion of this topic, see Guggenheim FG, Smith GR: Somatoform Disorders, Chap 18, p 1251; Jones RM: Factitious Disorders, Chap 19, p 1271; Mills MJ, Lipian MS: Malingering, Sec 28.2, p 1614, in CTP/VI.*

# 12

# Dissociative Disorders

## I. General introduction

**A. Definition.** Dissociative disorders are classified into five major types: (1) dissociative amnesia, (2) dissociative fugue, (3) dissociative identity disorder (also known as multiple personality disorder), (4) depersonalization disorder, and (5) dissociative disorder not otherwise specified (NOS). The common diagnostic feature is a psychologically induced loss of memory, consciousness, identity, or perception of the environment. Underlying brain disease is absent.

## II. Dissociative amnesia

**A. Definition.** Loss of important personal memory, usually stressful or traumatic, with preserved capacity to learn new material; not due to a medical condition or drug.

**B. Diagnosis, signs and symptoms.** See Table 12–1. Patient is alert usually and aware of loss of memory. Most common type of loss is localized amnesia in which the events of a short period of time are lost to memory. Apparent indifference to memory loss may be seen; mild clouding of consciousness may occur.

**C. Epidemiology.** See Table 12–2.

**D. Etiology.** See Table 12–2.

**E. Lab and psychological tests.** Must rule out organic pathology as indicated. Drug-assisted interview, e.g., amobarbital (Amytal), can help in distinguishing between amnestic disorder due to a general medical condition and dissociative amnesia; organically amnestic patients tend to worsen under amobarbital, whereas memory may return to psychogenically amnestic patients.

**F. Psychodynamics.** Memory loss is secondary to painful psychological conflict, in which the patient has limited emotional resources to confront. Defenses include repression (unconscious blocking of disturbing impulses from awareness), denial (external reality is ignored), and dissociation (separation and independent functioning of one group of mental processes from others). Similar defenses are used in all the dissociative disorders.

TABLE 12–1
**DSM-IV DIAGNOSTIC CRITERIA FOR DISSOCIATIVE AMNESIA**

A. The predominant disturbance is one or more episodes of inability to recall important personal information, usually of a traumatic or stressful nature, that is too extensive to be explained by ordinary forgetfulness.
B. The disturbance does not occur exclusively during the course of dissociative identity disorder, dissociative fugue, posttraumatic stress disorder, acute stress disorder, or somatization disorder and is not due to the direct physiological effects of a substance (e.g., a drug of abuse, a medication) or a neurological or other general medical condition (e.g., amnestic disorder due to head trauma).
C. The symptoms cause clinically significant distress or impairment in social, occupational, or other important areas of functioning.

Used with permission, APA.

**G. Differential diagnosis.** See Table 12–3.

**H. Course and prognosis.** See Table 12–2.

**I. Treatment.** Recovery generally is spontaneous without treatment.

1. **Hypnosis.** Relax patient enough to recall forgotten information.
2. **Drug-assisted interview.** Intermediate and short-acting barbiturates, e.g., thiopental (Pentothal) and sodium amobarbital given intravenously, and benzodiazepines may be used to help patients recover their forgotten memories.
3. **Psychotherapy.** Helps patients to incorporate the memories into their conscious states.

## III. Dissociative fugue

**A. Definition.** Unexpected sudden travel away from customary home or work and failure to remember important aspects of previous identity (name, family, occupation). A new identity often is assumed.

**B. Diagnosis, signs, and symptoms.** See Table 12–4. Sudden loss of memory associated with purposeful, unconfused travel, often for extended periods of time. Partial or complete loss of memory for past life, often without awareness of the loss. Assumption of apparently normal, nonbizarre new identity. However, perplexity and disorientation may occur.

**C. Epidemiology.** See Table 12–2.

**D. Etiology.** See Table 12–2.

**E. Lab and psychological tests.** Hypnosis and amobarbital interviews help in clarifying diagnosis.

**F. Differential diagnosis**

1. **Cognitive disorder.** Wandering is not as purposeful or complex.
2. **Temporal lobe epilepsy.** Generally no new identity is assumed.
3. **Dissociative amnesia.** No purposeful travel or new identity.
4. **Malingering.** Difficult to distinguish. Clear secondary gain should raise suspicion.

**G. Course and prognosis.** See Table 12–2.

**H. Treatment.** Recovery generally is spontaneous without treatment.

1. **Hypnosis and drug-assisted interviews.** May help reveal precipitating stressor.

TABLE 12-2
**SUMMARY OF DISSOCIATIVE DISORDERS**

| | Dissociative Amnesia | Dissociative Fugue | Dissociative Identity Disorder | Depersonalization Disorder |
|---|---|---|---|---|
| Signs and symptoms | Loss of memory, usually with abrupt onset<br>Patient aware of loss<br>Alert before and after loss | Purposeful wandering, often long distances<br>Amnesia for past life<br>Often unaware of loss of memory<br>Often assumes new identity<br>Normal behavior during fugue | More than one distinct personality within one person, each of which dominates person's behavior and thinking when it is present<br>Sudden transition from one personality to another<br>Generally amnesia for other personalities | Persistent sense of unreality about one's body and self<br>Intact reality testing<br>Ego-dynamic |
| Epidemiology | Most common dissociative disorder<br>More common following disasters or during war<br>Female>male<br>Adolescence, young adulthood | Rare<br>More common following disasters or during war<br>Variable sex ratio and age of onset | Not nearly as rare as once thought<br>Affects as many as 5% of psychiatric patients<br>Adolescence–young adulthood (although may begin much earlier)<br>Female>male<br>Increased in first-degree relatives | Although pure disorder is rare, intermittent episodes of depersonalization are common<br>Rare over age 40<br>May be more common in women |
| Etiology | Precipitating emotional trauma (e.g., domestic violence)<br>Rule out medical causes | Precipitating emotional trauma<br>Heavy alcohol abuse may predispose<br>Borderline, histrionic, schizoid personality disorders predispose<br>Rule out medical causes | Severe sexual and psychological abuse in childhood<br>Lack of support from significant others<br>Epilepsy may be involved<br>Rule out medical causes | Severe stress, anxiety, depression predispose<br>Rule out medical causes |
| Course and prognosis | Abrupt termination<br>Few recurrences | Usually brief, hours or days<br>Can last months and involve extensive travel<br>Recovery generally spontaneous and rapid<br>Recurrences are rare | Most severe and chronic of dissociative disorders<br>Incomplete recovery | Onset usually sudden<br>Tends to be chronic |

TABLE 12–3
**DIFFERENTIAL DIAGNOSTIC CONSIDERATIONS IN DISSOCIATIVE AMNESIA**

Dementia
Delirium
Amnestic disorder due to a general medical condition
  Anoxic amnesia
  Cerebral infections (e.g., herpes simplex affecting temporal lobes)
  Cerebral neoplasms (especially limbic and frontal)
  Epilepsy
  Metabolic disorders (e.g., uremia, hypoglycemia, hypertensive encephalopathy, porphyria)
  Postconcussion (posttraumatic) amnesia
  Postoperative amnesia
Electroconvulsive therapy (or other strong electric shock)
Substance-induced (e.g., ethanol, sedative-hypnotics, anticholinergics, steroids, lithium, β-adrenergic
  receptor antagonists, pentazocine, phencyclidine, hypoglycemic agents, cannabis, hallucinogens,
  methyldopa)
Transient global amnesia
Wernicke-Korsakoff syndrome
Sleep-related amnesia (e.g., sleepwalking disorder)
Other dissociative disorders
Posttraumatic stress disorder
Acute stress disorder
Somatoform disorders (somatization disorder, conversion disorder)
Malingering (especially when associated with criminal activity)

TABLE 12–4
**DSM-IV DIAGNOSTIC CRITERIA FOR DISSOCIATIVE FUGUE**

A. The predominant disturbance is sudden, unexpected travel away from home or one's customary place of work, with inability to recall one's past.
B. Confusion about personal identity or assumption of a new identity (partial or complete).
C. The disturbance does not occur exclusively during the course of dissociative identity disorder and is not due to the direct physiological effects of a substance (e.g., a drug of abuse, a medication) or a general medical condition (e.g., temporal lobe epilepsy).
D. The symptoms cause clinically significant distress or impairment in social, occupational, or other important areas of functioning.

Used with permission, APA.

    **2. Psychotherapy.** To help patients incorporate the precipitating stressors into their psyches in a healthy and integrated manner. Expressive-supportive psychodynamic psychotherapy is the treatment of choice.

## IV. Dissociative identity disorder

    **A. Definition.** Distinct personalities or identities within the same person, each of which when present may dominate the person's attitudes, behavior, and self-view, as though no other personality exists.

    **B. Diagnosis, signs, and symptoms.** See Table 12–5. Original personality is generally amnestic for and unaware of other personalities. Transition from one personality to another tends to be abrupt. Some personalities may be aware of aspects of other personalities; each personality may have its own set of memories and associations, and each generally has its own name or description. Different personalities may have different physiological characteristics, e.g., different eyeglass prescriptions, and different responses to psychometric testing, e.g., different intelligence quotient (I.Q.) scores. Personalities may be of different sexes, ages, or races. One or more of the personalities may exhibit signs of a coexisting psychiatric disorder, e.g., mood disorder, personality disorder.

TABLE 12-5
**DSM-IV DIAGNOSTIC CRITERIA FOR DISSOCIATIVE IDENTITY DISORDER**

A. The presence of two or more distinct identities or personality states (each with its own relatively enduring pattern of perceiving, relating to, and thinking about the environment and self).
B. At least two of these identities or personality states recurrently take control of the person's behavior.
C. Inability to recall important personal information that is too extensive to be explained by ordinary forgetfulness.
D. The disturbance is not due to the direct physiological effects of a substance (e.g., blackouts or chaotic behavior during alcohol intoxication) or a general medical condition (e.g., complex partial seizures). **Note:** In children, the symptoms are not attributable to imaginary playmates or other fantasy play.

Used with permission, APA.

C. **Epidemiology.** See Table 12-2.

D. **Etiology.** See Table 12-2.

E. **Lab and psychological tests.** Amobarbital interviews and hypnosis can help clarify diagnosis. In some studies, positron emission tomography (PET) scans and cerebral blood flow have revealed metabolic differences among different personalities in the same person.

F. **Psychodynamics.** Severe psychological and physical abuse (most often sexual) in childhood leads to a profound need to distance the self from horror and pain. The need to distance leads to an unconscious splitting off of different aspects of the original personality, each personality expressing some necessary emotion or state, e.g., rage, sexuality, flamboyance, competence, which the original personality does not dare express. During the abuse, the child attempts to protect the self from trauma by dissociating from the terrifying acts, becoming in essence another person or persons to whom abuse is not occurring and could not occur. The dissociated selves become a long-term, ingrained method of self-protection from perceived emotional threats.

G. **Differential diagnosis**

1. **Schizophrenia.** Patients may be delusional in believing that they have different identities or are being controlled by others, but the formal thought disorder and social deterioration distinguish schizophrenia from dissociative identity disorder.

2. **Malingering.** The most difficult differential diagnosis; clear secondary gain must raise suspicion. Drug-assisted interview may help.

3. **Borderline personality disorder.** Many patients with coexistent borderline personality disorder may be diagnosed as only having the personality disorder, because the different personalities are mistaken for the characteristic mood, behavior, and interpersonal instability of the borderline personality disorder patient.

4. **Bipolar disorder with rapid cycling.** Symptoms appear to be similar to those of dissociative identity disorder but without discrete personalities.

5. **Neurological disorders.** Complex partial epilepsy is the most likely to imitate the symptoms of dissociative identity disorder.

H. **Course and prognosis.** See Table 12-2.

TABLE 12–6
**DSM-IV DIAGNOSTIC CRITERIA FOR DEPERSONALIZATION DISORDER**

A. Persistant or recurrent experiences of feeling detached from, and as if one is an outside observer of, one's mental processes or body (e.g., feeling like one is in a dream).
B. During the personalization experience, reality testing remains intact.
C. The depersonalization causes clinically significant distress or impairment in social, occupational, or other important areas of functioning.
D. The depersonalization experience does not occur exclusively during the course of another mental disorder, such as schizophrenia, panic disorder, acute stress disorder, or another dissociative disorder, and is not due to the direct physiological effects of a substance (e.g., a drug of abuse, a medication) or a general medical condition (e.g., temporal lobe epilepsy).

Used with permission, APA.

I. **Treatment.** Intensive insight-oriented psychotherapy, often with hypnotherapy or drug-assisted interviewing. Pharmacotherapy has not been very useful. Goals of therapy include reconciliation of disparate, split-off affects by helping the patient to understand that the original reasons for the dissociation (overwhelming rage, fear, confusion secondary to abuse) no longer exist and that the affects can be expressed by one whole personality without destroying the self.

## V. Depersonalization disorder

A. **Definition.** Persistent, recurrent episodes of feeling detached from one's self or body, e.g., feeling mechanical or being in a dream.

B. **Diagnosis, signs, and symptoms.** See Table 12–6. Distortions in sense of time and space, extremities seeming too large or too small, and derealization (sense of strangeness about external world) are common. Patients may feel robotlike. Dizziness, depressive and obsessive ruminations, anxiety, and somatic preoccupations are common.

C. **Epidemiology.** See Table 12–2.

D. **Etiology.** See Table 12–2.

E. **Differential diagnosis.** Depersonalization as a symptom can occur in many syndromes, both psychiatric and medical. Mood disorders, anxiety disorders, schizophrenia, dissociative identity disorder, substance use, adverse medication, brain tumors or injury, and seizure disorders, e.g., temporal lobe epilepsy, must be ruled out. Depersonalization disorder describes the condition in which depersonalization is predominant.

F. **Course and prognosis.** See Table 12–2.

G. **Treatment.** Anxiety usually responds to anxiolytics and to both supportive and insight-oriented therapy. As anxiety is reduced episodes of depersonalization decrease.

## VI. Dissociative disorder NOS

A. **Definition.** Dissociative symptoms are prominent, but the clinical picture does not fully meet the specific criteria for dissociative disorder. Disorders in which the predominant feature is a dissociative symptom, i.e., a disturbance or alteration in the normally integrative functions of identity, memory, or consciousness, that does not meet the criteria for a specific dissociative disorder.

## B. Examples

1. Cases similar to dissociative identity disorder in which there is more than one personality state that can assume executive control of the person, but not more than one personality state is sufficiently distinct to meet the full criteria for dissociative identity disorder; or cases in which a second personality never assumes complete executive control; or cases without amnesia for important information.
2. Derealization unaccompanied by depersonalization.
3. Dissociated states that can occur in persons who have been subjected to periods of prolonged and intense coercive persuasion, e.g., brainwashing or indoctrination while the captive of terrorists or cultists.
4. Dissociative trance disorder—disturbances in consciousness, identity, or memory that are indigenous to particular locations and cultures, e.g., *amok* (rage reaction), *pibloktoq* (self-injurious behavior). Trance states are altered states of consciousness with markedly diminished or selectively focused responsiveness to environmental stimuli. In children, such states may follow physical abuse or trauma.
5. Coma, stupor, or loss of consciousness not due to a general medical condition. Cases in which sudden, unexpected travel and organized, purposeful behavior with inability to recall one's past are not accompanied by the assumption of a new identity, partial or complete.
6. Ganser's syndrome—the giving of approximate answers to questions, e.g., $2 + 2 = 5$, or talking past the point; commonly associated with other symptoms, such as amnesia, disorientation, perceptual disturbances, fugue, and conversion symptoms.

---

*For more detailed discussion of this topic, see Nemiah JC: Dissociative Disorders, Chap 20, p 1028, in* CTP/VI.

---

# 13

# Sexual Dysfunctions, Paraphilias, and Gender Identity Disorders

## I. Sexual dysfunctions

**A. Definition.** Sexual dysfunctions can be symptomatic of biological problems (biogenic), intrapsychic or interpersonal problems (psychogenic), or a combination of these factors. Sexual function can be adversely affected by stress of any kind, by emotional disorders, or by ignorance of sexual function and physiology. Regardless of etiology, the dysfunction is accompanied by and perpetuates anxiety regarding sexual performance. The dysfunctions can be **lifelong type** or **acquired type** (i.e., developing after a period of normal functioning), **generalized type** or **situational type** (i.e., limited to a certain partner or a specific situation), and **due to psychological factors** or **due to combined factors.** The seven major categories of sexual dysfunction listed in DSM-IV are (1) sexual desire disorders, (2) sexual arousal disorders, (3) orgasmic disorders, (4) sexual pain disorders, (5) sexual dysfunction due to a general medical condition, (6) substance-induced sexual dysfunction, and (7) sexual dysfunction not otherwise specified (NOS). Table 13–1 lists each of the DSM-IV phases of the sexual response cycle and the sexual functions usually associated with it.

**B. Sexual desire disorders.** Sexual desire disorders are divided into two classes: **hypoactive sexual desire disorder,** characterized by a deficiency or the absence of sexual fantasies and desire for sexual activity, and **sexual aversion disorder,** characterized by an aversion to and avoidance of genital sexual contact with a sexual partner.

Patients with desire problems may use inhibition of desire defensively to protect against unconscious fears about sex. Lack of desire can also accompany chronic anxiety or depression or the use of drugs that depress the central nervous system (CNS). In sex therapy clinic populations, lack of desire is one of the most common complaints among married couples, with women more affected than men.

**C. Sexual arousal disorders.** These disorders include male erectile disorder and female arousal disorder. Their diagnosis considers the focus, intensity, and duration of the sexual activity of the patient. If sexual stimulation is inadequate in focus, intensity, or duration, the diagnosis should not be made.

    **1. Women.** See Table 13–2. The prevalence of female sexual arousal disorder is generally underestimated. In one study of subjectively happily married couples, 33% of women described arousal problems.

        Difficulty in maintaining excitement can reflect psychological conflicts (e.g., anxiety, guilt, and fear) or physiological changes. Alterations

TABLE 13–1
**DSM-IV PHASES OF THE SEXUAL RESPONSE CYCLE AND ASSOCIATED SEXUAL DYSFUNCTIONS**[a]

| Phases | Characteristics | Dysfunction |
|---|---|---|
| 1. Desire | This phase is distinct from any identified solely through physiology and reflects the patient's motivations, drives, and personality. The phase is characterized by sexual fantasies and the desire to have sex. | Hypoactive sexual desire disorder; sexual aversion disorder; hypoactive sexual desire disorder due to a general medical condition (male or female); substance, induced sexual dysfunction with impaired desire |
| 2. Excitement | This phase consists of a subjective sense of sexual pleasure and accompanying physiological changes. All the physiological responses noted in Masters and Johnson's excitement and plateau phases are combined and occur in this phase. | Female sexual arousal disorder; male erectile disorder (may also occur in stage 3 and in stage 4); male erectile disorder due to a general medical condition; dyspareunia due to a general medical condition (male or female); substance-induced sexual dysfunction with impaired arousal |
| 3. Orgasm | This phase consists of a peaking of sexual pleasure, with release of sexual tension and rhythmic contraction of the perineal muscles and pelvic reproductive organs. | Female orgasmic disorder; male orgasmic disorder; premature ejaculation; other sexual dysfunction due to a general medical condition (male or female); substance-induced sexual dysfunction with impaired orgasm |
| 4. Resolution | This phase entails a sense of general relaxation, well-being, and muscle relaxation. During this phase men are refractory to orgasm for a period of time that increases with age, whereas women are capable of having multiple orgasms without a refractory period. | Postcoital dysphoria; postcoital headache |

[a]DSM-IV consolidates the William Masters and Virginia Johnson excitement and plateau phases into a single excitement phase, which is preceded by the desire (appetitive) phase. The orgasm and resolution phases remain the same as originally described by Masters and Johnson.

TABLE 13–2
**DSM-IV DIAGNOSTIC CRITERIA FOR FEMALE SEXUAL AROUSAL DISORDER**

A. Persistent or recurrent inability to attain, or to maintain until completion of the sexual activity, an adequate lubrication-swelling response of sexual excitement.
B. The disturbance causes marked distress or interpersonal difficulty.
C. The sexual dysfunction is not better accounted for by another Axis I disorder (except another sexual dysfunction) and is not due exclusively to the direct physiological effects of a substance (e.g., a drug of abuse, a medication) or a general medical condition.

*Specify* type:
   **Lifelong type**
   **Acquired type**

*Specify* type:
   **Generalized type**
   **Situational type**

*Specify:*
   **Due to psychological factors**
   **Due to combined factors**

Used with permission, APA.

TABLE 13–3
**DSM-IV DIAGNOSTIC CRITERIA FOR MALE ERECTILE DISORDER**

A. Persistent or recurrent inability to attain, or to maintain until completion of the sexual activity, an adequate erection.
B. The disturbance causes marked distress or interpersonal difficulty.
C. The erectile dysfunction is not better accounted for by another Axis I disorder (other than a sexual dysfunction) is not due exclusively to the direct physiological effects of a substance (e.g., a drug of abuse, a medication) or a general medical condition.

*Specify* type:
   **Lifelong type**
   **Acquired type**

*Specify* type:
   **Generalized type**
   **Situational type**

*Specify:*
   **Due to psychological factors**
   **Due to combined factors**

Used with permission, APA.

in testosterone, estrogen, prolactin, and thyroxin levels have been implicated in arousal disorders, as have antihistaminic medications.

**2. Men.**   (Also called erectile dysfunction and impotence). The prevalence of impotence in young men is estimated at 8%. However, this disorder may first appear later in life. See Table 13–3.

A number of procedures, from benign to invasive, are used to differentiate organically, i.e., medically, caused impotence from functional, i.e., psychological impotence. The most commonly used procedure is the monitoring of nocturnal penile tumescence (erections that occur during sleep), normally associated with rapid eye movement (REM).

A good history is invaluable in determining the cause. A history of spontaneous erections, morning erections, or good erections with masturbation or with partners other than the usual one indicates functional impotence.

Psychological causes of impotence include unresolved oedipal or preoedipal conflicts, which result in a punitive superego, an inability to trust, or feelings of inadequacy. Erectile dysfunction also may reflect relationship difficulties between partners.

**D. Orgasmic disorders**
   **1. Female.**   See Table 13–4. Female orgasmic disorder (anorgasmia) is the recurrent or persistent delay in or absence of orgasm following a normal sexual excitement phase. The estimated proportion of married women over age 35 who never have achieved orgasm is 5%. The proportion is higher in unmarried women and younger women. Overall prevalence of inhibited female orgasm is 30%.

Psychological factors associated with inhibited orgasm include fears of impregnation or rejection by the sex partner, hostility toward men, feelings of guilt about sexual impulses, or marital conflicts.

   **2. Male.**   In male orgasmic disorder (inhibited male orgasm), the man achieves ejaculation during coitus with great difficulty, if at all. Lifelong inhibited male orgasm usually indicates more severe psychopathology.

TABLE 13–4
**DSM-IV DIAGNOSTIC CRITERIA FOR FEMALE ORGASMIC DISORDER**

A.  Persistent or recurrent delay in, or absence of, orgasm following a normal sexual excitement phase. Women exhibit wide variability in the type or intensity of stimulation that triggers orgasm. The diagnosis of female orgasmic disorder should be based on the clinician's judgment that the woman's orgasmic capacity is less than would be reasonable for her age, sexual experience, and the adequacy of sexual stimulation she receives.
B.  The disturbance causes marked distress or interpersonal difficulty.
C.  The orgasmic dysfunction is not better accounted for by another Axis I disorder (except another sexual dysfunction) and is not due exclusively to the direct physiological effects of a substance (e.g., a drug of abuse, a medication) or a general medical condition.

*Specify* type:
  **Lifelong type**
  **Acquired type**

*Specify* type:
  **Generalized type**
  **Situational type**

*Specify:*
  **Due to psychological factors**
  **Due to combined factors**

Used with permission, APA.

Acquired ejaculatory inhibition frequently reflects interpersonal difficulties.

3. **Premature ejaculation.**   Premature ejaculation is the chief complaint of 35–40% of men treated for sexual disorders. The man persistently or recurrently achieves orgasm and ejaculation before he wishes to. It is more prevalent among young men, men with a new partner, and college-educated men than among men with less education; it is thought to be related to concern for partner satisfaction.

Premature ejaculation may be associated with unconscious fears about the vagina. It may also be the result of conditioning if the man's early sexual experiences occurred in situations in which discovery would be embarrassing. A stressful marriage exacerbates the disorder.

This dysfunction is the one most amenable to cure when behavioral techniques are used in treatment.

E.  **Sexual pain disorders**

1. **Vaginismus.**   Vaginismus is an involuntary muscle constriction of the outer third of the vagina that interferes with penile insertion and intercourse. This dysfunction most frequently afflicts women in higher socioeconomic groups. A sexual trauma, such as rape or childhood sexual abuse, can be the cause. Women with psychosexual conflicts may perceive the penis as a weapon. A strict religious upbringing that associates sex with sin or problems in the dyadic relationship are also noted in these cases.

2. **Dyspareunia.**   Dyspareunia is recurrent or persistent genital pain occurring before, during, or after intercourse. Organic etiologies (endometriosis, vaginitis, cervicitis, and other pelvic disorders) must be ruled out with this complaint.

Chronic pelvic pain is a common complaint in women with a history of rape or childhood sexual abuse. Painful coitus may result from tension

TABLE 13–5
**DISEASES AND OTHER MEDICAL CONDITIONS IMPLICATED IN MALE ERECTILE DISORDER**

**Infectious and parasitic diseases**
  Elephantiasis
  Mumps

**Cardiovascular disease[a]**
  Atherosclerotic disease
  Aortic aneurysm
  Leriche's syndrome
  Cardiac failure

**Renal and urological disorders**
  Peyronie's disease
  Chronic renal failure
  Hydrocele and varicocele

**Hepatic disorders**
  Cirrhosis (usually associated with alcohol
    dependence)

**Pulmonary disorders**
  Respiratory failure

**Genetics**
  Klinefelter's syndrome
  Congenital penile vascular and structural
    abnormalities

**Nutritional disorders**
  Malnutrition
  Vitamin deficiencies

**Endocrine disorders[a]**
  Diabetes mellitus
  Dysfunction of the pituitary-adrenal-testis axis
  Acromegaly
  Addison's disease
  Chromophobe adenoma
  Adrenal neoplasia
  Myxedema
  Hyperthyroidism

**Neurological disorders**
  Multiple sclerosis
  Transverse myelitis
  Parkinson's disease
  Temporal lobe epilepsy
  Traumatic and neoplastic spinal cord diseases[a]
  Central nervous system tumor
  Amyotrophic lateral sclerosis
  Peripheral neuropathy
  General paresis
  Tabes dorsalis

**Pharmacological contributants**
  Alcohol and other dependence-inducing
    substances (heroin, methadone, morphine,
    cocaine, amphetamines, and barbiturates)
  Prescribed drugs (psychotropic drugs,
    antihypertensive drugs, estrogens, and
    antiandrogens)

**Poisoning**
  Lead (plumbism)
  Herbicides

**Surgical procedures[a]**
  Perineal prostatectomy
  Abdominal-perineal colon resection
  Sympathectomy (frequently interferes with
    ejaculation)
  Aortoiliac surgery
  Radical cystectomy
  Retroperitoneal lymphadenectomy

**Miscellaneous**
  Radiation therapy
  Pelvic fracture
  Any severe systemic disease or debilitating
    condition

[a]In the United States an estimated two million men are impotent because they suffer from diabetes mellitus; an additional 300,000 are impotent because of other endocrine diseases; 1.5 million are impotent as a result of vascular disease; 180,000 because of multiple sclerosis; 400,000 because of traumas and fractures leading to pelvic fractures or spinal cord injuries; and another 650,000 are impotent as a result of radical surgery, including prostatectomies, colostomies, and cystectomies.

and anxiety. Dyspareunia is uncommon in men and is usually associated with an organic condition.

**F. Sexual dysfunction due to a general medical condition**

  **1. Male erectile disorder.**    Statistics indicate that erectile disorder is organically based in 20–50% of affected men. Organic causes of male erectile disorder are listed in Table 13–5.

  **2. Dyspareunia.**    30–40% of women with this complaint who are seen in sex therapy clinics have pelvic pathology. An estimated 30% of surgical procedures on the female pelvic or genital area also result in temporary dyspareunia. In most cases, however, dynamic factors are considered causative.

  Organic abnormalities leading to dyspareunia include irritated or infected hymenal remnants, episiotomy scars, Bartholin's gland infection, various forms of vaginitis and cervicitis, endometriosis, and Peyronie's disease.

3. **Hypoactive sexual desire disorder.**   Desire commonly decreases after major illness or surgery. Drugs that depress the CNS or decrease testosterone production can decrease desire.

4. **Other male sexual dysfunction.**   Male orgasmic disorder may have physiological causes and can occur after surgery on the genitourinary tract. It may also be associated with Parkinson's disease and other neurological disorders involving the lumbar or sacral sections of the spinal cord. Certain drugs, e.g., guanethidine monosulfate (Ismelin), have been implicated in retarded ejaculation (Table 13–6).

5. **Other female sexual dysfunctions.**   Some medical conditions—specifically, such endocrine diseases as hypothyroidism, diabetes mellitus, and primary hyperprolacetinemia—can affect a woman's ability to have orgasms. Table 13–7 lists psychiatric medications that may inhibit female orgasm.

G. **Substance-induced sexual dysfunction.**   Occurs within a month of significant substance intoxication or withdrawal. In small doses, many substances enhance sexual performance, but continued use impairs erectile, orgasmic, and ejaculatory capacities.

H. **Sexual dysfunction not otherwise specified.**   Includes sexual dysfunctions that do not meet the criteria for any specific dysfunction. Examples include postcoital headache, orgasmic anhedonia, and masturbatory pain.

I. **Treatment**   Methods that have proved effective singly or in combination include (1) training in behavioral-sexual skills, (2) systematic desensitization, (3) directive marital therapy, (4) psychodynamic approaches, (5) group therapy, (6) pharmacotherapy, (7) surgery, and (8) hypnotherapy. Evaluation and treatment must address the possibility of accompanying personality disorders and physical conditions.

1. **Analytically oriented sex therapy.**   One of the most effective treatment modalities is the integration of sex therapy (training in behavioral-sexual skills) with psychodynamic and psychoanalytically oriented psychotherapy. The addition of psychodynamic conceptualizations to the behavioral techniques used to treat sexual dysfunctions allows for the treatment of patients with sexual disorders associated with other psychopathology.

2. **Behavioral techniques.**   The aim of these techniques is to establish or reestablish verbal and sexual communication between partners. Specific exercises are prescribed to help the person or couple with their particular problem.

Beginning exercises focus on verbal interchange and then on heightening sensory awareness to sight, touch, and smell. Initially, intercourse is prohibited and partners caress each other, excluding stimulation of the genitalia. Performance anxiety is reduced because responses of genital excitement and orgasm are unnecessary for the completion of the initial exercises.

During these **sensate focus** exercises, patients receive encouragement and reinforcement to reduce their anxiety. They are urged to use fantasies

TABLE 13–6
**PHARMACOLOGICAL AGENTS IMPLICATED IN MALE SEXUAL DYSFUNCTIONS**

| Drug | Impairs Erection | Impairs Ejaculation |
|---|---|---|
| Psychiatric drugs | | |
| Cyclic drugs[a] | | |
| Imipramine (Tofranil) | + | + |
| Protriptyline (Vivactil) | + | + |
| Desipramine (Pertofrane) | + | + |
| Clomipramine (Anafranil) | + | + |
| Amitriptyline (Elavil) | + | + |
| Trazodone (Desyrel)[b] | – | – |
| Monoamine oxidase inhibitors | | |
| Tranylcypromine (Parnate) | + | |
| Phenelzine (Nardil) | + | + |
| Pargyline (Eutonyl) | – | + |
| Isocarboxazid (Marplan) | – | + |
| Other mood-active drugs | | |
| Lithium (Eskalith) | + | |
| Amphetamines | + | + |
| Fluoxetine (Prozac) | – | + |
| Antipsychotics[c] | | |
| Fluphenazine (Prolixin) | + | |
| Thioridazine (Mellaril) | + | + |
| Chlorprothixene (Taractan) | – | + |
| Mesoridazine (Serentil) | – | + |
| Perphenazine (Trilafon) | – | + |
| Trifluoperazine (Stelazine) | – | + |
| Reserpine (Serpasil) | + | + |
| Haloperidol (Haldol) | – | + |
| Antianxiety agent[d] | | |
| Chlordiazepoxide (Librium) | – | + |
| Antihypertensive drugs | | |
| Clonidine (Catapres) | + | |
| Methyldopa (Aldomet) | + | + |
| Spironolactone (Aldactone) | + | – |
| Hydrochlorothiazide (Hydrodiuril) | + | |
| Guanethidine (Ismelin) | + | + |
| Commonly abused substances | | |
| Alcohol | + | + |
| Barbiturates | + | + |
| Cannabis | + | – |
| Cocaine | + | + |
| Heroin | + | + |
| Methadone | + | – |
| Morphine | + | + |
| Miscellaneous drugs | | |
| Antiparkinsonian agents | + | + |
| Clofibrate (Atromid-S) | + | – |
| Digoxin (Lanoxin) | + | – |
| Glutethimide (Doriden) | + | + |
| Indomethacin (Indocin) | + | – |
| Phentolamine (Regitine) | – | + |
| Propranolol (Inderal) | + | – |

[a]The incidence of male erectile disorder associated with the use of tricyclic drugs is low.
[b]Trazodone has been causative in some cases of priapism.
[c]Impairment of sexual function is not a common complication of the use of antipsychotics. Priapism has occasionally occurred in association with the use of antipsychotics.
[d]Benzodiazepines have been reported to decrease libido, but in some patients the diminution of anxiety caused by those drugs enhances sexual function.
Table by Virginia A. Sadock, MD.

TABLE 13–7
**SOME PSYCHIATRIC DRUGS IMPLEMENTED IN INHIBITED FEMALE ORGASM**[a]

Tricyclic antidepressants
  Imipramine (Tofranil)
  Clomipramine (Anafranil)
  Nortriptyline (Aventyl)
Monoamine oxidase inhibitors
  Tranylcypromine (Parnate)
  Phenelzine (Nardil)
  Isocarboxazid (Marplan)
Dopamine receptor antagonists
  Thioridazine (Mellaril)
  Trifluoperazine (Stelazine)
Serotonin-specific reuptake inhibitors
  Fluoxetine (Prozac)
  Paroxetine (Paxil)
  Sertraline (Zoloft)

[a]The relation between female sexual dysfunction and pharmacological agents has been less extensively evaluated than have male reactions. Oral contraceptives are reported to decrease libido in some women, and some drugs with anticholinergic side effects may impair arousal as well as orgasm. Benzodiazepines have been reported to decrease libido, but in some patients the diminution of anxiety caused by those drugs enhances sexual function.

Both increase and decrease in libido have been reported with psychoactive agents. It is difficult to separate those effects from the underlying condition or from improvement of the condition. Sexual dysfunction associated with the use of a drug disappears when the drug is discontinued.

to distract them from obsessive concerns about performance (spectatoring). The expression of mutual needs is encouraged. Resistances, such as claims of fatigue or not enough time to complete the exercises, are common and must be dealt with by the therapist. Genital stimulation is eventually added to general body stimulation. Finally, intromission and intercourse are permitted. Therapy sessions follow each new exercise period, and problems and satisfactions, both sexual and in other areas of the patients' lives, are discussed.

a. **Dysfunction-specific techniques and exercises**—different techniques are used for specific dysfunctions.

i. **Vaginismus**—the woman is advised to dilate her vaginal opening with fingers or dilators.

ii. **Premature ejaculation**—the squeeze technique is used to raise the threshold of penile excitability. The patient or his partner forcibly squeezes the coronal ridge of the glans at the first sensation of impending ejaculation. The erection is diminished and ejaculation is inhibited. A variation is the **stop-start** technique. Stimulation is stopped as excitement increases, but no squeeze is used.

iii. **Male desire disorder**—the man is sometimes told to masturbate to demonstrate that full erection and ejaculation are possible.

iv. **Female orgasmic disorder (primary anorgasmia)**—the woman is instructed to masturbate, sometimes with the use of a vibrator. The use of fantasy is encouraged.

v. **Retarded ejaculation**—managed by extravaginal ejaculation initially and gradual vaginal entry after stimulation to the point of near ejaculation.

   b. **Behavioral techniques**—reported to be successful 40–85% of the time. 10% of refractory cases are estimated to need intensive individual psychotherapy. Approximately one third of dysfunctional couples refractory to behavioral techniques alone require some combination of marital and sex therapy.

   **3. Biological.**    These methods include pharmacotherapy (yohimbine, papaverine, psychotropics) and surgery (penile implants, revascularization).

## II. Gender identity disorders

A. **Definition.**    Characterized by persistent feelings of discomfort with one's biological sex or the gender role of one's sex. **Gender identity** is a psychological state that reflects the inner sense of oneself as being male or female. **Gender role** is the external behavioral pattern that reflects the person's inner sense of gender identity. **Sex** (or biological sex) is strictly the anatomical and physiological characteristics that indicate whether one is male or female, e.g., a penis or vagina. **Sexual orientation** is the person's erotic-response tendency, e.g., homosexual, heterosexual, bisexual, and takes into account one's object choice (men or women) and fantasy life. **Transsexuals** are persistently preoccupied with getting rid of primary and secondary sex characteristics and with acquiring the sex characteristics of the other sex and wish to dress and live as a member of the other sex.

B. **Diagnosis, signs, and symptoms.**    See Table 13–8.

C. **Epidemiology**
   1. Unknown, but rare.
   2. Male-to-female ratio—30:1–6:1
   3. About 1 per 30,000 men and 1 per 100,000 women seek sex-reassignment surgery.

D. **Etiology**
   **1. Biological.**    Testosterone affects brain neurons that contribute to the masculinization of the brain in such areas as the hypothalamus. Whether testosterone contributes to so-called masculine or feminine behavioral patterns in gender identity disorders remains controversial. Sex steroids influence the expression of sexual behavior in mature men and women, i.e., testosterone can increase libido and aggressiveness in women, and estrogen can decrease libido and aggressiveness in men.

   **2. Psychosocial.**    The absence of same-sex role models and explicit or implicit encouragement from caregivers to behave like the other sex contributes to gender identity disorder in childhood. Mothers may be depressed or withdrawn. Inborn temperamental traits sometimes result in sensitive, delicate boys and energetic, aggressive girls. Physical and sexual abuse may predispose.

E. **Differential diagnosis**
   **1. Transvestic fetishism.**    Cross-dressing for purpose of sexual excitement; can coexist (dual diagnosis).
   **2. Intersex conditions.**    See Table 13–9.
   **3. Schizophrenia.**    Rarely, true delusions of being other sex.

TABLE 13–8
**DSM-IV DIAGNOSTIC CRITERIA FOR GENDER IDENTITY DISORDER**

A.  A strong and persistent cross-gender identification (not merely a desire for any perceived cultural advantages of being the other sex).
 In children, the disturbance is manifested by four (or more) of the following:
 (1) repeatedly stated desire to be, or insistence that he or she is, the other sex
 (2) in boys, preference for cross-dressing or simulating female attire; in girls, insistence on wearing only stereotypical masculine clothing
 (3) strong and persistent preferences for cross-sex roles in make-believe play or persistent fantasies of being the other sex
 (4) intense desire to participate in the stereotypical games and pastimes of the other sex
 (5) strong preference for playmates of the other sex
 In adolescents and adults, the disturbance is manifested by symptoms such as a stated desire to be the other sex, frequent passing as the other sex, desire to live or be treated as the other sex, or the conviction that he or she has the typical feelings and reactions of the other sex.
B.  Persistent discomfort with his or her sex or sense of inappropriateness in the gender role of that sex.
 In children, the disturbance is manifested by any of the following: in boys, assertion that his penis or testes are disgusting or will disappear or assertion that it would be better not to have a penis, or aversion toward rough-and-tumble play and rejection of male stereotypical toys, games, and activities; in girls, rejection of urinating in a sitting position, assertion that she has or will grow a penis, or assertion that she does not want to grow breasts or menstruate, or marked aversion toward normative feminine clothing.
 In adolescents and adults, the disturbance is manifested by symptoms such as preoccupation with getting rid of primary and secondary sex characteristics (e.g., request for hormones, surgery, or other procedures to physically alter sexual characteristics to simulate the other sex) or belief that he or she was born the wrong sex.
C.  The disturbance is not concurrent with a physical intersex condition.
D.  The disturbance causes clinically significant distress or impairment in social, occupational, or other important areas of functioning.

*Code* based on current age:
 **Gender identity disorder in children**
 **Gender identity disorder in adolescents or adults**

*Specify* if (for sexually mature individuals):
 **Sexually attracted to males**
 **Sexually attracted to females**
 **Sexually attracted to both**
 **Sexually attracted to neither**

Used with permission, APA.

## F.  Course and prognosis.

**1. Children.**    Course varies. Symptoms may diminish spontaneously or with treatment. Prognosis depends on age of onset and intensity of symptoms. The disorder begins in boys before the age of 4 years, and peer conflict develops at about the age of 7 or 8 years. Tomboyism is generally better tolerated. The age of onset is also early for girls, but most give up masculine behavior by adolescence. Less than 10% of children go on to transsexualism.

**2. Adults.**    Course tends to be chronic.
**Transsexualism**—after puberty, there is distress with one's biological sex and a desire to eliminate one's primary and secondary sex characteristics and acquire those of the other sex. Most transsexuals have had gender identity disorder in childhood; cross-dressing is common; associated mental disorder is common, especially borderline personality disorder or depressive disorder; suicide is a risk, but persons may mutilate their sex organs to coerce surgeons to perform sex reassignment surgery.

TABLE 13–9
**CLASSIFICATION OF INTERSEXUAL DISORDERS[a]**

| Syndrome | Description |
| --- | --- |
| Virilizing adrenal hyperplasia (andrenogenital syndrome) | Results from excess androgens in fetus with XX genotype; most common female intersex disorder; associated with enlarged clitoris, fused labia, hirsutism in adolescence |
| Turner's syndrome | Results from absence of second female sex chromosome (XO); associated with web neck, dwarfism, cubitus valgus; no sex hormones produced; infertile; usually assigned as females because of female-looking genitals |
| Klinefelter's syndrome | Genotype is XXY; male habitus present with small penis and rudimentary testes because of low androgen production; weak libido; usually assigned as male |
| Androgen insensitivity syndrome (testicular-feminizing syndrome) | Congenital X-linked recessive disorder that results in inability of tissues to respond to androgens; external genitals look female and cryptorchid testes present; assigned as females, even though they have XY genotype; in extreme form patient has breasts, normal external genitals, short blind vagina, and absence of pubic and axillary hair |
| Enzymatic defects in XY genotype (e.g., 5-α-reductase deficiency, 17-hydroxysteroid deficiency) | Congenital interruption in production of testosterone that produces ambiguous genitals and female habitus; usually assigned as female because of female-looking genitalia |
| Hermaphroditism | True hermaphrodite is rare and characterized by both testes and ovaries in same person (may be 46 XX or 46 XY) |
| Pseudohermaphroditism | Usually the result of endocrine or enzymatic defect (e.g., adrenal hyperplasia) in persons with normal chromosomes; female pseudohermaphrodites have masculine-looking genitals but are XX; male pseudohermaphrodites have rudimentary testes and external genitals and are XY; assigned as males or females, depending on morphology of genitals |

[a]Intersexual disorders include a variety of syndromes that produce persons with gross anatomical or physiological aspects of the opposite sex.

### G. Treatment.

1. **Children.**  Improve existing role models or, in their absence, provide one from the family or elsewhere, e.g., big brother or sister. Caregivers are helped to encourage sex-appropriate behavior and attitudes. Any associated mental disorder is addressed.

2. **Adolescents.**  Difficult to treat because of the coexistence of normal identity crises and gender identity confusion. Acting out is common, and the adolescents rarely have a strong motivation to alter their stereotypical cross-gender roles.

3. **Adults**

   a. **Psychotherapy**—set the goal of helping patients become comfortable with the gender identity they desire; the goal is not to create a person with a conventional sexual identity. Therapy also explores sex-reassignment surgery and the indications and contraindications for such procedures, which are often impulsively decided on by severely distressed and anxious patients.

   b. **Sex-reassignment surgery**—definitive and irreversible. Patients must go through a 3- to 12-month trial of cross-dressing and receive hormone treatment. 70–80% of patients are satisfied by the results.

TABLE 13–10
**PARAPHILIAS**

| Disorder | Definition | General Considerations | Treatment |
|---|---|---|---|
| Exhibitionism | Exposing genitals in public; rare in females | Person wants to shock female—her reaction is affirmation to patient that penis is intact | Insight-oriented psychotherapy, aversive conditioning. Female should try to ignore exhibitionistic male, who is offensive but not dangerous, or call police |
| Fetishism | Sexual arousal with inanimate objects, e.g., shoes, hair, clothing | Almost always in men. Behavior often followed by guilt | Insight-oriented psychotherapy; aversive conditioning; implosion, i.e., patient masturbates with fetish until it loses its arousal effect (masturbatory satiation) |
| Frotteurism | Rubbing genitals against female to achieve arousal and orgasm | Occurs in crowded places, such as subways, usually by passive, nonassertive men | Insight-oriented psychotherapy; aversive conditioning; group therapy; antiandrogenic medication |
| Pedophilia | Sexual activity with children under age 13; most common paraphilia | 95% heterosexual. 5% homosexual. High risk of repeat behavior. Fear of adult sexuality in patient; low self-esteem. 10–20% of children have been molested by age 18 | Place patient in treatment unit; group therapy; insight-oriented psychotherapy; antiandrogen medication to diminish sexual urge |
| Sexual masochism | Sexual pleasure derived from being abused physically or mentally or from being humiliated (moral masochism) | Defense against guilt feelings related to sex—punishment turned inwards | Insight-oriented psychotherapy; group therapy |
| Sexual sadism | Sexual arousal resulting from causing mental or physical suffering to another person | Mostly seen in men. Named after Marquis de Sade. Can progress to rape in some cases | Insight-oriented psychotherapy; aversive conditioning |
| Transvestic fetishism | Cross-dressing | Most often used in heterosexual arousal. Most common is male-to-female cross-dressing. Do not confuse with transsexualism—wanting to be of opposite sex | Insight-oriented psychotherapy |
| Voyeurism | Sexual arousal by watching sexual acts, e.g., coitus or naked person. Can occur in women but more common in men. Variant is listening to erotic conversations, e.g., telephone sex | Masturbation usually occurs during voyeuristic activity. Usually arrested for loitering or peeping-tomism | Insight-oriented psychotherapy; aversive conditioning |
| **Other paraphilias** | | | |
| Excretory paraphilias | Defecating (coprophilia) or urinating (urophilia) on a partner or vice versa | Fixation at anal stage of development; klismaphilia (enemas) | Insight-oriented psychotherapy |
| Zoophilia | Sex with animals | More common in rural areas; may be opportunistic | Behavior modification, insight-oriented psychotherapy |

Dissatisfaction correlates with severity of preexisting psychopathology. A reported 2% commit suicide.

    **c. Hormonal treatments**—many patients are treated with hormones in lieu of surgery.

## III. Paraphilias

These are disorders characterized by sexual impulses, fantasies, or practices that are unusual, deviant, or bizarre. More common in men than in women. Etiology is unknown. There may be a biological predisposition (abnormal electroencephalogram [EEG], hormone levels), which is manifested by psychological factors, such as childhood abuse. Psychoanalytic theory holds that paraphilia results from fixation at one of the psychosexual phases of development or is an effort to ward off castration anxiety. Learning theory holds that the act was associated with sexual arousal during childhood and led to conditioned learning.

Paraphilic activity often is compulsive. Patients repeatedly engage in deviant behavior and are unable to control the impulse. When stressed, anxious, or depressed, the patient increases the deviant behavior. The patient may make numerous resolutions to stop the behavior but is generally unable to abstain for long, and acting out is followed by strong feelings of guilt. Treatment techniques result in only moderate success rates and include insight-oriented psychotherapy, behavior therapy, and pharmacotherapy alone or in combination. Table 13–10 lists the common paraphilias.

---

*For a more detailed discussion of this topic, see Sadock VA: Normal Human Sexuality and Sexual Dysfunctions, Sec 21.1a, p 1295; Meyer JK: Paraphilias, Sec 21.2, p 1334; Green R, Blanchard R: Gender Identity Disorders, Sec 21.3, p 1347, in CTP/VI.*

---

# 14

# Eating Disorders

## I. General introduction

Disorders characterized by a marked disturbance in eating behavior. The two major eating disorders are anorexia nervosa and bulimia nervosa.

## II. Anorexia nervosa

### A. Definition.
A serious and potentially fatal (in 5–18% of patients in studies) condition characterized by a disturbed body image and self-imposed severe dietary limitation, usually resulting in serious malnutrition.

### B. Diagnosis, signs, and symptoms.
See Table 14–1.

### C. Epidemiology
1. Prevalence—0.5–1% of adolescent girls.
2. Onset—usually 13–20 years; often associated with stressful life event.
3. Male-to-female ratio is 1:10–20.
4. Most common in professions that require thinness, e.g., modeling, ballet, and in developed countries.

### D. Etiology
1. **Biological.** Higher concordance rates in monozygotic (MZ) twins than in dizygotic twins (DZ). There is increased familial depression, alcohol dependence, or eating disorder. Some evidence of increased anorexia nervosa in sisters and a higher concordance in MZ than DZ twins. Neurobiologically, 3-methoxy-4-hydrozyphenylgylcol (MHPG) in urine and cerebrospinal fluid (CSF) is reduced, suggesting lessened norepinephrine turnover and activity. Endogenous opioid activity appears lessened as a consequence of starving. In one positron emission tomography (PET) scan study, caudate nucleus metabolism was higher during the anorectic state than after weight gain.
2. **Psychological.** Appears to be a reaction to demands for independence and social or sexual functioning in adolescence.
3. **Social.** Society's emphasis on thinness and exercise. Patient may have close but troubled relationship with parents.

### E. Psychodynamics
1. Patients are unable to separate psychologically from their mothers.
2. Pregnancy fear.
3. Repressed sexual or aggressive drives.

### F. Differential diagnosis
1. **Medical conditions and substance use disorders.** Medical illness, e.g., cancer, brain tumor, gastrointestinal (GI) disorders, drug abuse, that can account for weight loss.

TABLE 14-1
**DSM-IV DIAGNOSTIC CRITERIA FOR ANOREXIA NERVOSA**

A.  Refusal to maintain body weight at or above a minimally normal weight for age and height (e.g., weight loss leading to maintenance of body weight less than 85% of that expected; or failure to make expected weight gain during period of growth, leading to body weight less than 85% of that expected).
B.  Intense fear of gaining weight or becoming fat, even though underweight.
C.  Disturbance in the way in which one's body weight or shape is experienced, undue influence of body weight or shape on self-evaluation, or denial of the seriousness of the current low body weight.
D.  In postmenarcheal females, amenorrhea, i.e., the absence of at least three consecutive menstrual cycles. (A woman is considered to have amenorrhea if her periods occur only following hormone, e.g., estrogen, administration.)

*Specify* type:
   **Restricting type:** during the current episode of anorexia nervosa, the person has not regularly engaged in binge-eating or purging behavior (i.e., self-induced vomiting or the misuse of laxatives, diuretics, or enemas)
   **Binge-eating/purging type:** during the current episode of anorexia nervosa, the person has regularly engaged in binge-eating or purging behavior (i.e., self-induced vomiting or the misuse of laxatives, diuretics, or enemas)

Used with permission, APA.

2. **Depressive disorder.** Patient has a decreased appetite; anorexia nervosa patient claims to have a normal appetite and feel hungry (loss of appetite occurs only late in illness). No preoccupation with caloric content of food. No intense fear of obesity or disturbance of body image.

3. **Somatization disorder.** Weight loss not as severe; no morbid fear of becoming overweight; amenorrhea unusual.

4. **Bulimia nervosa.** Patient seldom has more than a 15% weight loss.

G. **Course and prognosis.** 40% recover, 30% improve, and 30% are chronic.

H. **Treatment**

1. May be outpatient or inpatient pediatric, medical, or psychiatric unit, depending on degree of weight loss and physical condition. Psychiatry unit is indicated, if physical condition permits, when there is depression, high suicide risk, or family crisis. Inpatient treatment of starvation provides for (1) assured weight gain and (2) the monitoring and treatment of the potentially life-threatening effects of starvation (and metabolic complications of bulimia nervosa, if present). A desired weight is set and a strategy devised, which may include supervised meals, food supplements, and nasogastric feedings for uncooperative patients.

2. **Pharmacological.** Anorexia nervosa patients often resist medication, and no drugs are of proven efficacy. Most promising is cyproheptadine (Periactin), and antidepressants are tried if major depressive disorder coexists. Serotonergic agents, as well as bupropion (Wellbutrin), may be useful.

3. **Psychological.** Psychotherapy is generally ineffective. Cognitive behavior therapy aimed at changing attitudes and habits concerning food, eating, and body image seems promising. Family therapy also is useful.

## III. Bulimia nervosa

**A. Definition.** Episodic, uncontrolled, compulsive, and rapid ingestion of large amounts of food over a short period of time (binge eating) followed by self-induced vomiting, use of laxatives or diuretics, fasting, or vigorous exercise in order to prevent weight gain (binge and purge).

**B. Diagnosis, signs, and symptoms.** See Table 14–2.

**C. Epidemiology**
1. Prevalence—1–3% of young women.
2. Onset usually $16\frac{1}{2}$–18 years.
3. Male-to-female ratio is 1:10.

**D. Etiology**
1. **Biological.** Metabolic studies indicate less norepinephrine and serotonin activity and turnover. Plasma levels are raised in some bulimia nervosa patients who vomit. Many are depressed; increased family history of depression and obesity.
2. **Social.** Reflects society's premium on thinness. Patients tend to be perfectionistic and achievement oriented. Family strife, rejection, and neglect are more common than in anorexia nervosa.
3. **Psychological.** Patients have difficulties with adolescent demands, but bulimia nervosa patients are more outgoing, angry, and impulsive than anorexia nervosa patients. Patients may fear leaving the family after school. Anxiety and depressive symptoms are common; suicide is a risk. Alcohol abuse occurs, and approximately one third shoplift food.

**E. Psychodynamics**
1. Struggle for separation from the maternal figure is played out in ambivalence toward food.
2. Sexual and aggressive fantasies are unacceptable and disgorged symbolically.

TABLE 14–2
**DSM-IV DIAGNOSTIC CRITERIA FOR BULIMIA NERVOSA**

A. Recurrent episodes of binge eating. An episode of binge eating is characterized by both of the following:
    (1) eating, in a discrete period of time (e.g., within any 2-hour period), an amount of food that is definitely larger than most people would eat during a similar period of time and under similar circumstances
    (2) a sense of lack of control over eating during the episode (e.g., a feeling that one cannot stop eating or control what or how much one is eating)
B. Recurrent inappropriate compensatory behavior in order to prevent weight gain, such as self-induced vomiting; misuse of laxatives, diuretics, enemas, or other medications; fasting; or excessive exercise.
C. The binge eating and inappropriate compensatory behaviors both occur, on average, at least twice a week for 3 months.
D. Self-evaluation is unduly influenced by body shape and weight.
E. The disturbance does not occur exclusively during episodes of anorexia nervosa.

*Specify* type:
    **Purging type:** during the current episode of bulimia nervosa, the person has regularly engaged in self-induced vomiting or the misuse of laxatives, diuretics, or enemas
    **Nonpurging type:** during the current episode of bulimia nervosa, the person has used other inappropriate compensatory behaviors, such as fasting or excessive exercise, but has not regularly engaged in self-induced vomiting or the misuse of laxatives, diuretics, or enemas

Used with permission, APA.

## F. Differential diagnosis

1. **Neurological disease.** For example, epileptic-equivalent seizures, central nervous system tumors, Klüver-Bucy syndrome, Kleine-Levin syndrome.
2. **Borderline personality disorder.** Patients sometimes binge eat, but the eating is associated with other signs of the disorder.
3. **Major depressive disorder.** Patients rarely have peculiar attitudes or idiosyncratic practices regarding food.

## G. Course and prognosis.
Course is usually chronic but not debilitating when not complicated by electrolyte imbalance and metabolic alkalosis.

## H. Treatment

1. **Hospitalization.** Electrolyte imbalance, metabolic alkalosis, and suicidality may necessitate hospitalization.
2. **Pharmacological.** Antidepressants appear to be more beneficial than in anorexia nervosa. Imipramine (Tofranil), desipramine (Norpramin), trazodone (Desyrel), and the monoamine oxidase inhibitors (MAOIs), e.g., phenelzine (Nardil), have reduced symptoms in studies. Fluoxetine (Prozac) is also of reported benefit in reducing binge eating and subsequent purging episodes.
3. **Psychological.** Lack of control over eating usually motivates desire for therapy, which may include individual psychotherapy, cognitive behavioral therapy, and group psychotherapy. Normalization of eating habits, attitudes about food, and the pursuit of the ideal body must be addressed.

---

*For a more detailed discussion of this topic, see Garfinkel PE: Eating Disorders, Chap 22, p 1361, in CTP/VI.*

# 15

# Sleep Disorders

## I. General introduction

Sleep disturbances are common in the general population and among patients with mental disorders. Insomnia is the most prevalent disorder. Up to 30% of the population suffers from insomnia and seeks help for it. Other conditions include excessive daytime sleepiness, difficulty sleeping during desired sleep time, and unusual nocturnal events, such as nightmares and sleepwalking.

In DSM-IV, sleep disorders are classified on the basis of clinical diagnostic criteria and presumed etiology. The three major categories are (1) primary sleep disorders, (2) sleep disorders related to another mental disorder, and (3) other sleep disorders (due to a general medical condition and substance-induced).

### A. Sleep stages.
Sleep is measured with a polysomnograph, which simultaneously measures brain activity—electroencephalogram (EEG), eye movement—electro-oculogram (EOG), and muscle tone—electromyogram (EMG). Other physiological tests can be applied during sleep and measured along with the above. EEG findings are used to describe sleep stages (Table 15–1).

It takes the average person 15–20 minutes to fall asleep. Over the next 45 minutes, one descends to stages 3 and 4 (deepest sleep, largest stimulus needed to arouse). Approximately 45 minutes after stage 4, reachs the first rapid eye movement (REM) period (average REM latency is 90 minutes). As the night progresses, each REM period gets longer and stages 3 and 4 disappear. Further into the night, persons sleep more lightly and dream (REM sleep).

### B. Characteristics of REM sleep
1. Tonic inhibition of skeletal muscle tone.
2. Reduced hypercapnic respiratory drive.
3. Relative poikilothermia (cold bloodedness).
4. Penile tumescence.

### C. Sleep and aging
1. Subjective reports of elderly
   a. Time in bed increases.
   b. Number of nocturnal awakenings increases.
   c. Total sleep time at night decreases.
   d. Time to fall asleep increases.
   e. Dissatisfaction with sleep.

TABLE 15–1
**SLEEP STAGES**

| | |
|---|---|
| Awake | Low voltage, random, very fast |
| Drowsiness | Alpha waves random and fast (8–12 cycles per second (CPS)) |
| Stage I | Slight slowing, 3–7 CPS, theta waves |
| Stage II | Further slowing, K complex (triphasic complexes), 12–14 CPS (sleep spindles); this stage marks the onset of true sleep |
| Stage III | High amplitude, slow waves (delta waves) at 0.5–2.5 CPS |
| Stage IV | At least 50% delta waves on EEG (stages 3 and 4 constitute delta sleep) |
| REM sleep | Sawtooth waves, similar to drowsy sleep on EEG |

TABLE 15–2
**NONSPECIFIC MEASURES TO INDUCE SLEEP (SLEEP HYGIENE)**

1. Arise at the same time daily.
2. Limit daily in-bed time to the usual amount present before the sleep disturbance.
3. Discontinue CNS-acting drugs (caffeine, nicotine, alcohol, stimulants).
4. Avoid daytime naps (except when sleep chart shows they induce better night sleep).
5. Establish physical fitness by means of a graded program of vigorous exercise early in the day.
6. Avoid evening stimulation; substitute radio or relaxed reading for television.
7. Try very hot, 20-minute, body temperature-raising bath soaks near bedtime.
8. Eat at regular times daily; avoid large meals near bedtime.
9. Practice evening relaxation routines, such as progressive muscle relaxation or meditation.
10. Maintain comfortable sleeping conditions.

Table from Regestein QR: Sleep disorders. In *Clinical Psychiatry for Medical Students*, A Stoudemire, editor, p 578. Lippincott, Philadelphia, 1990. Used with permission.

      f. Tired and sleepy in the daytime.

      g. More frequent napping.

  2. Objective evidence of age-related changes in sleep cycle

      a. Reduced total REM.

      b. Reduced stages 3 and 4.

      c. Frequent awakenings.

      d. Reduced duration of nocturnal sleep.

      e. Need for daytime naps.

      f. Propensity for phase advance.

  3. Sleep disorders that are more common in the elderly

      a. Nocturnal myoclonus.

      b. Restless legs syndrome.

      c. REM sleep behavior disturbance.

      d. Sleep apnea.

      e. Sundowning (confusion from sedation).

  4. Medications and medical disorders also contribute to the problem.

## II. Primary sleep disorders

### A. Dyssomnias.

  **1. Primary insomnia.** The term ''primary'' indicates that the insomnia occurs independently of any known physical or mental condition. It is characterized by difficulty in falling asleep and repeated awakenings, which continue for at least a month.

    a. Treatment can include deconditioning techniques, transcendental meditation, relaxation tapes, sedatives, or carefully administered hypnotics.

    b. Nonspecific measures (sleep hygiene) are discussed in Table 15–2.

2. **Primary hypersomnia.** Diagnosed when no other cause for excessive somnolence occurring for at least 1 month can be found. Treatment consists of stimulant drugs (such as amphetamines) given in the morning or evening.

3. **Narcolepsy**
   a. **Characterized by symptom tetrad**—(1) excessive daytime somnolence, (2) cataplexy, (3) sleep paralysis, and (4) hypnagogic hallucinations.
   
   i. **Excessive daytime somnolence**
      (a) Considered to be the primary symptom of narcolepsy; others are auxiliary.
      (b) Distinguished from fatigue by irresistible sleep attacks of short duration—less than 15 minutes.
      (c) Sleep attacks may be precipitated by monotonous or sedentary activity.
      (d) Naps are highly refreshing—effects last 30–120 minutes.
   
   ii. **Cataplexy**
      (a) Reported by 70–80% of narcoleptics.
      (b) Brief (seconds to minutes) episodes of muscle weakness or paralysis.
      (c) No loss of consciousness, if episode is brief.
      (d) When attack is over, the patient is completely normal.
      (e) Often triggered by:
         (1) Laughter (common).
         (2) Anger (common).
         (3) Athletic activity.
         (4) Excitement or elation.
         (5) Sexual intercourse.
         (6) Fear.
         (7) Embarrassment.
      (f) Some patients develop flat affect or lack of expressiveness as attempt to control emotions.
      (g) May manifest as partial loss of muscle tone (weakness, slurred speech, buckled knees, dropped jaw).
   
   iii. **Sleep paralysis**
      (a) Reported by 25–50% of general population.
      (b) Temporary partial or complete paralysis in sleep-wake transitions.
      (c) Most commonly occurs upon awakening.
      (d) Conscious but unable to move.
      (e) Generally lasts less than 1 minute.
   
   iv. **Hypnagogic hallucinations**
      (a) Dreamlike experience during transition from wakefulness to sleep.
      (b) Patient is aware of surroundings.
      (c) Vivid auditory or visual hallucinations or illusions.
      (d) Appear several years after the onset of sleep attacks.

**b. Sleep onset REM periods (SOREMPs)**
  i.   Narcolepsy can be distinguished from other disorders of excessive daytime sleepiness by SOREMPs.
  ii.  Defined as appearance of REM within 10–15 minutes of sleep onset.
  iii. Multiple Sleep Latency Test (MSLT) measures excessive sleepiness—patient given five 20-minute periods every 2 hours. More than one SOREMP is considered diagnostic of narcolepsy. (Seen in 70% of patients with narcolepsy, in fewer than 10% of patients with other hypersomnias.)

**c. Increased incidence of other clinical findings in narcolepsy**
  i.   Periodic leg movement.
  ii.  Sleep apnea—predominantly central.
  iii. Short sleep latency.
  iv.  Memory problems.
  v.   Ocular symptoms—blurring, diplopia, flickering.
  vi.  Depression.

**d. Onset and clinical course**
  i.   Insidious onset before age 15. Once established, condition is chronic without major remissions.
  ii.  Typically, full syndrome emerges in late adolescence or early 20s.
  iii. There may be long delay between the earliest symptoms (excessive somnolence) and the late appearance of cataplexy.

**e. HLA-DR2 and narcolepsy**
  i.   Strong association between narcolepsy and HLA-antigen DR2, a type of human lymphocyle antigen.
  ii.  Some experts maintain that the presence of HLA-antigen DR2 is necessary for the diagnosis of idiopathic narcolepsy.

**f. Treatment**
  i.   Regular bedtime.
  ii.  Daytime naps.
  iii. Safety considerations, such as caution in driving or avoiding having furniture with sharp edges.
  iv.  Stimulants for daytime sleepiness. High-dose propranolol (Inderal) may be effective.
  v.   Tricyclics and monoamine oxidase inhibitors (MAOIs) for REM-related symptoms, especially cataplexy (Table 15–3).

**4. Breathing-related sleep disorder.** Characterized by sleep disruption leading to excessive sleepiness or insomnia that is due to a sleep-related breathing disturbance. The three types of sleep apnea are (1) obstructive, (2) central, and (3) mixed.

**a. Obstructive sleep apnea**
  i.   Main symptoms—loud snoring with intervals of apnea.
  ii.  Extreme daytime sleepiness with long and unrefreshing daytime sleep attacks.
  iii. Patients unaware of apneas.
  iv.  Other symptoms include severe morning headaches, morning confusion, depression, and anxiety.

TABLE 15-3
**NARCOLEPSY DRUGS CURRENTLY AVAILABLE**

| Drug | Maximal Dosage (All Drugs Administered Orally) |
|---|---|
| *Treatment of excessive daytime somnolence (EDS)* | |
| Stimulants | |
| Amphetamine | ≤ 40 mg/day |
| Methylphenidate | ≤ 60 mg/day |
| Pemoline | ≤150 mg/day |
| Adjunct effect drugs (i.e., improve EDS if associated with stimulant) | |
| Protriptyline | ≤ 10 mg/day |
| *Treatment of cataplexy, sleep paralysis, and hypnagogic hallucinations* | |
| Tricyclic antidepressants (with atropinic side effects) | |
| Protriptyline | ≤ 20 mg/day |
| Imipramine | ≤200 mg/day |
| Clomipramine | ≤200 mg/day |
| Desipramine | ≤200 mg/day |
| Antidepressants (without major atropinic side effects) | |
| Bupropion | ≤300 mg/day |

Table adapted from Guilleminault C: Narcolepsy syndrome. In *Principles and Practice of Sleep Medicine*, MH Kryger, T Roth, WC Dement, eds. WB Saunders, Philadelphia, 1989, p 344.

    v.   Findings include hypertension, arrhythmias, right-sided heart failure, and peripheral edema; progressively worsens without treatment.

    vi.   Sleep lab evaluation reveals cessation of airflow in the presence of continued thoracic breathing movements.

    vii.   In severe cases, persons have over 500 apneas a night.

    viii.   Each lasts 10–20 seconds.

    ix.   Treatment consists of nasal continuous positive airway pressure (CPAP), uvulopharyngopalatoplasty, weight loss, or protriptyline (Vivactil). If a specific upper airway abnormality is found, surgical intervention is indicated.

**b. Central sleep apnea**

    i.   Rare.

    ii.   Cessation of air flow secondary to lack of respiratory effort.

    iii.   Treatment consists of mechanical ventilation or nasal CPAP.

**c. Central alveolar hypoventilation**—central apnea followed by an obstructive phase.

    i.   Impaired ventilation in which the respiratory abnormality appears or greatly worsens only during sleep and in which significant apneic episodes are absent.

    ii.   The ventilatory dysfunction is characterized by inadequate tidal volume or respiratory rate during sleep.

    iii.   Death may occur during sleep (Ondine's curse).

    iv.   Central alveolar hypoventilation is treated with some form of mechanical ventilation, e.g., nasal ventilation.

**5. Circadian rhythm sleep disorder.** Includes a wide range of conditions involving a misalignment between desired and actual sleep periods.

  a. Transient disturbances associated with jet lag and work shift changes.

    i.   Self-limited. Resolve as body readjusts to new sleep-wake schedule.

ii. Adjusting to an advance of sleep time is more difficult than adjusting to a delay.
  b. Disturbances include (1) delayed sleep-phase type, (2) jet lag type, (3) shift work type, and (4) unspecified type, e.g., advanced sleep phase, non-24 hour, and irregular or disorganized sleep-wake pattern.
    i. Quality of sleep basically is normal, but timing is off.
    ii. Patient can adjust through gradual delay of sleep time until new schedule is achieved.
  c. Most effective treatment of sleep-wake schedule disorders is a regular schedule of bright light therapy to entrain the sleep cycle. More useful in transient than in persistent disturbances. Melatonin, a natural hormone that induces sleep, produced by the pineal gland, has been used orally to alter sleep-wake cycles, but its effect is uncertain.

## 6. Dyssomnia not otherwise specified (NOS)

  a. **Nocturnal myoclonus**
    i. Stereotypical leg movements—periodic every 30 seconds.
    ii. No seizure activity.
    iii. Most prevalent in patients over age 55.
    iv. Frequent awakenings.
    v. Unrefreshing sleep.
    vi. Daytime sleepiness is a major symptom.
    vii. Patient is unaware of the myoclonic events.
    viii. Various drugs have been reported to help. These include clonazepam (Klonopin), opioids, and L-dopa (Larodopa).

  b. **Restless legs syndrome**
    i. Uncomfortable sensations in legs at rest.
    ii. Not limited to sleep, but can interfere with falling asleep.
    iii. Relieved by movement.
    iv. Patient may have associated sleep-related myoclonus.
    v. Benzodiazepines, e.g., clonazepam, are the treatment of choice. In severe cases, L-dopa or opioids may be used.

  c. **Kleine-Levin syndrome**
    i. Periodic disorder of hypersomnolence.
    ii. Usually affects young men who sleep excessively for several weeks.
    iii. Patient awakens only to eat (voraciously).
    iv. Associated with hypersexuality and extreme hostility.
    v. Amnesia follows attacks.
    vi. May resolve spontaneously after several years.
    vii. Patients are normal between episodes.
    viii. Treatment consists of stimulants (amphetamines, methylphenidate [Ritalin], and pemoline [Cylert]) for hypersomnia and preventive measures for other symptoms. Lithium also has been used successfully.

  d. **Menstrual-associated syndrome.** Some women experience intermittent marked hypersomnia, altered behavior patterns, and voracious eating at or shortly before the onset of menses.

e. **Insufficient sleep.** Characterized by complaints of daytime sleepiness, irritability, inability to concentrate, and impaired judgment by a person who persistently fails to sleep enough to support alert wakefulness.

f. **Sleep drunkenness**
   i. Inability to become fully alert for sustained period after awakening.
   ii. Most commonly seen with sleep apnea or after sustained sleep deprivation.
   iii. Can occur as an isolated disorder.
   iv. No specific treatment. Stimulants may be of limited value.

## B. Parasomnias

### 1. Nightmare disorder
a. Nightmares almost always occur during REM sleep.
b. Can occur at any time of night.
c. Good recall (quite detailed).
d. Long, frightening dream in which one awakens frightened.
e. Less anxiety, vocalization, motility, and autonomic discharge than in sleep terrors.
f. No specific treatment; benzodiazepines may be of help.

### 2. Sleep terror disorder
a. Especially common in children.
b. Sudden awakening with intense anxiety.
c. Autonomic overstimulation.
d. Movement.
e. Crying out.
f. Patient does not remember the event.
g. Occurs during deep non-REM sleep.
h. Often occurs within the first hour or two of sleep.
i. Treatment rarely is needed in childhood.
j. Awakening child prior to regular night terror for several days may eliminate terrors for extended periods.

### 3. Sleepwalking disorder
a. Also known as somnambulism.
b. Most common in children; generally disappears spontaneously with age.
c. Patients often have familial history of other parasomnias.
d. Complex activity—leaving bed and walking about without full consciousness.
e. Episodes are brief.
f. Amnesia for the event—patient does not remember the episode.
g. Occurs during deep non-REM sleep.
h. Initiated in first third of the night.
i. In adults and elderly persons, may reflect psychopathology—rule out central nervous system (CNS) pathology.
j. Can sometimes be initiated by placing a child who is in stage 4 sleep in the standing position.
k. Potentially dangerous.

l. Drugs that suppress stage 4 sleep, such as benzodiazepines, can be used to treat somnambulism.

m. Precautions include window guards and other measures to prevent injury.

### 4. Parasomnia NOS

**a. Sleep-related bruxism.**
   i.   Primarily occurs in stages 1 and 2 or during partial arousals or transitions.
   ii.  No EEG abnormality (no seizure activity).
   iii. Treatment consists of bite plates to prevent dental damage.

**b. REM sleep behavior syndrome**
   i.   Chronic and progressive, chiefly in elderly men.
   ii.  Loss of atonia during REM sleep with emergence of complex and violent behaviors.
   iii. Potential for serious injury.
   iv.  Neurological cause in many cases.
   v.   May occur during withdrawal REM rebound.
   vi.  Treat with clonazepam 0.5–2.0 mg a day, or carbamazepine (Tegretol), 100 mg 3 times a day.

**c. Sleeptalking (Somniloquy)**
   i.  Sometimes accompanies night terrors and sleepwalking.
   ii. Requires no treatment.

**d. Head banging (Jactatio capitis nocturnus)**
   i.   Rhythmic head or body rocking just before or during sleep; may extend into light sleep.
   ii.  Usually limited to childhood.
   iii. Usually observed in immediate presleep period and is sustained into light sleep.
   iv.  No treatment is required in most infants and young children. Crib padding or helmets may be used. Behavior modification, benzodiazepines, and tricyclic drugs may be effective.

**e. Familial sleep paralysis**
   i.   Isolated symptom.
   ii.  Not associated with narcolepsy.
   iii. Episode terminates with touch or noise (some external stimulus).

## III. Sleep disorders related to another mental disorder

A. Insomnia that is related to a mental disorder (such as major depressive disorder, panic disorder, schizophrenia) and that lasts for at least 1 month.

B. Hypersomnia related to a mental disorder usually found in a variety of conditions, such as the early stages of mild depressive disorder, grief, personality disorders, dissociative disorders, and somatoform disorders.

## IV. Other sleep disorders

### A. Sleep disorder due to a general medical condition.

1. Insomnia, hypersomnia, parasomnia, or combination can be caused by a general medical condition.

    **a. Sleep-related epileptic seizures**—seizures occur almost exclusively during sleep.

    **b. Sleep-related cluster headaches and chronic paroxysmal hemicrania**

        i.  Sleep-related cluster headaches are severe, unilateral, appear often during sleep, and are marked by an on-off pattern of attacks.

        ii.  Chronic paroxysmal hemicrania is a unilateral headache with frequent but short-lived onset without a preponderant sleep distribution.

        iii.  Both types appear in association with REM sleep periods.

    **c. Sleep-related abnormal swallowing syndrome**—inadequate swallowing results in aspiration of saliva, coughing, and choking.

    **d. Sleep-related cardiovascular symptoms**—associated with disorders of cardiac rhythm, myocardial incompetence, coronary artery insufficiency, and blood pressure variability, which may be induced or exacerbated by sleep-altered or sleep-stage-modified cardiovascular physiology.

    **e. Sleep-related gastroesophageal reflux**—Patient awakens from sleep with burning, substernal pain, feeling of tightness or pain in the chest, or a sour taste in the mouth. Often associated with hiatal hernia.

    **f. Sleep-related hemolysis (paroxysmal nocturnal hemoglobinuria)**—rare, acquired, chronic hemolytic anemia. The hemolysis and consequent hemoglobinuria are accelerated during sleep, coloring the morning urine brownish red.

  2.  Treatment, whenever possible, should be of the underlying medical condition.

**B. Substance-induced sleep disorder.** Insomnia, hypersomnia, parasomnia, or combination caused by a medication, intoxication, or withdrawal from drug of abuse.

  1.  Somnolence can be related to tolerance or withdrawal from a CNS stimulant, or to sustained use of CNS depressants.

  2.  Insomnia is associated with tolerance to or withdrawal from sedative-hypnotic drugs, CNS stimulants, or long-term alcohol consumption.

  3.  Sleep problems may occur as a side effect of many drugs, e.g., antimetabolites, thyroid preparations, anticonvulsant agents, antidepressants.

---

*For a more detailed discussion of this topic, see Gillin JC, Zoltoski RK, Salin-Pascual RJ: Basic Science of Sleep, Sec 1.9, p 89; Williams RL, Karacan I, Moore CA, Hirshkowitz M: Sleep Disorders, Chap 23, p 1373; Prinz PN, Vitiello MV, Borson S: Sleep Disorders, Sec 49.6f, p 2576, in CTP/VI.*

# 16

# Impulse-Control and Adjustment Disorders

## I. Impulse-control disorders

A. **Definition.** The inability to resist acting on an impulse or drive that is dangerous to others or to oneself and that is often characterized by a sense of pleasure when gratified. The six DSM-IV categories are:

1. **Intermittent explosive disorder**—episodes of aggression resulting in harm to others.
2. **Kleptomania**—repeated shoplifting or stealing.
3. **Pathological gambling**—repeated gambling episodes that result in socioeconomic disruption, indebtedness, illegal activities.
4. **Pyromania**—deliberate setting of fires.
5. **Trichotillomania**—compulsive hair pulling producing bald spots (alopecia areata).
6. **Impulse-control disorder not otherwise specified (NOS)**—residual category.

B. **Diagnosis, signs, and symptoms.** See Tables 16–1 through 16–5.

C. **Epidemiology**

1. Intermittent explosive disorder, pathological gambling, pyromania: affected men outnumber affected women.
2. Kleptomania, trichotillomania: women are affected more often than men.
3. Pathological gambling: affects 1–3% of adult United States population.

D. **Etiology.** Usually unknown. Some disorders may yield abnormal electroencephalogram (EEG) results, mixed cerebral dominance or soft neurological signs, e.g., intermittent explosive disorder. Alcohol reduces the patient's ability to control impulses (disinhibition).

E. **Psychodynamics.** Acting out of impulses related to the need to express sexual or aggressive drive. Gambling often is associated with underlying depression representing an unconscious need to lose and experience punishment.

F. **Differential diagnosis.** See Table 16–6.

1. **Temporal lobe epilepsy.** Characteristic temporal lobe abnormal EEG foci account for aggressive outbursts, kleptomania, or pyromania.
2. **Head trauma.** Brain imaging techniques will show residual signs of trauma.
3. **Bipolar I disorder.** Gambling may be an associated feature of manic episodes
4. **Substance-related disorder.** Will reveal history of drug or alcohol use.

TABLE 16-1
**DSM-IV DIAGNOSTIC CRITERIA FOR INTERMITTENT EXPLOSIVE DISORDER**

A. Several discrete episodes of failure to resist aggressive impulses that result in serious assaultive acts or destruction of property.
B. The degree of aggressiveness expressed during the episodes is grossly out of proportion to any precipitating psychosocial stressors.
C. The aggressive episodes are not better accounted for by another mental disorder (e.g., antisocial personality disorder, borderline personality disorder, a psychotic disorder, a manic episode, conduct disorder, or attention-deficit/hyperactivity disorder) and are not due to the direct physiological effects of a substance (e.g., a drug of abuse, a medication) or a general medical condition (e.g., head trauma, Alzheimer's disease).

Used with permission, APA.


TABLE 16-2
**DSM-IV DIAGNOSTIC CRITERIA FOR KLEPTOMANIA**

A. Recurrent failure to resist impulses to steal objects that are not needed for personal use or for their monetary value.
B. Increasing sense of tension immediately before committing the theft.
C. Pleasure, gratification, or relief at the time of committing the theft.
D. The stealing is not committed to express anger or vengeance and is not in response to a delusion or a hallucination.
E. The stealing is not better accounted for by conduct disorder, a manic episode, or antisocial personality disorder.

Used with permission, APA.


TABLE 16-3
**DSM-IV DIAGNOSTIC CRITERIA FOR PYROMANIA**

A. Deliberate and purposeful fire setting on more than one occasion.
B. Tension or affective arousal before the act.
C. Fascination with, interest in, curiosity about, or attraction to fire and its situational contexts (e.g., paraphernalia, uses, consequences).
D. Pleasure, gratification, or relief when setting fires, or when witnessing or participating in their aftermath.
E. The fire setting is not done for monetary gain, as an expression of sociopolitical ideology, to conceal criminal activity, to express anger or vengeance, to improve one's living circumstances, in response to a delusion or hallucination, or as a result of impaired judgment (e.g., in dementia, mental retardation, substance intoxication).
F. The fire setting is not better accounted for by conduct disorder, a manic episode, or antisocial personality disorder.

Used with permission, APA.


5. **Medical Condition.** Rule out organic disorder, brain tumor, degenerative disease, and endocrine disorder on basis of characteristic findings for each.

6. **Schizophrenia.** Shows delusions or hallucinations to account for acting out of impulse.

G. **Course and prognosis.** See Table 16–6. Course usually is chronic for all impulse-control disorders.

H. **Treatment**

1. **Intermittent explosive disorder.** Combined pharmacotherapy and psychotherapy. May have to try different medications, e.g., phenothiazines, imipramine (Tofranil), lithium (Eskalith) before result is achieved. If EEG findings are abnormal, carbamazepine (Tegretol) may be used. Benzodiazepines can aggravate the condition because of disinhi-

TABLE 16–4
**DSM-IV DIAGNOSTIC CRITERIA FOR PATHOLOGICAL GAMBLING**

A. Persistent and recurrent maladaptive gambling behavior as indicated by five (or more) of the following:
   (1) is preoccupied with gambling (e.g., preoccupied with reliving past gambling experiences, handicapping or planning the next venture, or thinking of ways to get money with which to gamble)
   (2) needs to gamble with increasing amounts of money in order to achieve the desired excitement
   (3) has repeated unsuccessful efforts to control, cut back, or stop gambling
   (4) is restless or irritable when attempting to cut down or stop gambling
   (5) gambles as a way of escaping from problems or of relieving a dysphoric mood (e.g., feelings of helplessness, guilt, anxiety, depression)
   (6) after losing money gambling, often returns another day to get even (''chasing'' one's losses)
   (7) lies to family members, therapist, or others to conceal the extent of involvement with gambling
   (8) has committed illegal acts such as forgery, fraud, theft, or embezzlement to finance gambling
   (9) has jeopardized or lost a significant relationship, job, or educational or career opportunity because of gambling
   (10) relies on others to provide money to relieve a desperate financial situation caused by gambling
B. The gambling behavior is not better accounted for by a manic episode.

Used with permission, APA.

TABLE 16–5
**DSM-IV DIAGNOSTIC CRITERIA FOR TRICHOTILLOMANIA**

A. Recurrent pulling out of one's hair resulting in noticeable hair loss.
B. An increasing sense of tension immediately before pulling out the hair or when attempting to resist the behavior.
C. Pleasure, gratification, or relief when pulling out the hair.
D. The disturbance is not better accounted for by another mental disorder and is not due to a general medical condition (e.g., a dermatological condition).
E. The disturbance causes clinically significant distress or impairment in social, occupational, or other important areas of functioning.

Used with permission, APA.

bition. Propranolol (Inderal) can be of help in selected cases. Other measures include supportive psychotherapy, limit-setting, family therapy if the patient is child or adolescent. Group therapy must be used cautiously if the patient is liable to attack fellow group members.

2. **Kleptomania.** Insight-oriented psychotherapy to understand motivation (e.g., guilt, need for punishment) and to control impulse. Behavior therapy to learn new patterns of behavior. Underlying depression responds to antidepressants drugs. Serotonin-specific reuptake inhibitors (SSRIs), e.g., fluoxetine (Prozac), may be effective in some kleptomania patients.

3. **Pathological gambling.** Insight-oriented psychotherapy coupled with peer support groups, especially Gamblers Anonymous (GA). Total abstinence is the goal. Treat associated depression, mania, substance abuse, or sexual dysfunction.

4. **Pyromania.** Insight-oriented therapy, behavior therapy. Patients require close supervision because of repeated fire-setting behavior and consequent danger to others. May need inpatient facility, night hospital, or other structured setting.

5. **Trichotillomania.** Supportive and insight-oriented psychotherapies are of value, but medications may also be required: benzodiazepines

TABLE 16–6
**DIFFERENTIAL DIAGNOSIS, COURSE, AND PROGNOSIS FOR IMPULSE CONTROL DISORDERS**

| Disorder | Differential Diagnosis | Course and Prognosis |
|---|---|---|
| Intermittent explosive disorder | Delirium, dementia<br>Personality change due to a general medical condition, aggressive type<br>Substance intoxication or withdrawal<br>Oppositional defiant disorder, conduct disorder, antisocial disorder, manic episode, schizophrenia<br>Purposeful behavior; malingering<br>Temporal lobe epilepsy | May increase in severity with time |
| Kleptomania | Ordinary theft<br>Malingering<br>Antisocial personality disorder, conduct disorder<br>Manic episode<br>Delusions, hallucinations, (e.g., schizophrenia)<br>Dementia<br>Temporal lobe epilepsy | Frequently arrested for shoplifting |
| Pyromania | Arson: profit, sabotage, revenge, political statement<br>Childhood experimentation<br>Conduct disorder<br>Manic episode<br>Antisocial personality disorder<br>Delusions, hallucinations (e.g., schizophrenia)<br>Dementia<br>Mental retardation<br>Substance intoxication<br>Temporal lobe epilepsy | Often produce increasingly larger fires over time |
| Pathological gambling | Social or professional gambling<br>Manic episode<br>Antisocial personality disorder | Progressive with increasing financial losses, writing bad checks, total deterioration |
| Trichotillomania | Alopecia areata, male-pattern baldness, chronic discoid lupus erythematosus, lichen planopilaris, or other cause of alopecia<br>Obsessive-compulsive disorder<br>Stereotypic movement disorder<br>Delusion, hallucination<br>Factitious disorder | Remissions and exacerbations |

for patients with high anxiety level; antidepressant drugs, especially serotonergic agents, e.g., SSRIs, clomipramine (Anafranil), for patients with or without depressed mood. Consider hypnosis and biofeedback in some cases.

## II. Adjustment disorders

**A. Definition.** Pathological behavioral response to a psychosocial stressor that results in impaired social or vocational functioning. Stressors are within the range of normal experience, e.g., birth of a baby, going away to school, marriage, job loss, divorce, illness.

TABLE 16–7
**DSM-IV DIAGNOSTIC CRITERIA FOR ADJUSTMENT DISORDERS**

A. The development of emotional or behavioral symptoms in response to an identifiable stressor(s) occurring within 3 months of the onset of the stressor(s).
B. These symptoms or behaviors are clinically significant as evidenced by either of the following:
   (1) marked distress that is in excess of what would be expected from exposure to the stressor
   (2) significant impairment in social or occupational (academic) functioning
C. The stress-related disturbance does not meet the criteria for another specific Axis I disorder and is not merely an exacerbation of a preexisting Axis I or Axis II disorder.
D. The symptoms do not represent bereavement.
E. Once the stressor (or its consequences) has terminated, the symptoms do not persist for more than an additional 6 months.

*Specify* if:
   **Acute:** if the disturbance lasts less than 6 months
   **Chronic:** if the disturbance lasts for 6 months or longer

Adjustment disorders are coded based on the subtype, which is selected to the predominant symptoms. The specific stressor(s) can be specified on Axis IV.
   **With depressed mood**
   **With anxiety**
   **With mixed anxiety and depressed mood**
   **With disturbance of conduct**
   **With mixed disturbance of emotions and conduct**
   **Unspecified**

Used with permission, APA.

**B. Diagnosis, signs, and symptoms.** See Table 16–7.

**C. Epidemiology.** Most frequent in adolescence, but can occur at any age.

**D. Etiology**
   **1. Genetic.** High anxiety temperament more prone to overreacting to a stressful event and experiencing subsequent adjustment disorders.
   **2. Biological.** Greater vulnerability with history of serious medical illness or disability.
   **3. Psychosocial.** Greater vulnerability in persons who lost a parent during infancy or who had poor mothering experiences. Ability to tolerate frustration in adult life correlates with gratification of basic needs in infant life.

**E. Differential diagnosis**
   **1. Posttraumatic stress disorder and acute stress disorder.** Psychosocial stressor determines diagnosis. Stressor is outside the range of normal human experience, e.g., war, rape, mass catastrophe, floods, being taken hostage.
   **2. Brief psychotic disorder.** Characterized by hallucinations and delusions.
   **3. Uncomplicated bereavement.** Occurs before, immediately, or shortly after death of a loved one; occupational or social functioning is impaired within expected bounds and remits spontaneously.

**F. Course and prognosis.** Most symptoms diminish over time without treatment, especially after stressor is removed; subgroup maintains chronic course with risk of secondary depression, anxiety, and substance use disorder.

**G. Treatment**
   **1. Psychological**
      **a. Psychotherapy**—the treatment of choice. Explore meaning of stres-

sor to the patient, provide support, encourage alternative ways of coping, offer empathy. Biofeedback, relaxation techniques, and hypnosis for anxious mood.

   **b. Crisis intervention**—aimed at helping the person resolve the situation quickly by supportive techniques, suggestion, reassurance, environmental modifications, and hospitalization, if necessary.

**2. Pharmacological.**    Patients can be treated with anxiolytic or antidepressant agents depending on the type of adjustment disorder, e.g., with anxiety, with depressed mood, but be careful to avoid drug dependency (especially if benzodiazepines are used).

---

*For more detailed discussion of this topic, see Impulse-Control Disorders Not Elsewhere Classified and Adjustment Disorders, Chap 24, pp 1409–1424, in CTP/VI.*

---

# 17

# Psychosomatic Disorders (Psychological Factors Affecting Medical Condition)

## I. Psychosomatic disorders

### A. Definition.
The term "psychosomatic disorder" refers to physical conditions caused or aggravated by psychological factors. Although most physical disorders are influenced by stress, conflict, or generalized anxiety, some disorders are more affected than others. In DSM-IV, psychosomatic disorders are subsumed under the classification of psychological factors affecting medical condition.

### B. Etiology

1. **Specificity theory.** This theory postulates specific stresses or personality types for each psychosomatic disease and is typified by the work of the following investigators:

   a. **Flanders Dunbar**—described personality traits that are specific for a psychosomatic disorder, e.g., coronary personality. Type A personality is hard-driving, aggressive, irritable, and susceptible to heart disease.

   b. **Franz Alexander**—described unconscious conflicts that produce anxiety, are mediated through the autonomic nervous system, and result in a specific disorder, e.g., repressed dependency needs result in peptic ulcer.

2. **Nonspecific theory.** This theory states that any prolonged stress can cause physiological changes that result in a physical disorder. Each person has a shock organ that is genetically vulnerable to stress: some patients are cardiac reactors, others are gastric reactors, and others are skin reactors. Persons who are chronically anxious or depressed are more vulnerable to physical or psychosomatic disease.

3. **Pathophysiology.** Hans Selye described the general adaption syndrome (GAS), which is the sum of all nonspecific systemic reactions of the body that follow prolonged stress. The hypothalamic-pituitary-adrenal axis is affected with excess secretion of cortisol, producing structural damage to various organ systems. George Engel postulated that in the stressed state, all neuroregulatory mechanisms undergo functional changes that depress the body's homeostatic mechanisms, leaving the body vulnerable to infection and other disorders.

   **Neurophysiological pathways** thought to mediate stress reactions include the cerebral cortex, limbic system, hypothalamus, adrenal medulla, and sympathetic and parasympathetic nervous systems. Neu-

romessengers include such hormones as cortisol, thyroxin, and epinephrine.

**C. Diagnosis.** To meet the diagnostic criteria for psychological factors affecting a medical condition, the following two criteria must be met: (1) a medical
condition is present, and (2) psychological factors adversely affect it, e.g.,
the psychologically meaningful environmental stimulus is temporally related
to the initiation or exacerbation of the specific physical condition or disorder.
The physical condition must show either demonstrable organic pathology,
e.g., rheumatoid arthritis, or a known pathophysiological process, e.g.,
migraine headache. A number of physical disorders meet these criteria and
are listed in Table 17–1.

**D. Medical, surgical, and neurological conditions that primarily
present with psychiatric symptoms.** A host of medical and neurological disorders, summarized in Table 17–2, may present with psychiatric
symptoms, which must be differentiated from primary psychiatric disorders.

**E. Differential diagnosis.** As outlined in Table 17–3, various psychiatric
syndromes and disorders can be confused with psychosomatic disorders.
Each lacks a demonstrable organic pathological lesion or known pathophysiological process.

**F. Treatment**

1. **Combined approach.** Necessary. Collaborate with internist or
   surgeon who manages physical disorder, with psychiatrist attending to
   psychiatric aspects.

2. **Supportive psychotherapy.** Of great value, especially when psychiatrist forms therapeutic alliance with patient. Psychiatrist allows
   patient to ventilate most fears of illness, especially death fantasies. Many
   patients have strong dependency needs, which are partially gratified
   in treatment.

3. **Dynamic insight-oriented psychotherapy.** Explore unconscious conflicts regarding sex and aggression. Anxiety associated with
   life stresses are examined and mature defenses are established.

4. **Group therapy.** Of use with patients who have similar physical
   conditions, e.g., colitis patients, hemodialysis patients.

5. **Family network therapy.** With patient's permission, the practitioner may see families, spouses, friends.

6. **Behavior therapy.** Behavior therapy, relaxation techniques, and
   biofeedback are useful when there is a strong autonomic nervous system
   component, e.g., asthma, allergies, hypertension.

7. **Pharmacotherapy**
   a. Use antipsychotic drugs when there is associated psychosis.
   b. Antianxiety drugs diminish harmful anxiety during period of acute
      stress. Limit use so as to avoid dependency.
   c. Antidepressants can be used with depression due to a medical condi-
      tion.

## II. Consultation-liaison (C-L) psychiatry

The C-L psychiatrist serves as a consultant to other fellow medical specialists
and usually operates directly in a surgical or medical setting, providing psychiat-

TABLE 17-1
**PHYSICAL CONDITIONS AFFECTED BY PSYCHOLOGICAL FACTORS**

| Disorder | Observations/Comments/Theory Approach |
|---|---|
| Angina, arrhythmias, coronary spasms | Type A person is aggressive, irritable, easily frustrated, and prone to coronary artery disease. Arrhythmias common in anxiety states. Sudden death from ventricular arrhythmia in some patients who experience massive psychological shock or catastrophe. Lifestyle changes: cease smoking, curb alcohol intake, lose weight, lower cholesterol to limit risk factors. Propranolol (Inderal) prescribed for patients who develop tachycardia as part of social phobia—protects against arrhythmia and decreases coronary blood flow. |
| Asthma | Attacks precipitated by stress, respiratory infection, allergy. Examine family dynamics, especially when child is the patient. Look for overprotectiveness and try to encourage appropriate independent activities. Propranolol and β-blockers contraindicated in asthma patients for anxiety. Psychological theories: strong dependency and separation anxiety; asthma wheeze is suppressed cry for love and protection. |
| Connective tissue diseases: systemic lupus erythematosus, rheumatoid arthritis | Disease can be heralded by major life stress, especially death of loved one. Worsens with chronic stress, anger, or depression. Important to keep patient as active as possible to minimize joint deformities. Treat depression with antidepressant medications or psychostimulants, and treat muscle spasm and tension with benzodiazepines. |
| Headaches | Tension headache results from contraction of strap muscles in neck constricting blood flow. Associated with anxiety, situational stress. Relaxation therapy, antianxiety medication useful. Migraine headaches are unilateral and can be triggered by stress, exercise, high tyramine foods. Manage with ergotamine (Cafergot). Propranolol prophylaxis can produce associated depression. Sumatriptan (Imitrex) can be used to treat nonhemiplegic and nonbasilar migraine attacks. |
| Hypertension | Acute stress produces catecholamines (epinephrine), raising systolic blood pressure. Chronic stress associated with essential hypertension. Look at lifestyle. Prescribe exercise, relaxation therapy, biofeedback. Benzodiazepines of use in acute stress if blood pressure rises as shock organ. Psychological theories: inhibited rage, guilt over hostile impulses, need to gain approval from authority. |
| Hyperventilation syndrome | Accompanies panic disorder, generalized anxiety disorder with associated hyperventilation, tachycardia, vasoconstriction. May be hazardous in patients with coronary insufficiency. Antianxiety agents of use; some patients respond to monoamine oxidase inhibitors, tricyclic antidepressants, or serotonergic agents. |
| Inflammatory bowel diseases: Crohn's disease, irritable bowel syndrome, ulcerative colitis | Depressed mood associated with illness; stress exacerbates symptoms. Onset after major life stress. Patients respond to stable doctor-patient relationship and supportive psychotherapy in addition to bowel medication. Psychological theories: passive personality, childhood intimidation, obsessive traits, fear of punishment, masked hostility. |
| Metabolic and endocrine disorders | Thyrotoxicosis following sudden severe stress. Glycosuria in chronic fear and anxiety. Depression alters hormone metabolism, especially adrenocorticotropic hormone (ACTH). |
| Neurodermatitis | Eczema in patients with multiple psychosocial stressors—especially death of loved one, conflicts over sexuality, repressed anger. Some respond to hypnosis in symptom management. |

*(continued on next page)*

TABLE 17–1 (continued)
**PHYSICAL CONDITIONS AFFECTED BY PSYCHOLOGICAL FACTORS**

| Disorder | Observations/Comments/Theory Approach |
|---|---|
| Obesity | Hyperphagia reduces anxiety. Night eating syndrome associated with insomnia. Failure to perceive appetite, hunger, and satiation. Psychological theories: conflicts about orality and pathologic dependency. Behavioral techiques, support groups, nutritional counseling, and supportive psychotherapy useful. Treat underlying depression. |
| Osteoarthritis | Lifestyle management induces weight reduction, isometric exercises to strengthen joint musculature, maintenance of physical activity, pain control. Treat associated anxiety or depression with supportive psychotherapy. |
| Peptic ulcer disease | Idiopathic type not related to specific bacterium or physical stimulus. Increased gastric acid and pepsin relative to mucosal resistance; both sensitive to anxiety, stress, coffee, alcohol. Lifestyle changes. Relaxation therapy. Psychological theories: strong frustrated dependency needs, cannot express anger, superficial self-sufficiency. |
| Raynaud's disease | Peripheral vasoconstriction associated with smoking, stress. Lifestyle changes: cessation of smoking, moderate exercise. Biofeedback can raise hand temperature by increased vasodilation. |
| Syncope, hypotension | Vaso-vagal reflex with acute anxiety or fear produces hypotension and fainting. More common in patients with hyperreactive autonomic nervous system. Aggravated by anemia, antidepressant medications (produces hypotension as side effect). |
| Urticaria, angioedema | Idiopathic type not related to specific allergens or physical stimulus. May be associated with stress, chronic anxiety, depression. Puritis worse with anxiety; self-excoriation associated with repressed hostility. Some phenothiazines have antipruritic effect. Psychological theories: conflict between dependence-independence, unconscious guilt feelings, itching as sexual displacement. |

ric consultation and management. Because 65% of medical inpatients have psychiatric problems and 50% are treatment problems, the C-L psychiatrist is important in the hospital setting. Table 17–4 lists the most common C-L problems encountered in general hospitals.

## III. Special medical settings

Besides the usual medical wards in a hospital, special settings produce uncommon, distinctive stress.

**A. Intensive Care Unit (ICU).** ICUs contains seriously ill patients who have life-threatening illnesses (coronary care units [CCUs] are good examples). Among the defensive reactions encountered are fear, anxiety, acting out, signing out against medical advice, hostility, dependency, depression, grief, and delirium.

**B. Hemodialysis.** Hemodialysis patients have a lifelong dependency on machines and health care providers. They have problems with prolonged dependency, regression to childhood states, hostility, and negativism in following the doctors' directions.

Dialysis dementia is a disorder characterized by loss of cognitive functions, dystonias, and seizures, which usually ends in death. It tends to occur in patients who have been on dialysis for long periods of time.

TABLE 17-2
MEDICAL CONDITIONS THAT PRESENT WITH PSYCHIATRIC SYMPTOMS

| Disease | Common Medical Symptoms | Psychiatric Symptoms and Complaints | Impaired Performance and Behavior | Laboratory Tests and Findings | Diagnostic Problems |
|---|---|---|---|---|---|
| AIDS | Fever Weight loss Ataxia Incontinence | Progressive dementia Personality changes Depression Loss of libido | Impaired memory Decreased concentration Seizures | HIV testing CT, MRI, lumbar puncture, CSF, and blood cultures | >60% of patients have neuropsychiatric symptoms; always consider in high-risk persons |
| Hyperthyroidism (thyrotoxicosis) | Heat intolerance Excessive sweating Diarrhea Weight loss Tachycardia Palpitations Vomiting | Nervousness Excitability Irritability Pressured speech Insomnia May express fear of impending death Psychosis | Fine tremor Impaired cognition Decreased concentration Hyperactivity Intrusiveness | Free $T_4$ increased $T_3$ increased TSH decreased $T_3$ uptake decreased ECG: Tachycardia Atrial fibrillation P and T wave changes | Full range of symptoms may not be present Hyperthyroidism and anxiety states may coexist Rule out occult malignancy, cardiovascular disease, amphetamine intoxication, cocaine intoxication, anxiety states, mania |
| Hypothyroidism (myxedema) | Cold intolerance Dry skin Constipation Weight gain Brittle hair Goiter | Lethargy Depressed affect Personality change Maniclike psychosis Paranoia Hallucinations | Muscle weakness Decreased concentration Psychomotor slowing Apathy Unusual sensitivity to barbiturates | TSH increased TSH low if pituitary disease Free $T_4$ ECG: Bradycardia | More common in women Associated with lithium carbonate therapy Rule out of pituitary disease, hypothalamic disease, major depressive disorder, bipolar I disorder |

(continued on next page)

TABLE 17-2 *(continued)*
**MEDICAL CONDITIONS THAT PRESENT WITH PSYCHIATRIC SYMPTOMS**

| Disease | Common Medical Symptoms | Psychiatric Symptoms and Complaints | Impaired Performance and Behavior | Laboratory Tests and Findings | Diagnostic Problems |
|---|---|---|---|---|---|
| Hyperparathyroidism | Constipation<br>Polydipsia<br>Nausea | Depression<br>Paranoia<br>Confusion | | Increased $Ca^{++}$<br>PTH variable<br>ECG: shortened QT interval | Causes hypercalcemia<br>Rule out major depressive disorder, schizoaffective disorder |
| Hypoparathyroidism | Headache<br>Paresthesias<br>Tetany<br>Carpopedal spasm<br>Laryngeal spasm<br>Abdominal pain | Anxiety<br>Agitation<br>Depression<br>Confusion | Impaired memory | Low $Ca^{++}$, normal albumin<br>Low blood pressure<br>ECG: QT prolongation, ventricular arrhythmias | Causes hypocalcemia<br>Rule out anxiety disorders, mood disorders |
| Cushing's syndrome | Central obesity<br>Purple striae<br>Easy bruising<br>Osteoporosis<br>Proximal muscle weakness<br>Hirsutism | Depression<br>Insomnia<br>Emotional lability<br>Suicidality<br>Euphoria<br>Mania<br>Psychosis<br>Delirium | Disturbed sleep<br>Decreased energy<br>Agitation<br>Difficulty in concentrating | Elevated blood pressure<br>Poor glucose tolerance<br>Dexamethasone-suppression test (may be falsely positive) | Must distinguish other causes—for example, cancer from exogenous steroid excess<br>Suicide rate in untreated cases is about 10%<br>Rule out major depressive disorder, bipolar I disorder |
| Adrenocortical insufficiency (Addison's disease) | Nausea<br>Vomiting<br>Anorexia<br>Stupor<br>Coma | Lethargy<br>Depression<br>Psychosis<br>Delirium | Fatigue | Decreased blood pressure<br>Decreased $Na^+$<br>Increased $K^+$<br>Eosinophilia | May be primary (Addison's disease) or secondary<br>Rule out eating disorders, mood disorders |

*(continued on next page)*

TABLE 17-2 *(continued)*
**MEDICAL CONDITIONS THAT PRESENT WITH PSYCHIATRIC SYMPTOMS**

| Disease | Common Medical Symptoms | Psychiatric Symptoms and Complaints | Impaired Performance and Behavior | Laboratory Tests and Findings | Diagnostic Problems |
|---|---|---|---|---|---|
| Acute intermittent porphyria | Abdominal pain Fever Nausea Vomiting Constipation Peripheral neuropathy Paralysis | Acute depression Agitation Paranoia Visual hallucinations | Restlessness Diaphoresis Weakness | Leukocytosis Elevated δ-aminoleuvulinic acid Elevated porphobilinogen Tachycardia | Autosomal dominant More common in women in the 20–40 age group May be precipitated by a variety of drugs Rule out acute abdominal disease, acute psychiatric episode, schizophreniform disorder, major depressive disorder |
| Wilson's disease | Kayser-Fleischer corneal ring Hepatitislike picture | Mood disturbances Delusions Hallucinations | Choreoathetoid movements Gait disturbance Clumsiness Rigidity | Decreased serum ceruloplasm Increased copper in urine | Hepatolenticular degeneration Autosomal recessive disorder of copper metabolism Often presents in adolescence, early adulthood Rule out extrapyramidal reactions, schizophreniform disorder, mood disorders |
| Hypoglycemia | Sweating Drowsiness Stupor Coma Tachycardia | Anxiety Confusion Agitation | Tremor Restlessness Seizures | Hypoglycemia Tachycardia | Excess insulin often complicated by exercise, alcohol, decreased food intake Rule out insulinoma, postictal states, agitated depression, paranoid psychosis |

*(continued on next page)*

TABLE 17–2 *(continued)*
**MEDICAL CONDITIONS THAT PRESENT WITH PSYCHIATRIC SYMPTOMS**

| Disease | Common Medical Symptoms | Psychiatric Symptoms and Complaints | Impaired Performance and Behavior | Laboratory Tests and Findings | Diagnostic Problems |
|---|---|---|---|---|---|
| Intracranial tumors | None early; headache, vomiting, papilledema later | Varied; depression, anxiety, personality changes | Loss of memory, judgment, self-criticism; clouding of consciousness | | Tumor location may not determine early symptoms |
| Pancreatic carcinoma | Weight loss Abdominal pain | Depression Lethargy Anhedonia | Apathy Decreased energy | Elevated amylase | Always consider in depressed middle-aged patients Rule out other GI illness, major depressive disorder |
| Pheochromocytoma | Paroxysmal hypertension Headache | Anxiety Apprehension Feeling of impending doom | Panic Diaphoresis Tremor | Hypertension Elevated VMA in 24-hr. urine Tachycardia | Adrenal medulla secreting catacholamines Rule out anxiety disorders |
| Multiple sclerosis | Sudden transient motor and sensory disturbances Impaired vision Diffuse neurological signs with remissions and exacerbations | Anxiety Euphoria Mania | Slurred speech Incontinence | CSF may show increased gamma globulin CT: degenerative patches in brain and spinal cord | Onset usually in young adults Rule out tertiary syphilis, other degenerative diseases, hysteria, mania (late) |

*(continued on next page)*

TABLE 17-2 *(continued)*
**MEDICAL CONDITIONS THAT PRESENT WITH PSYCHIATRIC SYMPTOMS**

| Disease | Common Medical Symptoms | Psychiatric Symptoms and Complaints | Impaired Performance and Behavior | Laboratory Tests and Findings | Diagnostic Problems |
|---|---|---|---|---|---|
| Systemic lupus erythematosus | Fever Photosensitivity Butterfly rash Joint pains Headache | Depression Mood disturbances Psychosis Delusions Hallucinations | Fatigue | Positive ANA Positive lupus erythematosus test Anemia Thrombocytopenia Chest X-ray: pleural effusion, pericarditis | Multisystemic autoimmune disease most frequent in women Psychiatric symptoms are present in 50% of cases Steroid treatment can cause psychiatric symptoms Rule out depressive disorders, paranoid psychosis, psychotic mood disorder |

Table adapted from Maurice J. Martin, MD.

TABLE 17–3
**CONDITIONS MIMICKING PSYCHOSOMATIC DISORDERS**

| Diagnosis | Definition and Example |
|---|---|
| Conversion disorder | There is an alteration of physical function that suggests a physical disorder but is an expression of psychological conflict, e.g., psychogenic aphonia. The symptoms are falsely neurologic-anatomic in distribution, are symbolic in nature, and allow much secondary gain. |
| Body dysmorphic disorder | Preoccupation with an imagined physical defect in appearance in a normal appearing person, e.g., preoccupation with facial hair. |
| Hypochondriasis | Imaged overconcern about physical disease when objective examination reveals none to exist, e.g., angina pectoris with normal heart functioning. |
| Somatization disorder | Recurrent somatic and physical complaints with no demonstrable physical disorder despite repeated physical examinations and no organic basis. |
| Pain disorder | Preoccupation with pain with no physical disease to account for intensity. It does not follow a neuroanatomical distribution. There may be a close correlation between stress and conflict and the initiation or exacerbation of pain. |
| Physical complaints associated with classic psychological disorders | Somatic accompaniment of depression, e.g., weakness, asthenia. |
| Physical complaints with substance abuse disorder | Bronchitis and cough associated with nicotine and tobacco dependence. |

C. **Surgery.**   Patients who have undergone severe surgical procedures have a variety of psychological reactions, depending on their premorbid personality and the nature of the surgery. These reactions are summarized in Table 17–5.

## IV. Pain

Pain is a complex symptom consisting of a sensation underlying potential disease and an associated emotional state. Acute pain is a reflex biological response to injury. By definition, chronic pain consists of pain that lasts at least 6 months. A physiological classification of pain is listed in Table 17–6, and characteristics of pain are listed in Table 17–7.

## V. Analgesia

Analgesia is the loss or absence of pain. Most effective are the narcotics (drugs derived from opium or an opiumlike substance that relieves pain, alters mood and behavior, and produces the potential for dependence and tolerance). *Opioids* is a generic term that includes drugs that bind to opioid receptors and produce a narcotic effect. They are most useful in the short-term management of severe, acute, serious pain. A goal should be to lower the pain level so that the patient can eat and sleep with minimal upset. A guideline should be to give the drug at the request of the patient but not more than hourly for the two first doses. It can then be reduced to a frequency of every 3 hours. Self-administration of measured amounts of narcotics through an intravenous pump by patients with

TABLE 17–4
**COMMON CONSULTATION-LIAISON PROBLEMS**

| Reason for Consultation | Comments |
|---|---|
| Suicide attempt or threat | High-risk factors are males over 45, no social support, alcoholism, previous attempt, incapacitating medical illness with pain, and suicidal ideation. If risk is present, transfer to psychiatric unit or start 24-hour nursing care. |
| Depression | Suicidal risks must be assessed in every depressed patient (see above); presence of cognitive defects in depression may cause diagnostic dilemma with dementia (pseudodementia); check for history of substance abuse or depressant drugs, e.g., reserpine, propranolol; use antidepressants cautiously in cardiac patients because of conduction side effects, orthostatic hypotension. |
| Agitation | Often related to medical condition, withdrawal from drugs, e.g., opioids, alcohol, sedative-hypnotics; haloperidol most useful drug for excessive agitation; use physical restraints with great caution; examine for command hallucinations or paranoid ideation to which patient is responding in agitated manner; rule out toxic reaction to medication, e.g., cortisol paranoia, anticholinergic delirium. |
| Hallucinations | Most common cause in hospital is delirium tremens; onset 3–4 days after hospitalization. In intensive care units, check for sensory isolation; rule out brief psychotic disorder, schizophrenia, associated medical condition, drug intoxication or withdrawal. Treat with antipsychotic medication. |
| Sleep disorder | Common cause is pain; early morning awakening associated with depression; difficulty falling asleep associated with anxiety. Use antianxiety or antidepressant agent depending on cause. Those drugs have no analgesic effect, so prescribe adequate pain killers. Rule out early drug withdrawal reaction. |
| No organic basis for symptoms | Rule out conversion disorder, somatization disorder, factitious disorder, malingering; glove and stocking anesthesia with autonomic nervous system symptoms seen in conversion; multiple body complaints seen in somatization; wish to be hospitalized seen in factitious disorder; obvious secondary gain in malingering, e.g., compensation case. |
| Disorientation | Delirium versus dementia; review metabolic status, neurologic findings, drug history. Prescribe small dose of antipsychotics for major agitation; benzodiazepines may worsen condition and cause sundowner syndrome (ataxia, confusion); modify environment so patient does not experience sensory deprivation. |
| Noncompliance or refusal to consent to procedure | Explore relationship of patient and treating doctor; negative transference is most common cause of noncompliance; fears of medication or procedure require education and reassurance. Refusal to give consent is issue of judgment; if impaired, patient can be declared incompetent, but only by court; associated medical or neurological condition is main cause of impaired judgment in hospitalized patients. |

pain, when carried out in a hospital, is a new approach to pain control that is proving effective. The major opioid analgesics are:

1. **Morphine**—10 mg intramuscularly; 60 mg orally.
2. **Meperidine (Demerol)**—75 mg intramuscularly; 300 mg orally; meperidine is a synthetic opioid analgesic.
3. **Methadone**—10 mg intramuscularly; 20 mg orally. Methadone is used as short-term treatment for heroin withdrawal and long-term maintenance of opioid addiction and for analgesia in cancer patients. Methadone has

TABLE 17–5
**TRANSPLANTATION AND SURGICAL PROBLEMS**

| Organ | Biological Factor | Psychological Factor |
|---|---|---|
| Kidney | 50–90% success rate. May not be done if patient over age 55. Increasing use of cadaver kidneys rather than those from living donors. | Living donors must be emotionally stable; parents are best donors, siblings may be ambivalent; donors are subject to depression. Patients who panic before surgery may have poor prognosis; altered body image with fear of organ rejection is common. Group therapy for patients is helpful. |
| Bone marrow | Used in aplastic anemias and immune system disease. | Patients are usually very ill and must deal with death and dying; compliance important. Commonly done in children who present problems of prolonged dependency; siblings are often donors who may be angry or ambivalent about procedure. |
| Heart | End-stage coronary artery disease and cardiomyopathy. | Donor is legally dead; relatives of deceased may refuse permission or be ambivalent. No fall-back position if organ rejected; kidney rejection can go on hemodialysis. Some patients seek transplant hoping to die. Postcardiotomy delirium in 25% of patients. |
| Breast | Radical mastectomy versus lumpectomy. | Reconstruction of breast at time of surgery leads to better postoperative adaptation; veteran patients used to counsel new patients; lumpectomy patients more open about surgery and sex than are mastectomy patients; group support helpful. |
| Uterus | Hysterectomy performed on 10% of women over 20. | Fear of loss of sexual attractiveness with sexual dysfunction may occur in small percentage of women; loss of childbearing capacity upsetting. |
| Brain | Anatomic location of lesion determines behavioral change. | Environmental dependency syndrome in frontal lobe tumors characterized by inability to show initiative; memory disturbances involved in periventricular surgery; hallucinations in parieto-occipital area. |
| Prostate | Cancer surgery has more negative psychobiological effects and is more technically difficult than is surgery for benign hypertrophy. | Sexual dysfunction common except in transurethral prostatectomy (TUP). Perineal prostatectomy produces absence of emission, ejaculation, and erection; penile implant may be of use. |
| Colon and rectum | Common outcome is colostomy, especially for cancer. | One-third of patients with colostomy feel worse about themselves than before bowel surgery; shame and self-consciousness about stoma can be alleviated by self-help groups that deal with those issues. |
| Limbs | Amputation performed for massive injury, diabetes, or cancer. | Phantom limb phenomenon occurs in 98% of cases; experience can last for years; sometimes sensation can be painful, and neuroma at stump should be ruled out; no known cause or treatment, can stop spontaneously. |

TABLE 17–6
**PHYSIOLOGICAL CLASSIFICATION OF PAIN**

| Type | Subtypes | Example | Comment |
|---|---|---|---|
| Nociceptive | Somatic<br>Visceral | Bone metastasis<br>Intestinal obstruction | Due to activation of pain-sensitive fibers; usually aching or pressure |
| Neuropathic | Peripheral<br>Central<br>Somatic<br>Visceral<br><br>Sympathetic dependent<br>Nonsympathetic dependent | Causalgia<br>Thalamic pain<br>Causalgia<br>Visceral pain in paraplegics<br>Postherpetic pain<br>Phamtom pain | Due to interruption of afferent pathways. Pathophysiology poorly understood, with most syndromes probably involving both peripheral and central nervous system changes. Usually dysesthetic, often burning and lancinating |
| Psychogenic | Somatization disorder<br>Psychogenic pain<br>Hypochondriasis<br>Specific pain diagnoses, with organic contribution | Failed low back<br>Atypical facial pain<br>Chronic headache | Does not include factitious disorders (i.e., malingering, Munchausen's syndrome) |

Table adapted from Berkow R, ed: *Merck Manual*, ed 15, p 1341. Merck, Sharp & Dohme Research Laboratories, Rahway, NJ, 1987.

TABLE 17–7
**CHARACTERISTICS OF SOMATIC AND NEUROPATHIC PAIN**

| Somatic pain | Neuropathic pain: |
|---|---|
| Nociceptive stimulus usually evident | No obvious nociceptive stimulus |
| Usually well localized; visceral pain may be referred | Often poorly localized |
| Similar to other somatic pains in patient's experience | Unusual, dissimilar from somatic pain |
| Relieved by anti-inflammatory or narcotic analgesics | Only partially relieved by narcotic analgesics |

Table adapted from Braunwald E, Isselbacher K, Petersdorf RG, Wilson JD, Martin JB, Fauci AS: *Harrison's Principles of Internal Medicine-II, Companion Handbook*. McGraw-Hill, New York, 1988, p 1. Modified from Maciewicz R, Martin JB: HPIM-11, p 15.

a long duration of action, oral effectiveness, and less sedation than morphine.

A. **Nonnarcotic analgesics.** Typical of this group is aspirin, or acetylsalicylic acid (ASA). Unlike narcotic analgesics that act on the central nervous system, salicylates act at the peripheral or local level—the site of the origin of the pain. Usually prescribed every 3 hours.

For most analgesics, peak plasma concentrations occur in 45 minutes, with analgesic effects lasting 3–4 hours. Nonsteroidal anti-inflammatory drugs (NSAIDs) also have analgesic use: ibuprofen 200–400 mg every 4 hours. Drug equivalents: 650 mg of ASA = 32 mg of codeine = 65 mg of propoxyphene (Darvon) = 50 mg of oral pentazocine (Talwin).

B. **Placebos.** Substances with no known pharmacological activity that act through suggestion rather than biological action. It has recently been demonstrated, however, that naloxone (Narcan), an opioid antagonist, can block the analgesic effects of a placebo, thus suggesting that a release of endogenous opioids may explain some placebo effects.

Chronic treatment with placebos should never be undertaken when patients have clearly stated an objection to such treatment. Furthermore, deceptive treatment with placebos seriously undermines patients' confidence in their physicians. Finally, placebos should not be used when an effective therapy is available.

## VI. Alternative (or unconventional) medicine

Being used increasingly today. One in three persons use such therapies at some point for such common ailments as depression, anxiety, chronic pain, low back pain, headaches, and digestive problems.

**A. Approach.**   Practitioners of holistic medicine use a total approach to the patient, evaluating psychosocial, environmental, and lifestyle parameters that have been subsumed under the psychosomatic approach in previous years.

**B. Treatment evaluation.**   Only hypnosis and biofeedback have entered the mainstream of psychiatry. Each treatment method requires exhaustive evaluation, but most methods appear to work through the power of suggestion. 70% of patients do not tell their physicians that they are using alternative medicine.

---

*For a more detailed discussion of this topic, see Psychological Factors Affecting Medical Condition (Psychosomatic Disorders), Chap 26, pp 1463–1606; Mamelok AE: Psychiatry and Surgery, Sec 29.3, p 1680, in CTP/VI.*

---

# 18

# Personality Disorders

## I. General introduction

**A. Definition.** Pervasive, persistent maladaptive patterns of behavior that are deeply ingrained and that are not attributable to Axis I disorders, Axis III disorders, or cultural role difficulties. Disorders of trait, rather than state. Maladaptive traits can be behavioral, emotional, cognitive, perceptual, or psychodynamic.

**B. Diagnosis, signs, and symptoms**
1. Requires history of long-term difficulties in various spheres of life.
2. Egosyntonic, i.e., acceptable to the ego.
3. Rigidity.
4. Underneath protective armor—anxiety.
5. Lacks empathy with others.
6. Developmental fixation; immature.
7. Interpersonal difficulties in love and work.

**C. Epidemiology**
1. Prevalence—6–9%.
2. Early analogue is a disorder of temperament. Usually, personality disorder is first evident in late adolescence or early adulthood.
3. Overall, women and men are affected equally.
4. Family history—nonspecific history of psychiatric disorders is common. With some personality disorders, a partial genetic transmission is established.

**D. Etiology**
1. Multifactorial.
2. Biological determinants are sometimes evident (genetics, perinatal injury, encephalitis, head trauma). High concordance rate in monozygotic (MZ) twins.
3. Developmental histories frequently reveal individual difficulties and family problems, sometimes severe (abuse, incest).

**E. Psychological tests**
1. Neuropsychological test can reveal organicity (electroencephalogram [EEG], computed tomography [CT] scan, and electrophysiologic mapping can be useful).
2. Projective tests can reveal preferred personality patterns and styles (Minnesota Multiphasic Personality Inventory [MMPI], Thematic Apperception Test [TAT], Rorschach, Draw-A-Person).

**F. Pathophysiology**
1. **Frontal lobe**—impulsivity, poor judgment, abulia.

TABLE 18–1
**DSM-IV DIAGNOSTIC CRITERIA FOR PARANOID PERSONALITY DISORDER**

A.  A pervasive distrust and suspiciousness of others such that their motives are interpreted as malevolent, beginning by early adulthood and present in a variety of contexts, as indicated by four (or more) of the following:
    (1) suspects, without sufficient basis, that others are exploiting, harming, or deceiving him or her
    (2) is preoccupied with unjustified doubts about the loyalty or trustworthiness of friends or associates
    (3) is reluctant to confide in others because of unwarranted fear that the information will be used maliciously against him or her
    (4) reads hidden demeaning or threatening meanings into benign remarks or events
    (5) persistently bears grudges, i.e., is unforgiving of insults, injuries, or slights
    (6) perceives attacks on his or her character or reputation that are not apparent to others and is quick to react angrily or to counterattack
    (7) has recurrent suspicions, without justification, regarding fidelity of spouse or sexual partner
B.  Does not occur exclusively during the course of schizophrenia, a mood disorder with psychotic features, or another psychotic disorder and is not due to the direct physiological effects of a general medical condition.

**Note:** If criteria are met prior to the onset of schizophrenia, add ``premorbid,'' e.g., ``paranoid personality disorder (premorbid)''

Used with permission, APA.

      **2. Temporal lobe**—Klüver-Bucy traits, religiosity, possible violence.
      **3. Parietal lobe**—denial or euphoric features.

**G. Psychodynamics.**   Vary with different disorders.

**H. Course and prognosis.**   Varies—usually stable or deteriorating, but some patients improve.

**I. Treatment.**   Usually, patients are not motivated. Otherwise, multiple and mixed modalities are employed: psychoanalysis, psychoanalytic psychotherapy, supportive psychotherapy, group therapy, family therapy, milieu therapy, hospitalization (short- and long-term), pharmacotherapy.

**J. Classification.**   DSM-IV groups the personality disorders into three clusters. The first (cluster A) is the **odd, eccentric cluster** and consists of the paranoid, schizoid, and schizotypal personality disorders; the second (cluster B) is the **dramatic, emotional, and erratic cluster** and includes the histrionic, narcissistic, antisocial, and borderline personality disorders; the third (cluster C) is the **anxious, fearful cluster** and includes the avoidant, dependent, and obsessive-compulsive personality disorders.

## II. Odd and eccentric cluster

### A. Paranoid personality disorder

    **1. Definition.**   Tendency to attribute malevolent motives to others.
    **2. Diagnosis, signs, and symptoms.**   See Table 18–1.
    **3. Epidemiology**
      a. Prevalence—0.5–2.5%.
      b. Increased incidence in families of probands with schizophrenia and delusional disorders.
      c. More common in men than in women.
    **4. Etiology**
      a. Genetic component.
      b. Nonspecific early family difficulties; childhood abuse.
      c. Rule out drug abuse, e.g., amphetamines.

TABLE 18-2
**DSM-IV DIAGNOSTIC CRITERIA FOR SCHIZOID PERSONALITY DISORDER**

A.  A pervasive pattern of detachment from social relationships and a restricted range of expression of emotions in interpersonal settings, beginning by early adulthood and present in a variety of contexts, as indicated by four (or more) of the following:
    (1) neither desires nor enjoys close relationships, including being part of a family
    (2) almost always chooses solitary activities
    (3) has little, if any, interest in having sexual experiences with another person
    (4) takes pleasure in few, if any, activities
    (5) lacks close friends or confidants other than first-degree relatives
    (6) appears indifferent to the praise or criticism of others
    (7) shows emotional coldness, detachment, or flattened affectivity
B.  Does not occur exclusively during the course of schizophrenia, a mood disorder with psychotic features, another psychotic disorder, or a pervasive developmental disorder and is not due to the direct physiological effects of a general medical condition.

**Note:** If criteria are met prior to the onset of schizophrenia, add ''premorbid,'' e.g., ''schizoid personality disorder (premorbid)''

Used with permission, APA.

### 5. Psychodynamics
    a. Projection, denial, rationalization.
    b. Shame.
    c. Defensive, masochistic, hypochondriacal features.
    d. Unresolved separation and autonomy issues.
    e. Identification with aggressor.

### 6. Differential diagnosis
    **a. Delusional disorder**—patient has fixed delusions.
    **b. Paranoid schizophrenia**—presence of hallucinations and formal thought disorder.
    **c. Schizoid, borderline, and antisocial personality disorders**—patient does not show similar active involvement with others.

### 7. Course and prognosis.
Varies, depending on individual ego strengths and life circumstances; possible complications of delusional disorders, schizophrenia, depression, anxiety disorders. In general, patient has lifelong problems living and working with others.

### 8. Treatment
    a. Rarely low-dose antipsychotics, e.g., haloperidol (Haldol) 2 mg a day; antianxiety agent, e.g., diazepam (Valium), to deal with agitation and anxiety.
    b. Usually supportive psychotherapy
        i.   Openness, consistency, avoidance of humor.
        ii.  Support healthy parts of the ego.
        iii. Emphasize reality.
    c. Patient does not do well in group psychotherapy.

## B. Schizoid personality disorder
### 1. Definition.
Isolated life-style without overt longing for others.
### 2. Diagnosis, signs, and symptoms.
See Table 18–2.
### 3. Epidemiology
    a. May affect 7.5% of the general population.
    b. Increased incidence among family members of schizophrenic probands.
    c. Greater incidence among men than women.

TABLE 18–3
**DSM-IV DIAGNOSTIC CRITERIA FOR SCHIZOTYPAL PERSONALITY DISORDER**

A.  A pervasive pattern of social and interpersonal deficits marked by acute discomfort with, and reduced capacity for, close relationships as well as by cognitive or perceptual distortions and eccentricities of behavior, beginning by early adulthood and present in a variety of contexts, as indicated by five (or more) of the following:

  (1)  ideas of reference (excluding delusions of reference)
  (2)  odd beliefs or magical thinking that influences behavior and is inconsistent with subcultural norms (e.g., superstitiousness, belief in clairvoyance, telepathy, or "sixth sense"; in children and adolescents, bizarre fantasies or preoccupations)
  (3)  unusual perceptual experiences, including bodily illusions
  (4)  odd thinking and speech (e.g., vague, circumstantial, metaphorical, overelaborate, or stereotyped)
  (5)  suspiciousness or paranoid ideation
  (6)  inappropriate or constricted affect
  (7)  behavior of appearance that is odd, eccentric, or peculiar
  (8)  lack of close friends or confidants other than first-degree relatives
  (9)  excessive social anxiety that does not diminish with familiarity and tends to be associated with paranoid fears rather than negative judgments about self

B.  Does not occur exclusively during the course of schizophrenia, a mood disorder with psychotic features, another psychotic disorder, or a pervasive developmental disorder.

**Note:** If criteria are met prior to the onset of schizophrenia, add "premorbid," e.g., "schizotypal personality disorder (premorbid)"

Used with permission, APA.

### 4. Etiology
  a. Genetic factors likely.
  b. Theories regarding etiology of schizophrenia apply.
  c. History of disturbed early family relationships often is elicited.

### 5. Psychodynamics
  a. Social inhibition.
  b. Restriction of affect and denial are defenses used most prominently against aggression.

### 6. Differential diagnosis
  a. **Paranoid personality disorder**—patient is involved with others.
  b. **Schizotypal personality disorder**—patient has oddities and eccentricities of manners.
  c. **Avoidant personality disorder**—patient is isolated but wants to be involved with others.

### 7. Course and prognosis
  a. Varies.
  b. Possibility of complications of delusional disorder, schizophrenia, other psychoses.

### 8. Treatment
  a. Low-dose antipsychotics may be of some benefit in some patients, e.g., haloperidol (Haldol) 2 mg a day.
  b. Supportive psychotherapy—focus on relatedness, identification of emotions.
  c. Group psychotherapy.
  d. Possible milieu therapy in some patients.

## C. Schizotypal personality disorder
  ### 1. Definition.   Multiple oddities and eccentricities of behavior, thought, affect, speech, appearance.
  ### 2. Diagnosis, signs, and symptoms.   See Table 18–3.

### 3. Epidemiology
   a. 3% prevalence.
   b. Increased prevalence in families of schizophrenic probands.
   c. More common in men than in women.
### 4. Etiology.   Etiological models of schizophrenia apply.
### 5. Psychological tests.   Thought disorder is common.
### 6. Pathophysiology
   a. Possible diminished monoamine oxidase (MAO).
   b. Possible impairments in smooth pursuit eye tracking.
   c. Possible diminished brain mass, especially temporal.
### 7. Psychodynamics.   Dynamics of psychosis and schizophrenia apply.
### 8. Differential diagnosis
   a. **Paranoid personality disorder**—no eccentricities.
   b. **Schizoid personality disorder**—no eccentricities.
   c. **Borderline personality disorder**—prominent affect, anger, impulsiveness.
   d. **Schizophrenia**—reality testing is lost.
### 9. Course and prognosis
   a. Prognosis probably is guarded; about 10% commit suicide.
   b. Possible schizophrenic decompensation.
### 10. Treatment
   a. Pharmacological—use guidelines for treating residual schizophrenia (low-dose antipsychotics, e.g., haloperidol 2–5 mg a day; pimozide [Orap] 2–5 mg a day; adjunctive benzodiazepines, e.g., diazepam 2–10 mg a day).
   b. Supportive psychotherapy.
   c. Group psychotherapy.
   d. Milieu therapy.

## III. Dramatic, emotional, and erratic cluster

### A. Antisocial personality disorder
#### 1. Definition.   Maladaptive behavior that does not recognize the rights of others.
#### 2. Diagnosis, signs, and symptoms.   See Table 18–4.
#### 3. Epidemiology
   a. Prevalence—3% of men, 1% of women.
   b. Increased incidence of antisocial personality disorder, somatization disorder, and alcoholism in families.
   c. Adoptive studies demonstrate genetic factors.
   d. More common in lower socioeconomic groups.
   e. Predisposing conditions—attention-deficit/hyperactivity disorder (ADHD), conduct disorder.
#### 4. Etiology
   a. Genetic factors.
   b. Organicity can be due to such conditions as perinatal brain injury, head trauma, encephalitis.
   c. Parental abandonment or abuse.
   d. Repeated, arbitrary, or harsh punishment by parents.

TABLE 18–4
**DSM-IV DIAGNOSTIC CRITERIA FOR ANTISOCIAL PERSONALITY DISORDER**

A. There is a pervasive pattern of disregard for and violation of the rights of others occurring since age 15 years, as indicated by three (or more) of the following:
   (1) failure to conform to social norms with respect to lawful behaviors as indicated by repeatedly performing acts that are grounds for arrest
   (2) deceitfulness, as indicated by repeated lying, use of aliases, or conning others for personal profit or pleasure
   (3) impulsivity or failure to plan ahead
   (4) irritability and aggressiveness, as indicated by repeated physical fights or assaults
   (5) reckless disregard for safety of self or others
   (6) consistent irresponsibility, as indicated by repeated failure to sustain consistent work behavior or honor financial obligations
   (7) lack of remorse, as indicated by being indifferent to or rationalizing having hurt, mistreated, or stolen from another
B. The individual is at least age 18 years.
C. There is evidence of conduct disorder with onset before age 15 years.
D. The occurrence of antisocial behavior is not exclusively during the course of schizophrenia or a manic episode.

Used with permission, APA.

### 5. Pathophysiology
   a. If organicity is present, impulsivity usually is due to frontal lobe injury.
   b. Other brain lesions, e.g., amygdala or possibly other temporal lesions, can predispose to violence.

### 6. Psychodynamics
   a. Impulse-ridden with associated ego deficits in planning, judgment.
   b. Superego deficits or lacunae; primitive or poorly formed conscience.
   c. Object relation deficits—failure in empathy, love, basic trust.
   d. Prominence of aggression.
   e. Features of sadomasochism, narcissism, depression.

### 7. Differential diagnosis
   **a. Adult antisocial behavior**—does not meet all criteria in Table 18–4.
   **b. Substance use disorders**—may exhibit antisocial behavior as a consequence of substance abuse and dependence; may coexist.
   **c. Mental retardation**—antisocial behavior as a consequence of impaired intellect and judgment; may coexist.
   **d. Psychoses**—may exhibit antisocial behavior as a consequence of psychotic delusions; may coexist.
   **e. Borderline personality disorder**—common are suicide attempts, self-loathing, and intense, ambivalent attachments.
   **f. Narcissistic personality disorder**—patient is law abiding in the service of narcissistic needs.

### 8. Course and prognosis
   a. Diagnosis usually is not made before age 18.
   b. Prognosis varies.
   c. Condition often significantly improves after early or middle adulthood.
   d. Complications include death by violence, substance abuse, suicide, physical injury, legal and financial difficulties.

### 9. Treatment
   a. Difficult.

TABLE 18–5
**DSM-IV DIAGNOSTIC CRITERIA FOR BORDERLINE PERSONALITY DISORDER**

A pervasive pattern of instability of interpersonal relationships, self-image, and affects, and marked impulsivity beginning by early adulthood and present in a variety of contexts, as indicated by five (or more) of the following:

(1) frantic efforts to avoid real or imagined abandonment. **Note:** Do not include suicidal or self-mutilating behavior, covered in criterion 5

(2) a pattern of unstable and intense interpersonal relationships characterized by alternating between extremes of idealization and devaluation

(3) identity disturbance: markedly and persistently unstable self-image or sense of self

(4) impulsivity in at least two areas that are potentially self-damaging (e.g., spending, sex, substance abuse, reckless driving, binge eating). **Note:** Do not include suicidal or self-mutilating behavior covered in criterion 5

(5) recurrent suicidal behavior, gestures, or threats, or self-mutilating behavior

(6) affective instability due to a marked reactivity of mood (e.g., intense episodic dysphoria, irritability, or anxiety usually lasting a few hours and only rarely more than a few days)

(7) chronic feelings of emptiness

(8) inappropriate, intense anger or difficulty controlling anger (e.g., frequent displays of temper, constant anger, recurrent physical fights)

(9) transient, stress-related paranoid ideation or severe dissociative symptoms

Used with permission, APA.

    b. Treatment of substance abuse often effectively treats antisocial traits.

    c. Long-term hospitalization or therapeutic community sometimes is effective.

    d. Usually, effective treatment is behavioral, e.g., behavior may be modified by the threat of legal sanctions or the fear of punishment.

## B. Borderline personality disorder

### 1. Definition

    a. Multiple complexities and controversies in defining this disorder. Often confused with neurosis, psychosis, mood disorders, other personality disorders, cognitive disorders.

    b. Manifestations of separation-individuation problems, affective control problems, and intense, personal attachments appear central.

### 2. Diagnosis, signs, and symptoms. See Table 18–5.

### 3. Epidemiology

    a. Prevalence—about 2% of general population.

    b. More common in women than in men.

    c. Increased prevalence of mood and substance-related disorders in families.

    d. Increased prevalence of borderline personality disorder in mothers of borderline persons.

### 4. Etiology

    a. Organicity can be due to perinatal brain injury, encephalitis, head injury, and other brain disorders.

    b. Physical and sexual abuse, abandonment, or overinvolvement.

### 5. Psychological tests. Projective tests reveal impaired reality testing.

### 6. Pathophysiology

    a. Frontal lesions can impair judgment and affective control.

    b. Temporal lesions can produce Klüver-Bucy traits.

### 7. Psychodynamics

    a. Splitting—manifests rage without a consciousness of ambivalent or positive emotions toward someone. Usually transient. Associated ability to divide persons into those who like and those who hate patient.

b. Primitive idealization.

c. Projective identification—attributes idealized features to another, then seeks to engage the other in various interactions that may resolve the patient's ambivalence. Also, patient tries, unconsciously, to make the therapist feel as the patient feels.

d. Both intense aggressive needs and intense object hunger, often alternating.

e. Fear of abandonment.

f. Rapprochement subphase of separation-individuation is unresolved; object constancy is impaired.

g. Turning against the self—self-hate, self-loathing.

h. Generalized ego dysfunction results in identity disturbance.

## 8. Differential diagnosis

a. **Psychotic disorder**—reality testing impairment persists.

b. **Mood disorders**—mood disturbance is usually nonreactive.

   Major depressive disorder with atypical features—often a difficult differential diagnosis. At times, only a treatment trial will tell. Atypical patients often have sustained episodes of depression, however.

c. **Personality change due to a general medical condition**—testing for significant organicity.

d. **Schizotypal personality disorder**—affective features are less severe.

e. **Antisocial personality disorder**—defect in conscience, and attachment is more severe.

f. **Histrionic personality disorder**—suicide and self-mutilation are less common. More stable interpersonal relationships.

g. **Narcissistic personality disorder**—more stable identity formation.

h. **Dependent personality disorder**—attachments are stable.

i. **Paranoid personality disorder**—extreme suspiciousness.

## 9. Course and prognosis

a. Varies; may improve in later years.

b. Suicide, self-injury, depression, somatoform disorders, psychosis, substance abuse are possible.

c. Usually diagnosed before age 40.

## 10. Treatment

a. Usually mixed supportive and exploratory psychotherapy. Management of transference psychosis, countertransference, acting out, and suicide threats and wishes are problematic. Therapist functions as auxiliary ego and uses limit-setting.

b. Behavior therapy to control impulses and angry outbursts and to reduce sensitivity to criticism and rejection; social skills training is used.

c. Frequent use of medications—antidepressants; lithium; low-dose antipsychotics, e.g., haloperidol 2 mg a day; carbamazepine (Tegretol) at therapeutic levels.

TABLE 18-6
**DSM-IV DIAGNOSTIC CRITERIA FOR HISTRIONIC PERSONALITY DISORDER**

A pervasive pattern of excessive emotionality and attention seeking, beginning by early adulthood and present in a variety of contexts, as indicated by five (or more) of the following:

(1) is uncomfortable in situations in which he or she is not the center of attention
(2) interaction with others is often characterized by inappropriate sexually seductive or provocative behavior
(3) displays rapidly shifting and shallow expression of emotions
(4) consistently uses physical appearance to draw attention to self
(5) has a style of speech that is excessively impressionistic and lacking in detail
(6) shows self-dramatization, theatricality, and exaggerated expression of emotion
(7) is suggestible, i.e., easily influenced by others or circumstances
(8) considers relationships to be more intimate than they actually are

Used with permission, APA.

    d. Hospitalization is usually brief; some patients require long-term hospitalization.

## C. Histrionic personality disorder

1. **Definition.** Dramatic, emotional, impressionistic style.
2. **Diagnosis, signs, and symptoms.** See Table 18-6.
3. **Epidemiology**
   a. Prevalence—2–3%.
   b. Greater prevalence in women than in men.
   c. Underdiagnosed in men.
4. **Etiology.** Suggestion that early interpersonal difficulties were resolved by dramatic behavior.
5. **Psychodynamics**
   a. Fantasy, emotionality, and dramatic style are typical.
   b. Common defenses—regression, identification, somatization, conversion, dissociation, denial, externalization.
   c. Faulty identification with and ambivalent relationship to opposite-sex parent.
   d. Fixation at early genital level.
   e. Prominent oral traits.
   f. Fear of sexuality, despite seductiveness.
6. **Differential diagnosis**
   a. **Borderline personality disorder**—more overt despair, suicidal and self-mutilating features; can coexist.
   b. **Somatization disorder**—physical complaints predominate.
   c. **Conversion disorder**—apparent physical deficits are present.
   d. **Dependent personality disorder**—lacks the emotional style.
7. **Course and prognosis**
   a. Varies.
   b. Possible complications of somatization disorders, conversion disorders, dissociative disorders, sexual disorders, depressive disorders.
8. **Treatment**
   a. Usually individual psychotherapy, insight-oriented or supportive, depending on ego strength.
   b. Psychoanalysis is appropriate for some patients.
   c. Group therapy can be useful.

TABLE 18-7
**DSM-IV DIAGNOSTIC CRITERIA FOR NARCISSISTIC PERSONALITY DISORDER**

A pervasive pattern of grandiosity (in fantasy or behavior), need for admiration, and lack of empathy, beginning by early adulthood and present in a variety of contexts, as indicated by five (or more) of the following:
- (1) has a grandiose sense of self-importance (e.g., exaggerates achievements and talents, expects to be recognized as superior without commensurate achievements)
- (2) is preoccupied with fantasies of unlimited success, power, brilliance, beauty, or ideal love
- (3) believes that he or she is "special" and unique and can only be understood by, or should associate with, other special or high-status people (or institutions)
- (4) requires excessive admiration
- (5) has a sense of entitlement, i.e., unreasonable expectations of especially favorable treatment or automatic compliance with his or her expectations
- (6) is interpersonally exploitative, i.e., takes advantage of others to achieve his or her own ends
- (7) lacks empathy: is unwilling to recognize or identify with the feelings and needs of others
- (8) is often envious of others or believes that others are envious of him or her
- (9) shows arrogant, haughty behaviors or attitudes

Used with permission, APA.

   d. Adjunctive use of medications, usually anxiolytic, for transient emotional states, e.g., diazepam 5–10 mg a day.
## D. Narcissistic personality disorder
1. **Definition.** Pervasive pattern of grandiosity and overconcern with issues of self-esteem.
2. **Diagnosis, signs, and symptoms.** See Table 18–7.
3. **Epidemiology.** Less than 1% in the general population.
4. **Etiology.** Failure in maternal empathy, early rejection or loss.
5. **Psychodynamics**
   a. Defense versus deficit controversy—are narcissistic traits developmental arrests or defenses?
   b. Grandiosity and empathic failure defend against primitive aggression.
   c. Sense of entitlement.
   d. Compensation for sense of inferiority.
   e. Difficulty in making meaningful attachments to others.
6. **Differential diagnosis**
   a. **Antisocial personality disorder**—more flagrant disregard of the law and the rights of others.
   b. **Substance-related disorders**—patient can manifest narcissistic traits. Conditions can coexist (dual diagnosis).
   c. **Paranoid schizophrenia**—overt delusions are present.
   d. **Borderline personality disorder**—higher anxiety, greater chaos.
   e. **Histrionic personality disorder**—more emotional display than with narcissistic personality.
7. **Course and prognosis.** The disorder is chronic and difficult to treat. Possible complications of mood disorders, transient psychoses, somatoform disorders, substance use disorders. Guarded prognosis.
8. **Treatment**
   a. Individual psychotherapy, supportive or insight-oriented, depending on ego strength.
   b. Milieu therapy for severe disorders.
   c. Treatment challenge is preservation of self-esteem, threatened by psychiatric interventions.

TABLE 18–8
**DSM-IV DIAGNOSTIC CRITERIA FOR OBSESSIVE-COMPULSIVE PERSONALITY DISORDER**

A pervasive pattern of preoccupation with orderliness, perfectionism, and mental and interpersonal control, at the expense of flexibility, openness, and efficiency, beginning by early adulthood and present in a variety of contexts, as indicated by four (or more) of the following:

    (1) is preoccupied with details, rules, lists, order, organization, or schedules to the extent that the major point of the activity is lost
    (2) shows perfectionism that interferes with task completion (e.g., is unable to complete a project because his or her own overly strict standards are not met)
    (3) is excessively devoted to work and productivity to the exclusion of leisure activities and friendships (not accounted for by obvious economic necessity)
    (4) is overconscientious, scrupulous, and inflexible about matters of morality, ethics, or values (not accounted for by cultural or religious identification)
    (5) is unable to discard worn-out or worthless objects even when they have no sentimental value
    (6) is reluctant to delegate tasks or to work with others unless they submit to exactly his or her way of doing things
    (7) adopts a miserly spending style toward both self and others; money is viewed as something to be hoarded for future catastrophes
    (8) shows rigidity and stubbornness

Used with permission, APA.

## IV. Anxious or fearful cluster

### A. Obsessive-compulsive personality disorder

    **1. Definition.** Perfectionism and inflexibility predominate.

    **2. Diagnosis, signs, and symptoms.** See Table 18–8.

    **3. Epidemiology**

        a. Greater prevalence in men than in women.

        b. Likely familial transmission.

        c. Increased concordance in MZ twins.

        d. Diagnosed most often in oldest children.

    **4. Etiology.** Patients often have backgrounds characterized by harsh discipline.

    **5. Psychodynamics**

        a. Isolation, reaction formation, undoing, intellectualization, rationalization.

        b. Distrust of emotions.

        c. Issues of defiance and submission.

        d. Fixation during anal period.

    **6. Differential diagnosis.** Obsessive-compulsive disorder has true obsessions or compulsions, compared with obsessive-compulsive personality disorder, which does not. If obsessions and compulsions appear, obsessive-compulsive disorder should be diagnosed.

    **7. Course and prognosis.** Possible complications of depressive disorders and somatoform disorders.

    **8. Treatment**

        a. Individual psychotherapy, supportive or insight-oriented, depending on ego strengths.

        b. Group therapy can be beneficial.

        c. Therapeutic issues include those of control, submission, intellectualization.

        d. Pharmacotherapy may be useful, e.g., clonazepam (Klonopin), clomipramine (Anafranil), fluoxetine (Prozac).

TABLE 18–9
**DSM-IV DIAGNOSTIC CRITERIA FOR AVOIDANT PERSONALITY DISORDER**

A pervasive pattern of social inhibition, feelings of inadequacy, and hypersensitivity to negative evaluation, beginning by early adulthood and present in a variety of contexts, as indicated by four (or more) of the following:
  (1) avoids occupational activities that involve significant interpersonal contact, because of fears of criticism, disapproval, or rejection
  (2) is unwilling to get involved with people unless certain of being liked
  (3) shows restraint within intimate relationships because of the fear of being shamed or ridiculed
  (4) is preoccupied with being criticized or rejected in social situations
  (5) is inhibited in new interpersonal situations because of feelings of inadequacy
  (6) views self as socially inept, personally unappealing, or inferior to others
  (7) is unusually reluctant to take personal risks or to engage in any new activities because they may prove embarrassing

Used with permission, APA.

## B. Avoidant personality disorder

1. **Definition.** Shy or timid personality.
2. **Diagnosis, signs, and symptoms.** See Table 18–9.
3. **Epidemiology**
   a. Prevalence—0.05–1% of general population.
   b. Possible predisposing factors—avoidant disorder of childhood or adolescence, deforming physical illness.
4. **Etiology.** Possible overt parental deprecation.
5. **Psychodynamics**
   a. Avoidance and inhibition are defensive.
   b. Deep-seated fears of rejection.
   c. Underlying aggression, either oedipal or preoedipal.
6. **Differential diagnosis**
   a. **Schizoid personality disorder**—no overt desire for involvement with others.
   b. **Social phobia**—specific social situations, rather than personal relationships, are avoided. May coexist (dual diagnosis).
   c. **Dependent personality disorder**—patient does not avoid attachments, has greater fear of abandonment.
7. **Course and prognosis.** Patient functions best in a protected environment. Possible complication of social phobia.
8. **Treatment**
   a. Individual psychotherapy, supportive or insight-oriented, depending on ego strength.
   b. Group therapy is often helpful.
   c. Social skills and assertiveness training.
   d. Pharmacotherapy to manage anxiety or depression when present.

## C. Dependent personality disorder

1. **Definition.** Predominantly dependent and submissive.
2. **Diagnosis, signs, and symptoms.** See Table 18–10.
3. **Epidemiology**
   a. More prevalent in women than in men.
   b. Common.
   c. Possible predispositions include chronic physical illness in childhood and separation anxiety disorder.

TABLE 18–10
**DSM-IV DIAGNOSTIC CRITERIA FOR DEPENDENT PERSONALITY DISORDER**

A pervasive and excessive need to be taken care of that leads to submissive and clinging behavior and fears of separation, beginning by early adulthood and present in a variety of contexts, as indicated by five (or more) of the following:

    (1) has difficulty making everyday decisions without an excessive amount of advice and reassurance from others
    (2) needs others to assume responsibility for most major areas of his or her life
    (3) has difficulty expressing disagreement with others because of fear of loss of support or approval. **Note:** Do not include realistic fears of retribution
    (4) has difficulty initiating projects or doing things on his or her own (because of a lack of self-confidence in judgment or abilities rather than a lack of motivation or energy)
    (5) goes to excessive lengths to obtain nurturance and support from others, to the point of volunteering to do things that are unpleasant
    (6) feels uncomfortable or helpless when alone because of exaggerated fears of being unable to care for himself or herself
    (7) urgently seeks another relationship as a source of care and support when a close relationship ends
    (8) is unrealistically preoccupied with fears of being left to take care of himself or herself

Used with permission, APA.

TABLE 18–11
**DSM-IV RESEARCH CRITERIA FOR PASSIVE-AGGRESSIVE PERSONALITY DISORDER**

A.  A pervasive pattern of negativistic attitudes and passive resistance to demands for adequate performance, beginning by early adulthood and present in a variety of contexts, as indicated by four (or more) of the following:
    (1) passively resists fulfilling routine social and occupational tasks
    (2) complains of being misunderstood and unappreciated by others
    (3) is sullen and argumentative
    (4) unreasonably criticizes and scorns authority
    (5) expresses envy and resentment toward those apparently more fortunate
    (6) voices exaggerated and persistent complaints of personal misfortune
    (7) alternates between hostile defiance and contrition
B.  Does not occur exclusively during major depressive episodes and is not better accounted for by dysthymic disorder.

Used with permission, APA.

    **4. Etiology.**   Early childhood parental loss in some patients.
    **5. Psychodynamics**
        a. Unresolved separation issues.
        b. Possible defense against aggressive wishes.
    **6. Differential diagnosis.**   Agoraphobia—fear of leaving or being away from home.
    **7. Course and prognosis.**   Varies. Possible depressive complications. Prognosis is favorable with treatment.
    **8. Treatment**
        a. Insight-oriented psychotherapy.
        b. Behavior therapy, assertiveness training, family therapy, and group therapy also are useful.
        c. Pharmacotherapy is useful for treating specific symptoms, e.g., anxiety, depression.

**V. Other personality disorders**
    **A. Passive-aggressive personality disorder**
        **1. Definition.**   Covert obstructionism, procrastination, stubbornness, and inefficiency.
        **2. Diagnosis, signs, and symptoms.**   See Table 18–11.

TABLE 18–12
**DSM-IV RESEARCH CRITERIA FOR DEPRESSIVE PERSONALITY DISORDER**

A. A pervasive pattern of depressive cognitions and behaviors beginning by early adulthood and present in a variety of contexts, as indicated by five (or more) of the following:
    (1) usual mood is dominated by dejection, gloominess, cheerlessness, joylessness, unhappiness
    (2) self-concept centers around beliefs of inadequacy, worthlessness, and low self-esteem
    (3) is critical, blaming, and derogatory toward self
    (4) is brooding and given to worry
    (5) is negativistic, critical, and judgmental toward others
    (6) is pessimistic
    (7) is prone to feeling guilty or remorseful
B. Does not occur exclusively during major depressive episodes and is not better accounted for by dysthymic disorder.

Used with permission, APA.

3. **Epidemiology.** Oppositional defiant disorder may predispose.
4. **Etiology.** Learned behavior—parental modeling.
5. **Psychodynamics**
    a. Conflicts regarding authority, submission, and defiance.
    b. Conflicts regarding autonomy and dependence.
    c. Fear of aggression.
6. **Differential diagnosis**
    a. **Histrionic and borderline personality disorders**—behavior is more flamboyant, dramatic, and openly aggressive than in passive-aggressive personality.
    b. **Antisocial personality disorder**—defiance is overt.
    c. **Obsessive-compulsive personality disorder**—usually involves perfectionism, which limits overt opposition.
7. **Course and prognosis.** Possible complications of depressive disorders and alcohol abuse.
8. **Treatment**
    a. Major difficulty lies in opposition to intervention by psychiatrist.
    b. Supportive psychotherapy may be useful if patient is willing.
    c. Assertiveness training.

B. **Depressive personality disorder**
  1. **Definition.** Persons are pessimistic, anhedonic, duty-bound, self-doubting, and chronically unhappy.
  2. **Diagnosis, signs, and symptoms.** See Table 18–12.
  3. **Epidemiology.** Common, but no hard data.
  4. **Etiology.** Unknown. May involve early loss, poor parenting, punitive superego, extreme guilt feelings.
  5. **Psychodynamics**
    a. Low self-esteem.
    b. Self-punishing.
    c. Early loss of love object.
  6. **Differential diagnosis**
    a. **Dysthymic disorder**—greater fluctuation in mood than in depressive personality.
    b. **Avoidant personality disorder**—persons tend to be more anxious than depressed.

7. **Course and prognosis.**    Patient may be at risk for dysthymic disorder and major depressive disorder.

8. **Treatment**

   a. Insight-oriented psychotherapy.

   b. Cognitive therapy, group therapy, and interpersonal therapy are useful.

   c. Pharmacotherapy—serotonin-specific reuptake inhibitors, e.g., fluoxetine 20 mg a day, or sympathomimetics, e.g., amphetamine 5–15 mg a day (but use with caution).

C. **Sadistic personality disorder**    Relationships are dominated by cruel or demeaning behavior. Clinically rare; common in forensic settings. Often caused by parental abuse.

D. **Self-defeating personality disorder.**    Patients direct their lives toward bad outcomes; reject help or good outcomes; have dysphoric responses to good outcomes.

---

*For a more detailed discussion of this topic, see Gunderson JG, Phillips KA: Personality Disorders, Chap 25, p 1425; Bleiberg E: Identity Problem and Borderline Disorders, Sec 49.6e, p 2574, in CTP/VI.*

# 19

# Suicide, Violence, and Other Psychiatric Emergencies

## I. General introduction

A psychiatric emergency is a disturbance in thoughts, feelings, or actions that requires immediate treatment.

A. Common examples include imminent violence, suicide, self-mutilation, and injury to self or others by errors in judgment or passive neglect.

B. Such disturbances can occur in any location—home, office, street, medical or psychiatric unit, psychiatric emergency room.

C. General interventions of emergency management:
   1. Physical restraint.
   2. Pharmacotherapy.
   3. Hospitalization.
   4. Management of medical problems.
   5. Crisis intervention.
      a. Supportive psychotherapy.
      b. Environmental manipulation.
      c. Dealing with support systems—spouse, friends.

D. Social service resources, referral centers, and availability of medical backup are important.

E. General strategy in evaluating the patient:
   1. Protect self.
   2. Prevent harm.
      a. Prevent suicide and self-injury.
      b. Prevent violence toward others.

## II. Self-protection

A. Know as much as possible about the patient before meeting him or her.

B. Leave physical restraint procedures to those who are trained to use them.

C. Be alert to risks of impending violence.

D. Attend to the safety of the physical surroundings, e.g., door access, room objects.

E. Have others present during your assessment if needed.

F. Have others in the vicinity.

G. Attend to developing an alliance with the patient, e.g., do not confront or threaten patients with paranoid psychoses.

## III. Prevent harm

### A. Prevent self-injury and suicide

1. **Self-injury.** Use whatever methods are necessary to prevent the patient from hurting himself or herself during the evaluation (see section

on violence below). Always err in the direction of caution, e.g., admit to hospital when in doubt.

## 2. Suicide

**a. Incidence**—tends to cluster in the spring, summer, and with media exposure. There are 30,000 suicides per year in the United States.

**b. Age**

    i.  Risk increases starting at age 40–50; especially high in elderly persons.

    ii.  High risk also in adolescence and early adulthood.

**c. Sex**

    i.  Men commit suicide more often than women.

    ii.  Women attempt suicide more often than men.

    iii.  Men often use more violent methods than women.

    iv.  The risk of successful suicide among women is increasing, especially elderly women.

    v.  The risk among widowers is high.

**d. Race**—risk is less in non-whites. High risk in Native Americans and Inuits.

**e. Nationality**

    i.  Eastern Europeans, Scandinavians, Japanese—high rates.

    ii.  Immigrants—rates are higher than among native born.

**f. Climate**—Suicide does not correlate with season. Suicides increase slightly in the spring and fall, but contrary to popular belief, suicides do not increase during December and holiday periods.

**g. Other risk factors**

    i.  Recent attempt or gesture.

    ii.  Violence of method, e.g., gun, pills, gun possession.

    iii.  Little possibility of rescue.

    iv.  Thoroughness and implementation of plan.

    v.  Number of lifetime attempts or gestures: 2% succeed within 1 year of recent attempt; 50% repeat the attempt; 10% of those who attempt suicide eventually succeed.

    vi.  Intent to die.

    vii.  Reunion fantasy.

    viii.  Bizarre method (suggests psychosis).

    ix.  Diagnosis—major depressive disorder (15% will succeed); bipolar disorder (10% will succeed); psychotic disorder (> 10% of schizophrenic persons will succeed); substance-related disorders (15% will succeed); antisocial personality disorder, cyclothymic disorder, borderline personality disorder (10% will succeed); attempts are common early in the course of delirium and dementia; also may occur with panic disorder.

    x.  Medical history—illness, especially if of recent onset; chronic; terminal; painful; debilitating; neoplasms with pain; involving high drug use.

    xi.  Recent stressor, e.g., loss of spouse, especially with impulse-control disorder.

    xii. Living situation—urban, isolated, extremes of social class, recent geographic move, in prison.

   xiii. Conjugal status—separated, divorced, widowed, single.

   xiv. Vocational status—unemployed (especially recently), professionals.

    xv. Family history—suicide, early parental loss, mood disorder, chaotic family background.

   xvi. Mental status signs—command auditory hallucinations, hopelessness, suicidal ideation (assess intention, plan, method, means, lethality, implementation, violence).

## Prevent violence toward others

1. During the evaluation, briefly assess the patient for risk of violence. If risk is deemed significant, consider the following options:
   a. Inform the patient that violence is not acceptable.
   b. Approach the patient in a nonthreatening manner.
   c. Reassure, calm, or assist patient's reality testing.
   d. Offer medication.
   e. Inform the patient that restraint (or seclusion) will be used if necessary.
   f. Show of force—have teams ready to restrain.
   g. When patient is restrained, always closely observe him or her, and frequently check vital signs. Isolate the restrained patient from surrounding agitating stimuli. Immediately plan a further approach—medication, reassurance, medical evaluation.

2. Signs of impending violence:
   a. Very recent acts of violence; also property violence.
   b. Menacing verbal or physical threats.
   c. Carrying weapons or other objects that might be used as such, e.g., forks, ashtrays.
   d. Progressive psychomotor agitation.
   e. Alcohol or drug intoxication.
   f. Paranoid features in a psychotic patient.
   g. Violent command auditory hallucinations.
   h. Brain disease, e.g., tumors, dementia, global or with frontal lobe findings; less commonly with temporal lobe findings (controversial).
   i. Patients with catatonic excitement.
   j. Mania.
   k. Agitated depression.
   l. Personality disorder patients prone to rage, violence, or impulsivity.

3. Assess the risk of violence:
   a. Consider violent ideation, wish, intention, plan, availability of means, implementation of plan, wish for help.

   b. Consider demographics—sex (male), age (15–24), socioeconomic status (low), social supports (few).
   c. Consider past history: violence, nonviolent antisocial acts, impulse-dyscontrol problems, e.g., gambling, substance abuse, suicide or self-injury, psychosis.
   d. Consider overt stressors, e.g., marital conflict.
4. Management
   a. Hospitalization:
      i.   Locked unit may be necessary.
      ii.  Involuntary admission may be necessary (see Chapter 26).
      iii. 1-to-1 precautions often are required to prevent assault, arson, elopement.
   b. Crisis intervention—requires the following:
      i.   Reliable and motivated patient.
      ii.  Reliable accessory persons.
      iii. Immediate follow-up.
      iv.  Avoidance of provocative situations.
      v.   Possible medications, electroconvulsive therapy (ECT).

## IV.  Other psychiatric emergencies

Common psychiatric emergencies are listed in Table 19–1.

---

*For a more detailed discussion of this topic, see Psychiatric Emergencies, Chap 30, pp 1739–1765 in* CTP/VI.

---

TABLE 19–1
**COMMON PSYCHIATRIC EMERGENCIES**

| Syndrome | Emergency Manifestations | Treatment Issues |
|---|---|---|
| Abuse of child or adult | Signs of physical trauma | Management of medical problems; psychiatric evaluation |
| Acquired immunodeficiency syndrome (AIDS) | Changes in behavior secondary to organic causes; changes in behavior secondary to fear and anxiety; suicidal behavior | Management of neurological illness; management of psychological concomitants; reinforcement of social support |
| Adolescent crises | Suicidal attempts and ideation; substance abuse, truancy, trouble with law, pregnancy, running away; eating disorders; psychosis | Evaluation of suicidal potential, extent of substance abuse, family dynamics; crisis-oriented family and individual therapy; hospitalization if necessary; consultation with appropriate extrafamilial authorities |
| Agoraphobia | Panic; depression | Alprazolam (Xanax), 0.25–2 mg; propranolol (Inderal); antidepressant medication |
| Agranulocytosis (Clozapine (Clozaril)-induced) | High fever, pharyngitis, oral and perianal ulcerations | Discontinue medication immediately; administer granulocyte-colony stimulating factor |
| Akathisia | Agitation, restlessness, muscle discomfort; dysphoria | Reduce antipsychotic dosage; propranolol (30–120 mg a day); benzodiazepines; diphenhydramine (Benadryl) orally or IV; benztropine (Cogentin) IM |
| Alcohol-related emergencies | | |
| Alcohol-induced delirium | Confusion, disorientation, fluctuating consciousness and perception, autonomic hyperactivity; may be fatal | Chlordiazepoxide; haloperidol (Haldol) for psychotic symptoms may be added if necessary |
| Alcohol intoxication | Disinhibited behavior, sedation at high doses | With time and protective environment, symptoms abate |
| Alcohol-induced persisting amnestic disorder | Confusion, loss of memory even for all personal identification data | Hospitalization; hypnosis; amobarbital (Amytal) interview; rule out other causes |
| Alcohol-induced persisting dementia | Confusion, agitation, impulsivity | Rule out other causes for dementia; no effective treatment; hospitalization if necessary |
| Alcohol-induced psychotic disorder with hallucinations | Vivid auditory (at times visual) hallucinations with affect appropriate to content (often fearful); clear sensorium | Haloperidol for psychotic symptoms |
| Alcohol seizures | Grand mal seizures; rarely status epilepticus | Diazepam (Valium), phenytoin (Dilantin); prevent by using chlordiazepoxide (Librium) during detoxification |
| Alcohol withdrawal | Irritability, nausea, vomiting, insomnia, malaise, autonomic hyperactivity, shakiness | Fluid and electrolytes maintained; sedation with benzodiazepines; restraints; monitoring of vital signs; 100 mg thiamine IM |
| Idiosyncratic alcohol intoxication | Marked aggressive or assaultive behavior | Generally no treatment required other than protective environment |
| Korsakoff's syndrome | Alcohol stigmata, amnesia, confabulation | No effective treatment; institutionalization often needed. |

*(continued on next page)*

TABLE 19–1 *(continued)*
**COMMON PSYCHIATRIC EMERGENCIES**

| Syndrome | Emergency Manifestations | Treatment Issues |
|---|---|---|
| Wernicke's encephalopathy | Oculomotor disturbances, cerebellar ataxia; mental confusion | Thiamine, 100 mg IV or IM, with $MgSO_4$ given before glucose loading |
| Amphetamine (or amphetaminelike) intoxication | Delusions, paranoia; violence; depression (from withdrawal); anxiety, delirium | Antipsychotics; restraints; hospitalization if necessary; no need for gradual withdrawal; antidepressants may be necessary |
| Anorexia nervosa | Loss of 25% of body weight of the norm for age and sex | Hospitalization; electrocardiogram (EKG), fluid and electrolytes; neuroendocrine evaluation |
| Anticholinergic intoxication | Psychotic symptoms, dry skin and mouth, hyperpyrexia, midriasis, tachycardia, restlessness, visual hallucinations | Discontinue drug, IV physostigmine (Antilirium), 0.5–2 mg, for severe agitation or fever, benzodiazepines; antipsychotics contraindicated |
| Anticonvulsant intoxication | Psychosis; delirium | Dosage of anticonvulsant is reduced |
| Benzodiazepine intoxication | Sedation, somnolence, and ataxia | Supportive measures; flumazenil (Romazicon), 7.5–45 mg a day; titrated as needed, should be used only by skilled personnel with resuscitative equipment available |
| Bereavement | Guilt feelings; irritability; insomnia; somatic complaints | Must be differentiated from major depressive disorder; antidepressants not indicated; benzodiazepines for sleep; encouragement of ventilation |
| Borderline personality disorder | Suicidal ideation and gestures; homicidal ideations and gestures; substance abuse; micropsychotic episodes; burns, cut marks on body | Suicidal and homicidal evaluation (if great, hospitalization; small dosages of antipsychotics; clear follow-up plan |
| Brief psychotic disorder | Emotional turmoil, extreme lability; acutely impaired reality testing after obvious psychosocial stress | Hospitalization often necessary; low dosage of antipsychotics may be necessary but often resolves spontaneously |
| Bromide intoxication | Delirium; mania; depression; psychosis | Serum concentrations obtained (> 50 mg a day); bromide intake discontinued; large quantities of sodium chloride IV or orally; if agitation, paraldehyde or antipsychotic is used |
| Caffeine intoxication | Severe anxiety, resembling panic disorder; mania; delirium; agitated depression; sleep disturbance | Cessation of caffeine-containing substances; benzodiazepines |
| Cannabis intoxication | Delusions; panic; dysphoria; cognitive impairment | Benzodiazepines and antipsychotics as needed; evaluation of suicidal or homicidal risk; symptoms usually abate with time and reassurance |
| Catatonic schizophrenia | Marked psychomotor disturbance (either excitement or stupor); exhaustion, can be fatal | Rapid tranquilization with antipsychotics; monitor vital signs; amobarbital may release patient from catatonic mutism or stupor but can precipitate violent behavior |

*(continued on next page)*

TABLE 19–1 (continued)
**COMMON PSYCHIATRIC EMERGENCIES**

| Syndrome | Emergency Manifestations | Treatment Issues |
|---|---|---|
| Cimetidine psychotic disorder | Delirium; delusions | Reduce dosage or discontinue drug |
| Clonidine withdrawal | Irritability; psychosis; violence; seizures | Symptoms abate with time, but antipsychotics may be necessary; gradual lowering of dosage |
| Cocaine intoxication and withdrawal | Paranoia and violence; severe anxiety; manic state, delirium; schizophreniform psychosis; tachycardia, hypertension, myocardial infarction, cerebrovascular disease; depression and suicidal ideation | Antipsychotics and benzodiazepines; antidepressants or ECT for withdrawal depression if persistent; hospitalization |
| Delirium | Fluctuating sensorium; suicidal and homicidal risk; cognitive clouding; visual, tactile, and auditory hallucinations; paranoia | Evaluate all potential contributing factors and treat each accordingly; reassurance, structure, clues to orientation; benzodiazepines and low-dosage, high-potency antipsychotics must be used with extreme care because of their potential to act paradoxically and increase agitation |
| Delusional disorder | Most often brought in to emergency room involuntarily; threats directed toward others | Antipsychotics if patient will comply (IM if necessary); intensive family intervention; hospitalization if necessary |
| Dementia | Unable to care for self; violent outbursts; psychosis; depression and suicidal ideation; confusion | Small dosages of high-potency antipsychotics; clues to orientation; organic evaluation, including medication use; family intervention |
| Depressive disorders | Suicidal ideation and attempts; self-neglect; substance abuse | Assessment of danger to self; hospitalization if necessary; nonpsychiatric causes of depression must be evaluated |
| L-Dopa intoxication | Mania; depression; schizophreniform psychosis; may induce rapid cycling in patients with bipolar I disorder | Lower dosage or discontinue drug |
| Dystonia, acute | Intense involuntary spasm of muscles of neck, tongue, face, jaw, eyes, or trunk | Decrease dosage of antipsychotic; benztropine or diphenhydramine IM |
| Group hysteria | Groups of people exhibit extremes of grief or other disruptive behavior | Group is dispersed with help of other health care workers; ventilation, crisis-oriented therapy; if necessary, small dosages of benzodiazepines |
| Hallucinogen-induced psychotic disorder with hallucinations | Symptom picture is result of interaction of type of substance, dose taken, duration of action, user's premorbid personality, setting; panic; agitation; atropine psychosis | Serum and urine screens; rule out underlying medical or mental disorder; benzodiazepines (2–20 mg) orally; reassurance and orientation; rapid tranquilization; often responds spontaneously |
| Homicidal and assaultive behavior | Marked agitation with verbal threats | Seclusion, restraints, medication |

(continued on next page)

TABLE 19–1 *(continued)*
**COMMON PSYCHIATRIC EMERGENCIES**

| Syndrome | Emergency Manifestations | Treatment Issues |
|---|---|---|
| Homosexual panic | Not seen with men or women who are comfortable with their sexual orientation; occurs in those who adamantly deny having any homoerotic impulses; impulses are aroused by talk, a physical overture, or play among same-sex friends, such as wrestling, sleeping together, or touching each other in a shower or hot tub; panicked person sees others as sexually interested in him or her and defends against them | Ventilation, environmental structure, and, in some instances, medication for acute panic (e.g., alprazolam, 0.25–2 mg) or antipsychotics may be required; opposite-sex clinician should evaluate the patient whenever possible, and the patient should not be touched save for the routine examination; patients have attacked physicians who were examining an abdomen or performing a rectal examination (e.g., on a man who harbors thinly veiled unintegrated homosexual impulses) |
| Hypertensive crisis | Life-threatening hypertensive reaction secondary to ingestion of tyramine-containing foods in combination with MAOIs; headache, stiff neck, sweating, nausea, vomiting | α-Adrenergic blockers (e.g., phentolamine (Regitine)); nifedipine (Procardia) 10 mg orally; chlorpromazine (Thorazine); make sure symptoms are not secondary to hypotension (side effect of monoamine oxidase inhibitors (MAOIs) alone) |
| Hyperthermia | Extreme excitement or catatonic stupor or both; extremely elevated temperature; violent hyperagitation | Hydrate and cool; may be drug reaction, so discontinue any drug; rule out infection |
| Hyperventilation | Anxiety, terror, clouded consciousness; giddiness, faintness; blurring vision | Shift alkalosis by having patient breathe into paper bag; patient education; antianxiety agents |
| Hypothermia | Confusion; lethargy; combativeness; low body temperature and shivering; paradoxical feeling of warmth | IV fluids and rewarming; cardiac status must be carefully monitored; avoidance of alcohol |
| Incest and sexual abuse of a child | Suicidal behavior; adolescent crises; substance abuse | Corroboration of charge; protection of victim; contact social services; medical and psychiatric evaluation; crisis intervention |
| Insomnia | Depression and irritability; early morning agitation; frightening dreams; fatigue | Hypnotics only in short term; e.g., triazolam (Halcion), 0.25–0.5 mg, at bedtime; treat any underlying mental disorder; sleep hygiene |
| Intermittent explosive disorder | Brief outbursts of violence; periodic episodes of suicide attempts | Benzodiazepines or antipsychotics for short term; long-term evaluation with computed tomography (CT) scan, sleep-deprived electroencephalogram (EEG), glucose tolerance curve |
| Jaundice | Uncommon complication of low-potency phenothiazine use (e.g., chlorpromazine) | Change drug to low dosage of a low-potency agent in a different class |
| Leukopenia and agranulocytosis | Side effects within the first two months of treatment with antipsychotics | Patient should call immediately for sore throat, fever, etc., and obtain immediate blood count; discontinue drug; hospitalize if necessary |

*(continued on next page)*

TABLE 19–1 *(continued)*
**COMMON PSYCHIATRIC EMERGENCIES**

| Syndrome | Emergency Manifestations | Treatment Issues |
|---|---|---|
| Lithium toxicity | Vomiting; abdominal pain; profuse diarrhea; severe tremor, ataxia; coma; seizures; confusion; dysarthria; focal neurological signs | Lavage with wide-bore tube; osmotic diuresis; medical consultation; may require ICU treatment |
| Major depressive episode with psychotic features | Major depressive episode symptoms with delusions; agitation, severe guilt; ideas of reference; suicide and homicide risk | Antipsychotics plus antidepressants; evaluation of suicide and homicide risk; hospitalization and ECT if necessary |
| Manic episode | Violent, impulsive behavior; indiscriminate sexual or spending behavior; psychosis; substance abuse | Hospitalization; restraints if necessary; rapid tranquilization with antipsychotics; restoration of lithium levels |
| Marital crises | Precipitant may be discovery of an extramarital affair, onset of serious illness, announcement of intent to divorce, or problems with children or work; one or both members of the couple may be in therapy or may be psychiatrically ill; one spouse may be seeking hospitalization for the other | Each should be questioned alone regarding extramarital affairs, consultations with lawyers regarding divorce, and willingness to work in crisis-oriented or long-term therapy to resolve the problem; sexual, financial, and psychiatric treatment histories from both, psychiatric evaluation at the time of presentation; may be precipitated by onset of untreated mood disorder or affective symptoms caused by medical illness or insidious-onset dementia; referral for management of the illness reduces immediate stress and enhances the healthier spouse's coping capacity; children may give insights available only to someone intimately involved in the social system |
| Migraine | Throbbing, unilateral headache | Sumatriptan (Imitrex) 6 mg IM |
| Mitral valve prolapse | Associated with panic disorder, dyspnea and palpitations; fear and anxiety | Echocardiogram; alprazolam or propranolol |
| Neuroleptic malignant syndrome | Hyperthermia; muscle rigidity; autonomic instability; parkinsonian symptoms; catatonic stupor; neurological signs; 10–30% fatality; elevated creatine phosphokinase | Discontinue antipsychotic; IV dantrolene (Dantrium); bromocriptine (Parlodel) orally; hydration and cooling; monitor CPK levels |
| Nitrous oxide toxicity | Euphoria and light-headedness | Symptoms abate without treatment within hours of use |
| Nutmeg intoxication | Agitation; hallucinations; severe headaches; numbness in extremities | Symptoms abate within hours of use without treatment |
| Opioid intoxication and withdrawal | Intoxication can lead to coma and death; withdrawal is not life-threatening | IV naloxone, narcotic antagonist; urine and serum screens; psychiatric and medical illnesses (e.g., AIDS) may complicate picture |

*(continued on next page)*

TABLE 19-1 (continued)
**COMMON PSYCHIATRIC EMERGENCIES**

| Syndrome | Emergency Manifestations | Treatment Issues |
| --- | --- | --- |
| Panic disorder | Panic, terror; acute onset | Must differentiate from other anxiety-producing disorders, both medical and psychiatric; EKG to rule out mitral valve prolapse; propranolol (10-30 mg); alprazolam (0.25-2.0 mg); long-term management may include an antidepressant |
| Paranoid schizophrenia | Command hallucinations; threat to others or themselves | Rapid tranquilization; hospitalization; long-acting depot medication; threatened persons must be notified and protected |
| Parkinsonism | Stiffness, tremor, bradykinesia, flattened affect, shuffling gait, salivation, secondary to antipsychotic medication | Oral antiparkinsonian drug for four weeks to three months; decrease dosage of the antipsychotic |
| Perioral (rabbit) tremor | Perioral tremor (rabbitlike facial grimacing) usually appearing after long-term therapy with antipsychotics | Decrease dosage or change to a medication in another class |
| Phencyclidine (or phencyclidinelike) intoxication | Paranoid psychosis; can lead to death; acute danger to self and others | Serum and urine assay; benzodiazepines may interfere with excretion; antipsychotics may worsen symptoms because of anticholinergic side effects; medical monitoring and hospitalization for severe intoxication |
| Phenelzine-induced psychotic disorder | Psychosis and mania in predisposed people | Reduce dosage or discontinue drug |
| Phenylpropanolamine toxicity | Psychosis; paranoia; insomnia; restlessness; nervousness; headache | Symptoms abate with dosage reduction or discontinuation (found in over-the-counter diet aids and oral and nasal decongestants) |
| Phobias | Panic, anxiety; fear | Treatment same as for panic disorder |
| Photosensitivity | Easy sunburning secondary to use of antipsychotic medication | Patient should avoid strong sunlight and use high-level sunscreens |
| Pigmentary retinopathy | Reported with dosages of thioridazine (Mellaril) equal to or greater than 800 mg a day | Remain below 800 mg a day of thioridazine |
| Postpartum psychosis | Childbirth can precipitate schizophrenia, depression, reactive psychoses, mania, and depression; affective symptoms are most common; suicide risk is reduced during pregnancy but increased in the postpartum period | Danger to self and others (including infant) must be evaluated and proper precautions taken; medical illness presenting with behavioral aberrations is included in the differential diagnosis and must be sought and treated; care must be paid to the effects on father, infant, grandparents, and other children |

(continued on next page)

TABLE 19–1 *(continued)*
**COMMON PSYCHIATRIC EMERGENCIES**

| Syndrome | Emergency Manifestations | Treatment Issues |
|---|---|---|
| Posttraumatic stress disorder | Panic, terror; suicidal ideation; flashbacks | Reassurance; encouragement of return to responsibilities; avoid hospitalization if possible to prevent chronic invalidism; monitor suicidal ideation |
| Priapism (trazodone (Desyrel)-induced) | Persistent penile erection accompanied by severe pain | Intracorporeal epinephrine; mechanical or surgical drainage |
| Propranolol toxicity | Profound depression; confusional states | Reduce dosage or discontinue drug; monitor suicidality |
| Rape | Not all sexual violations are reported; silent rape reaction is characterized by loss of appetite, sleep disturbance, anxiety, and, sometimes, agoraphobia; long periods of silence, mounting anxiety, stuttering, blocking, and physical symptoms during the interview when the sexual history is taken; fear of violence and death and of contracting a sexually transmitted disease or being pregnant | Rape is a major psychiatric emergency; victim may have enduring patterns of sexual dysfunction; crisis-oriented therapy, social support, ventilation, reinforcement of healthy traits, and encouragement to return to the previous level of functioning as rapidly as possible; legal counsel; thorough medical examination and tests to identify the assailant (e.g., obtaining samples of pubic hairs with a pubic hair comb, vaginal smear to identify blood antigens in semen); if a woman, methoxyprogesterone or diethylstilbestrol orally for five days to prevent pregnancy; if menstruation does not commence within one week of cessation of the estrogen, all alternatives to pregnancy, including abortion, should be offered; if the victim has contracted a venereal disease, appropriate antibiotics; witnessed written permission is required for the physician to examine, photograph, collect specimens, and release information to the authorities; obtain consent, record the history in the patient's own words, obtain required tests, record the results of the examination, save all clothing, defer diagnosis, and provide protection against disease, psychic trauma, and pregnancy; men's and women's responses to rape affectively are reported similarly, although men are more hesitant to talk about the assault, particularly if it was homosexual, for fear they will be assumed to have consented |
| Reserpine intoxication | Major depressive episode; suicidal ideation; nightmares | Evaluation of suicidal ideation; lower dosage or change drug; antidepressants or ECT may be indicated |

*(continued on next page)*

TABLE 19–1 *(continued)*
**COMMON PSYCHIATRIC EMERGENCIES**

| Syndrome | Emergency Manifestations | Treatment Issues |
|---|---|---|
| Schizoaffective disorder | Severe depression; manic symptoms; paranoia | Evaluation of dangerousness to self or others; rapid tranquilization if necessary; treatment of depression (antidepressants alone can enhance schizophrenic symptoms); use of antimanic agents |
| Schizophrenia | Extreme self-neglect; severe paranoia; suicidal ideation or assaultiveness; extreme psychotic symptoms | Evaluation of suicidal and homicidal potential; identification of any illness other than schizophrenia; rapid tranquilization |
| Schizophrenia in exacerbation | Withdrawn; agitation; suicidal and homicidal risk | Suicide and homocide evaluation; screen for medical illness; restraints and rapid tranquilization if necessary; hospitalization if necessary; reevaluation of medication regimen |
| Sedative, hypnotic, or anxiolytic intoxication and withdrawal | Alterations in mood, behavior, thought—delirium; derealization and depersonalization; untreated, can be fatal; seizures | Naloxone (Narcan) to differentiate from opioid intoxication; slow withdrawal with phenobarbital (Luminal) or sodium thiopental or benzodiazepine; hospitalization |
| Seizure disorder | Confusion; anxiety, derealization and depersonalization; feelings of impending doom; gustatory or olfactory hallucinations; fuguelike state | Immediate EEG; admission and sleep-deprived and 24-hour EEG; rule out pseudoseizures; anticonvulsants |
| Substance withdrawal | Abdominal pain; insomnia, drowsiness; delirium; seizures; symptoms of tardive dyskinesia may emerge; eruption of manic or schizophrenic symptoms | Symptoms of psychotropic drug withdrawal disappear with time and disappear with reinstitution of the substance; symptoms of antidepressant withdrawal can be successfully treated with anticholinergic agents, such as atropine; gradual withdrawal of psychotropic substances over two to four weeks generally obviates development of symptoms |
| Sudden death associated with antipsychotic medication | Seizures; asphyxiation; cardiovascular causes; postural hypotension; laryngeal-pharyngeal dystonia; suppression of gag reflex | Specific medical treatments |
| Sudden death of psychogenic origin | Myocardial infarction after sudden psychic stress; voodoo and hexes; hopelessness, especially associated with serious physical illness | Specific medical treatments; folk healers |
| Suicide | Suicidal ideation; hopelessness | Hospitalization, antidepressants |
| Sympathomimetic withdrawal | Paranoia; confessional states; depression | Most symptoms abate without treatment; antipsychotics; antidepressants if necessary |

*(continued on next page)*

TABLE 19–1 *(continued)*
**COMMON PSYCHIATRIC EMERGENCIES**

| Syndrome | Emergency Manifestations | Treatment Issues |
|---|---|---|
| Tardive dyskinesia | Dyskinesia of mouth, tongue, face, neck, and trunk; choreoathetoid movements of extremities; usually but not always appearing after long-term treatment with antipsychotics, especially after a reduction in dosage; incidence highest in the elderly and brain-damaged; symptoms are intensified by antiparkinsonian drugs and masked but not cured by increased dosages of antipsychotic | No effective treatment reported; may be prevented by prescribing the least amount of drug possible for as little time as is clinically feasible and using drug-free holidays for patients who need to continue taking the drug; decrease or discontinue drug at first sign of dyskinetic movements |
| Thyrotoxicosis | Tachycardia; gastrointestinal dysfunction; hyperthermia; panic, anxiety, agitation; mania; dementia; psychosis | Thyroid function test ($T_3$, $T_4$, thyroid-stimulating hormone (TSH)); medical consultation |
| Toluene abuse | Anxiety; confusion; cognitive impairment | Neurological damage is nonprogressive and reversible if toluene use is discontinued early |
| Vitamin $B_{12}$ deficiency | Confusion, mood and behavior changes; ataxia | Treatment with vitamin $B_{12}$ |
| Volatile nitrates | Alternations of mood and behavior; light-headedness; pulsating headache | Symptoms abate with cessation of use |

# 20

# Infant, Child, and Adolescent Disorders

## I. Principles of child and adolescent diagnostic assessment

A. Supplement data from patient interviews with information from family members, guardians, teachers, outside agencies.

B. Understand normal development in order to fully understand what constitutes abnormality at a given age. Table 20–1 presents developmental milestones.

C. Be familiar with the current diagnostic criteria of disorders to guide anamnesis on mental status examination.

D. Understand family psychiatric history, which is necessary given the genetic predispositions and environmental influences of many disorders (Table 20–1).

## II. Child development

Development results from the interplay of **maturation** of the central nervous system (CNS), neuromuscular apparatus, and endocrine system, and **environmental influences,** e.g., parents, teachers, who can either facilitate or thwart the child's attainment of his or her developmental potential. This potential is specific to each person's given genetic predispositions to (1) intellectual level and (2) mental disorder, temperament, and, probably, certain personality traits.

Development is continual and lifelong but most rapid in early life. The neonatal brain weighs 350 grams, almost triples in weight by 18 months, and at 7 years is close to 90% of the adult 1,350 grams. Cytogenetic changes, such as neuronal differentiation, axonal growth, synapse formation, and myelination, which begin during embryonic and fetal development, continue after birth.

For decades, the most cited theorists in child development have been Sigmund Freud, Margaret Mahler, Erik Erikson, and Jean Piaget; their work is outlined in Table 20–2.

A. **Sigmund Freud.** First to discover and submit to theoretical frameworks the importance of early childhood in the development of personality and psychopathology. His data, however, came from the psychoanalyses of late adolescent or adult patients. He did not systematically observe or treat normal or abnormal children. Those who have done so have added to and revised his theory. Moreover, concerning psychopathogenesis, Freud focused on the Oedipus complex. According to Freud, neurosis resulted from the inability to resolve rivalries and unconscious libidinal and aggressive feelings toward parents within the oedipal triangle. Today this theory accounts for some, but certainly not all, of psychopathology.

TABLE 20-1
**LANDMARKS OF NORMAL BEHAVIORAL DEVELOPMENT**

| Age | Motor and Sensory Behavior | Adaptive Behavior | Personal and Social Behavior |
|---|---|---|---|
| Birth to 4 weeks | Hand to mouth reflex, grasping reflex<br>Rooting reflex (puckering lips in response to perioral stimulation), Moro reflex (digital extension when startled); sucking reflex, Babinski reflex (toes spread when sole of foot is touched)<br>Differentiates sounds (orients to human voice) and sweet and sour tastes<br>Visual tracking<br>Fixed focal distance of 8 inches<br>Makes alternating crawling movements<br>Moves head laterally when placed in prone position | Anticipatory feeding-approach behavior at 4 days<br>Responds to sound of rattle and bell<br>Regards moving objects momentarily | Responsiveness to mother's face, eyes, and voice within first few hours of life<br>Endogenous smile<br>Independent play (until 2 years)<br>Quiets when picked up<br>Impassive face |
| 4 weeks | Tonic neck reflex positions predominate<br>Hands fisted<br>Head sags but can hold head erect for a few seconds<br>Visual fixation, stereoscopic vision (12 weeks) | Follows moving objects to the midline<br>Shows no interest and drops objects immediately | Regards face and diminishes activity<br>Responds to speech<br>Smiles preferentially to mother |
| 16 weeks | Symmetrical postures predominate<br>Holds head balanced<br>Head lifted 90 degrees when prone on forearm<br>Visual accommodation | Follows a slowly moving object well<br>Arms activate on sight of dangling object | Spontaneous social smile (exogenous)<br>Aware of strange situations |
| 28 weeks | Sits steadily, leaning forward on hands<br>Bounces actively when placed in standing position | One-hand approach and grasp of toy<br>Bangs and shakes rattle<br>Transfers toys | Takes feet to mouth<br>Pats mirror image<br>Starts to imitate mother's sounds and actions |
| 40 weeks | Sits alone with good coordination<br>Creeps<br>Pulls self to standing position<br>Points with index finger | Matches two objects at midline<br>Attempts to imitate scribble | Separation anxiety manifest when taken away from mother<br>Responds to social play, such as pat-a-cake and peekaboo<br>Feeds self cracker and holds own bottle |

(continued on next page)

TABLE 20–1 (continued)
LANDMARKS OF NORMAL BEHAVIORAL DEVELOPMENT

| Age | Motor and Sensory Behavior | Adaptive Behavior | Personal and Social Behavior |
|---|---|---|---|
| 52 weeks | Walks with one hand held<br>Stands alone briefly | Seeks novelty | Cooperates in dressing |
| 15 months | Toddles<br>Creeps up stairs | | Points or vocalizes wants<br>Throws objects in play or refusal |
| 18 months | Coordinated walking, seldom falls<br>Hurls ball<br>Walks up stairs with one hand held | Build a tower of three or four cubes<br>Scribbles spontaneously and imitates a writing stroke | Feeds self in part, spills<br>Pulls toy on string<br>Carries or hugs a special toy, such as a doll<br>Imitates some behavioral patterns with slight delay |
| 2 years | Runs well, no falling<br>Kicks large ball<br>Goes up and down stairs alone<br>Fine motor skills increase | Builds a tower of six or seven cubes<br>Aligns cubes, imitating train<br>Imitates vertical and circular strokes<br>Develops original behaviors | Pulls on simple garment<br>Domestic mimicry<br>Refers to self by name<br>Says "no" to mother<br>Separation anxiety begins to diminish<br>Organized demonstrations of love and protest<br>Parallel play (plays side by side but does not interact with other children) |
| 3 years | Rides tricycle<br>Jumps from bottom steps<br>Alternates feet going up stairs | Builds tower of 9 or 10 cubes<br>Imitates a three-cube bridge<br>Copies a circle and a cross | Puts on shoes<br>Unbuttons buttons<br>Feeds self well<br>Understands taking turns |
| 4 years | Walks down stairs one step to a tread<br>Stands on one foot for five to eight seconds | Copies a cross<br>Repeats four digits<br>Counts three objects with correct pointing | Washes and dries own face<br>Brushes teeth<br>Associative or joint play (plays cooperatively with other children) |
| 5 years | Skips, using feet alternately<br>Usually has complete sphincter control<br>Fine coordination improves | Copies a square<br>Draws a recognizable man with a head, a body, limbs<br>Counts 10 objects accurately | Dresses and undresses self<br>Prints a few letters<br>Plays competitive exercise games |
| 6 years | Rides two-wheel bicycle | Prints name<br>Copies triangle | Ties shoelaces |

Table adapted from Arnold Gessell, M.D., and Stella Chess, MD.

TABLE 20-2
**A SYNTHESIS OF DEVELOPMENTAL THEORISTS**

| Age (Years) | Margaret Mahler | Sigmund Freud | Erik Erikson | Jean Piaget | Comments |
|---|---|---|---|---|---|
| 0–1 | Normal autistic phase (birth to 4 weeks)<br>• State of half-sleep, half-wake<br>• Major task of phase is to achieve homeostatic equilibrium with the environment<br><br>Normal symbiotic phase (3–4 weeks to 4–5 months)<br>• Dim awareness of caretaker, but infant still functions as if he and caretaker are in state of undifferentiation or fusion<br>• Social smile characteristic (2–4 months)<br><br>The subphases of separation-individuation proper<br><br>First subphase: differentiation (5–10 months)<br>• Process of hatching from autistic shell, i.e., developing more alert sensorium that reflects cognitive and neurological maturation | Oral phase (birth to 1 year)<br>• Major site of tension and gratification is the mouth, lips, tongue<br>—includes biting and sucking activities | Basic trust vs. basic mistrust (oral sensory) (birth to 1 year)<br>• Social mistrust demonstrated via ease of feeding, depth of sleep, bowel relaxation<br>• Depends on consistency and sameness of experience provided by caretaker<br>• Second 6-months teething and biting moves infant "from getting to taking"<br>• Weaning leads to "nostalgia for lost paradise"<br>• If basic trust is strong, child maintains hopeful attitude | Sensorimotor phase (birth to 2 years)<br>• Intelligence rests mainly on actions and movements coordinated under "schemata." (Schema is a pattern of behavior in response to a particular environmental stimulus.)<br>• Environment is mastered through *assimilation* and *accommodation*. (Assimilation is the incorporation of new environmental stimuli. Accommodation is the modification of behavior to adapt to new stimuli.)<br>• *Object permanence* is achieved by age 2 yrs. Object still exists in mind if disappears from view; search for hidden object<br>• Reversibility in action begins | In contrast to Mahler, other observers of mother-infant pairs are impressed with a mutuality and complementarity (not autism or fusion), which provides a groundwork for relatedness and language development as if there were a prewiring for these abilities. Piaget and others emphasize the infant actively striving to manipulate the inanimate environment. This supplements Freud's work because the infant and young child's motivation for behavior is not simply to relieve drive tension and attain oral, anal, and phalic gratification. |

(continued on next page)

TABLE 20–2 (continued)
**A SYNTHESIS OF DEVELOPMENTAL THEORISTS**

| Age (Years) | Margaret Mahler | Sigmund Freud | Erik Erikson | Jean Piaget | Comments |
|---|---|---|---|---|---|
| | • Beginning of comparative scanning, i.e., comparing what is and what is not mother<br>• Characteristic anxiety: stranger anxiety, which involves curiosity and fear (most prevalent around 8 months) | | | | Supplementing the work of Freud and Mahler, theorists have postulated that severe problems in mother-infant/ toddler interactions contribute to the formation of pathological character traits, gender identity disorder, or personality disorders. Angry, frustrating, narcissistic caretakers often produce angry, needy children and adults who cannot tolerate the normal frustrations and disappointments in relationships and whose character formation is grossly deformed. |
| 1–2 | Second subphase, practicing (10–16 months)<br>• Beginning of this phase marked by upright locomotion—child has new perspective and also mood of elation<br>• Mother used as home base<br>• Characteristic anxiety: separation anxiety<br>Third subphase: rapprochement (16–24 months)<br>• Infant now a toddler—more aware of physical separateness, which dampens mood of elation<br>• Child tries to bridge gap between himself and mother—concretely seen as bringing objects to mother | Anal phase (1 year to 3 years)<br>• Anus and surrounding area is major source of interest<br>• Acquisition of voluntary sphincter control (toilet training) | Autonomy vs. shame and doubt (muscular-anal) (1–3 years)<br>• Biologically includes learning to walk, feed self, talk<br>• Muscular maturation sets stage for "holding on and letting go"<br>• Need for outer control, firmness of caretaker prior to development of autonomy<br>• Shame occurs when child is overtly self-conscious via negative exposure<br>• Self-doubt can evolve if parents overtly shame child (e.g., about elimination) | Preoperational phase (2–7 years)<br>• Appearance of symbolic functions, associated with language acquisition<br>• Egocentrism: child understands everything exclusively from own perspective<br>• Thinking is illogical and magical<br>• Nonreversible thinking with absence of conversation<br>—Animism: belief that inanimate objects are alive (i.e. have feelings and intentions)<br>—"Imminent justice": belief that punishment for bad deeds is inevitable | |

(continued on next page)

TABLE 20–2 (continued)
**A SYNTHESIS OF DEVELOPMENTAL THEORISTS**

| Age (Years) | Margaret Mahler | Sigmund Freud | Erik Erikson | Jean Piaget | Comments |
|---|---|---|---|---|---|
| | • Mother's efforts to help toddler often not perceived as helpful; temper tantrums typical<br>• Characteristic event: rapprochement crisis: wanting to be soothed by mother and yet not be able to accept her help<br>• Symbol of rapprochement: child standing on threshold of door not knowing which way to turn to helpless frustration<br>• Resolution of crisis occurs as child's skills improve and child able to get gratification from doing things himself | | | | |
| 2–3 | Fourth subphase: consolidation and object constancy (24–36 months)<br>• Child better able to cope with mother's absence and engage substitutes<br>• Child can begin to feel comfortable with mother's absences by knowing she will return | | | | |

(continued on next page)

TABLE 20-2 *(continued)*
**A SYNTHESIS OF DEVELOPMENTAL THEORISTS**

| Age (Years) | Margaret Mahler | Sigmund Freud | Erik Erikson | Jean Piaget | Comments |
|---|---|---|---|---|---|
| | • Gradual internalization of image of mother as reliable and stable<br>• Through increasing verbal skills and better sense of time, child can tolerate delay and endure separations | | | | |
| 3–4 | | Phallic-oedipal phase (3–5 years)<br>• Genital focus of interest, stimulation, and excitement<br>• Penis is organ of interest for both sexes<br>• Genital masturbation common<br>• Intense preoccupation with *castration anxiety* (fear of genital loss or injury)<br>• *Penis envy* (discontent with one's own genitals and wish to possess genitals of male) seen in girls in this phase<br>• *Oedipus complex* universal: child wishes to have sex and marry parent of opposite sex and simultaneously be rid of parent of same sex | Initiative vs. guilt (locomotor genital) (3–5 years)<br>• *Initiative* arises in relation to tasks for the sake of activity, both motor and intellectual<br>• *Guilt* may arise over goals contemplated (especially aggressive)<br>• Desire to mimic adult world; involvement in oedipal struggle leads to resolution via social role identification<br>• Sibling rivalry frequent | | Researchers have amended Freud's work. Children of both sexes explore and are aware of their own genitals during the second year of life and, with proper parental reinforcement, begin to correctly identify themselves as girls or boys. Penis envy is neither universal nor normative. |
| 4–5 | | | | | |

*(continued on next page)*

TABLE 20–2 (continued)
**A SYNTHESIS OF DEVELOPMENTAL THEORISTS**

| Age (Years) | Margaret Mahler | Sigmund Freud | Erik Erikson | Jean Piaget | Comments |
|---|---|---|---|---|---|
| 5–6 | | Latency phase (from 5–6 years to 11–12 years) <br>• State of relative quiescence of sexual drive with resolution of Oedipal complex <br>• Sexual drives channeled into more socially appropriate aims (i.e., schoolwork and sports) | | | Contrary to Freud, the onset of latency (school age or middle childhood) is now considered primarily due to changes in the central nervous system (CNS) and less dependent on the nondemonstrable quiescence and sublimation of sexual drive. Changes in the CNS are reflected in developmental progress, during the years 6–8, of perceptual-sensory-motor functioning and thought processes. In Piaget's framework, it is the transition from the preoperational to the concrete (operational) phase. Compared with preschoolers, latency children are capable of greater learning, independent functioning, and socialization. Friendships develop with less dependence on parents (and less preoccupation with intrafamilial oedipal rivalries). Superego development is today considered more prolonged, gradual, and less related to oedipal resolution. |
| 6–11 | | • Formation of *superego*: one of three psychic structures in mind which is responsible for moral and ethical development, including conscience <br>• (Other two psychic structures are *ego*, which is a group of functions mediating between the drives and the external environment, and <br>• the *id*, repository of sexual and aggressive drives <br>• The id is there at birth and the ego develops gradually from rudimentary structure present at birth) | Industry vs. inferiority (latency) (6–11 years) <br>• Child is busy building, creating, accomplishing <br>• Receives systematic instruction as well as fundamentals of technology <br>• Danger of sense of inadequacy and inferiority if child despairs of his tools/ skills and status among peers <br>• Socially decisive age | Concrete (operational) phase (7–11 years) <br>• Emergence of logical (cause–effect) thinking, including reversibility and ability to sequence and serialize <br>• Understanding of part/ whole relationships and classifications <br>• Child able to take other's point of view <br>• Conservation of number, length, weight, and volume | |

(continued on next page)

TABLE 20–2 (continued)
A SYNTHESIS OF DEVELOPMENTAL THEORISTS

| Age (Years) | Margaret Mahler | Sigmund Freud | Erik Erikson | Jean Piaget | Comments |
|---|---|---|---|---|---|
| 11+ | | Genital phase (from 11–12 years and beyond)<br>• Final stage of psychosexual development—begins with puberty and the biological capacity for orgasm but involves the capacity for true intimacy | Identity vs. role diffusion (11 years through end of adolescence)<br>• Struggle to develop *ego identity* (sense of inner sameness and continuity)<br>• Preoccupation with appearance, hero worship, ideology<br>• *Group identity* (peers) develops<br>• Danger of *role confusion,* doubts about sexual and vocational identity<br>• *Psychosocial moratorium,* stage between morality learned by the child and the ethics to be developed by the adult | Formal (abstract) phase (11 years through end of adolescence)<br>• Hypothetical-deductive reasoning, not only on basis of objects but also on basis of hypotheses or of propositions<br>• Capable of thinking about one's thoughts<br>• Combinative structures emerge, permitting flexible grouping of elements in a system<br>• Ability to use two systems of reference simultaneously<br>• Ability to grasp concept of probabilities | |

Table by Richard Perry, MD. Adapted from Sylvia Karasu, MD, and Richard Oberfield, MD.

TABLE 20–3
**DSM-IV DIAGNOSTIC CRITERIA FOR MENTAL RETARDATION**

A. Significantly subaverage intellectual functioning: an I.Q. of approximately 70 or below on an individually administered I.Q. test (for infants, a clinical judgment of significantly subaverage intellectual functioning).

B. Concurrent deficits or impairments in present adaptive functioning (i.e., the person's effectiveness in meeting the standards expected for his or her age by his or her cultural group) in at least two of the following areas: communication, self-care, home living, social/interpersonal skills, use of community resources, self-direction, functional academic skills, work, leisure, health, and safety.

C. The onset is before age 18 years.

*Code* based on degree of severity reflecting level of intellectual impairment:

| | |
|---|---|
| **Mild mental retardation:** | IQ level 50–55 to approximately 70 |
| **Moderate mental retardation:** | IQ level 35–40 to 50–55 |
| **Severe mental retardation:** | IQ level 20–25 to 35–40 |
| **Profound mental retardation:** | IQ level below 20 or 25 |

**Mental retardation, severity unspecified:** when there is strong presumption of mental retardation but the person's intelligence is untestable by standard tests

Used with permission, APA.

**B. Margaret Mahler.** Observed children and their mothers and evolved a theory of separation-individuation. This is generally accepted today, with the exception of her theory of phases during the first months of life, which emphasizes that infants lack alertness and responsivity.

**C. Erik Erikson.** Extended development throughout life. At each stage, there is a conflict and resolution, e.g., basic trust versus mistrust in the first stage. His work emphasizes the individual's adaptation to society.

**D. Jean Piaget.** A genetic epistemologist who studied the behaviors, from birth, of his three children and evolved a comprehensive, respected theory of cognitive development. His work reveals the infant as an active problem solver.

## III. Mental retardation (MR)

(Code on Axis II.) Occurs in 3% of live births and 1% of the population. The male-to-female ratio is 1.5:1.

**A. Diagnosis.** See Table 20–3. About 85% of persons with MR have mild MR and are considered educable, being able to attain about a grade 6 education; about 10% have moderate type and are consider trainable, being able to attain about a grade 2 education; about 3–4% have severe type; and about 1–2% have profound type.

**B. Etiology.** Organic or psychosocial; known in 50–70% of cases.

  **1. Genetic**

  a. Inborn errors of metabolism, e.g., phenylketonuria (PKU), Tay-Sachs disease.

  b. Chromosomal abnormalities, foremost: Down's syndrome (trisomy 21), 1 per 7,000 live births. Typical facies, hypotonia, hyperreflexia, cardiac malformations, gastrointestinal anomalies. Fragile X syndrome, 1 per 1,000 male births. Postpubertal macroorchidism, large head and ears, long, narrow face. (Some female carriers have facial features and cognitive dysfunction.)

  **2. Psychosocial.** Mild MR often is caused by chronic lack of intellectual stimulation.

**3. Other.**  Sequelae of infection, toxin, or brain trauma sustained prenatally, perinatally, or later, e.g., congenital rubella or fetal alcohol syndrome (microcephaly, midfacial hypoplasia, short palpebral fissure, pectus excavatum, possible cardiac defects, short stature).

**C. General considerations.**  There is no typical behavior or personality type. Poor self-esteem is common. Thinking tends to be concrete and egocentric. One third to two thirds of MR patients have concomitant mental disorder running the gamut of DSM-IV disorders.

**D. Treatment**

**1. Educational.**  Special schools or classes, remediation, tutoring.

**2. Pharmacological.**  See Table 20–4.

    a. Concomitant mental disorder, such as attention-deficit/hyperactivity disorder (ADHD) or depression, may need stimulants or antidepressants, respectively.

    b. Agitation, aggression, and tantrums often respond to antipsychotics. High-dosage, low-potency drugs, e.g., chlorpromazine (Thorazine) or thioridazine (Mellaril), are more cognitively dulling than low-dosage, high-potency ones, e.g., haloperidol (Haldol). Many institutionalized mentally retarded persons are poorly monitored on medication.

    c. Lithium (Eskalith) is useful for aggressive or self-abusive behaviors.

    d. Carbamazepine (Tegretol), valproate (Depakene), and propranolol (Inderal) can be tried for aggressive behavior or tantrums. Efficacy is less proven than for antipsychotics and lithium.

**3. Psychological**

    a. Behavior therapy.

    b. Parental and family counseling.

    c. Individual supportive psychotherapy. Awareness of inadequacies can breed low self-esteem.

    d. Mildly impaired persons with good verbal skills may profit from insight-oriented psychotherapy for concomitant disorders.

    e. Activity groups help to improve socialization.

**IV. Pervasive developmental disorders (PDDs)**

(Code on Axis I.) Autistic disorder that occurs in 4 per 10,000 persons. The male-to-female ratio is 3:1. Asperger's disorder is characterized by autisticlike behavior without delays in language or cognitive development; it may affect a subgroup of highly functioning autistic children. Rett's disorder is neurodegenerative and only affects girls. Childhood disintegrative disorder (Heller's syndrome) is distinguished by at least 2 years of normal development before deterioration to the clinical picture of autistic disorder.

**A. Diagnosis, signs, and symptoms.**  See Tables 20–5 through 20–8.

**B. General considerations.**

**1. Autistic disorder.**  Children with autistic disorder can be high or low functioning depending on I.Q., amount and communicativeness of language, and severity of other symptoms. 70% have I.Q.s below 70, and 50% have I.Q.s below 50–55. Autistic disorder is an organic disorder.

TABLE 20–4
**COMMON PSYCHOACTIVE DRUGS IN CHILDHOOD AND ADOLESCENCE**

| Drugs | Indications | Dosage | Adverse Reactions and Monitoring |
|---|---|---|---|
| **Antipsychotics**—also known as major tranquilizers, neuroleptics Divided into (1) high-potency, low-dosage, e.g. haloperidol (Haldol), trifluoperazine (Stelazine), Thiothixene (Navane); (2) low-potency, high-dosage (more sedating), e.g., chlorpromazine (Thorazine), thioridazine (Mellaril); and (3) clozapine (Clozaril); and (4) risperidone (Risperdal) | Psychoses: agitated, aggressive, self-injurious behaviors in mental retardation (MR), pervasive developmental disorders (PDD), and conduct disorder (CD) Studies support following indications: haloperidol—schizophrenia, PDD, CD with severe aggression, Tourette's disorder Clozapine—refractory schizophrenia in adolescence | All can be given in two to four divided doses or combined into one dose after gradual buildup Haloperidol—child 0.5–6 mg a day, adolescent 0.5–16 mg a day Thiothixene—5–42 mg a day Chlorpromazine and thioridazine—child 10–200 mg a day, adolescent 50–600 mg a day, over 16 years of age 100–700 mg a day Clozapine—dosage not determined in children; <600 mg/day in adolescents Risperidone—1–3 mg a day in several children with PDD | Sedation, weight gain, hypotension, lowered seizure threshold, constipation, extrapyramidal symptoms, jaundice, agranulocytosis, dystonic reaction, tardive dyskinesia; with clozapine no extrapyramidal adverse effects Monitor: blood pressure, complete blood count (CBC), liver function tests (LFTs), electroencephalogram (EEG). If indicated; with thioridazine pigmentary retinopathy is rare but dictates ceiling of 800 mg in adults and proportionately lower in children; with clozapine, weekly white blood counts (WBCs) for development of agranulocytosis and EEG monitoring due to lowering of seizure threshold |
| **Stimulants** Dextroamphetamine (Dexedrine) FDA-approved for children 3 years and older Methylphenidate (Ritalin) and pemoline (Cylert) FDA-approved for children 6 years and older | In attention-deficit/hyperactivity disorder (ADHD) for hyperactivity, impulsivity, and inattentiveness | Dextroamphetamine and methylphenidate are generally given at 8 AM and noon (the usefulness of sustained release preparations is not proved) Dextroamphetamine—2.5–40 mg a day up to 0.5 mg per kg a day Methylphenidate—10–60 mg a day or up to 1.0 mg per kg a day Pemoline—37.5–112.5 mg given at 8 AM | Insomnia, anorexia, weight loss (and possibly growth delay), headache, tachycardia, precipitation or exacerbation of tic disorders With pemoline, monitor LFTs, as hepatoxicity is possible |

(continued on next page)

TABLE 20–4 *(continued)*
**COMMON PSYCHOACTIVE DRUGS IN CHILDHOOD AND ADOLESCENCE**

| Drugs | Indications | Dosage | Adverse Reactions and Monitoring |
|---|---|---|---|
| **Lithium**—considered an antipsychotic drug, also has antiaggression properties | Studies support use in MR and CD for aggressive and self-injurious behaviors; can be used for same in PDD; also indicated for early-onset bipolar I disorder | 600–2.100 mg in two or three divided doses; keep blood levels to 0.4–1.2 mEq per L | Nausea, vomiting, enuresis, headache, tremor, weight gain, hypothyroidism Experience with adults suggests renal function monitoring |
| **Tricyclic drugs** Imipramine (Tofranil) has been used in most child studies Nortriptyline (Pamelor) has been studied in children Clomipramine (Anafranil) is effective in child obsessive-compulsive disorder (OCD) | Major depressive disorder, separation anxiety disorder, bulimia nervosa, enuresis; sometimes used in ADHD, sleepwalking disorder, and sleep terror disorder Clomipramine is effective in child OCD and sometimes in PDD | Imipramine—start with divided dosages totalling about 1.5 mg per kg a day; can build up to not more than 5 mg per kg a day and eventually combine in one dose; not FDA-approved for children except for enuresis; dosage is usually 50–100 mg before sleep Clomipramine—start at 50 mg a day; can raise to not more than 3 mg per kg a day or 200 mg a day | Dry mouth, constipation, tachycardia, drowsiness, postural hypotension, hypertension, mania Electrocardiogram (ECG) monitoring is needed because of risk for cardiac conduction slowing; consider lowering dosage if PR interval >0.20 seconds or QRS interval >0.12 seconds; baseline EEG is advised, as it can lower seizure threshold (especially with clomipramine); blood levels of drug are sometimes useful |
| **Serotonin-specific reuptake inhibitors**— fluoxetine (Prozac), sertraline (Zoloft) and fluvoxamine (Luvox) | OCD; (may be useful in major depressive disorder, anorexia, bulimia nervosa, repetitive behaviors in MR or PDD | Appears less than adult dosages | Nausea, headache, nervousness, insomnia, dry mouth, diarrhea, drowsiness |
| **Carbamazepine** (Tegretol)—an anticonvulsant | Aggression or dyscontrol in MR or CD, bipolar disorder | Start with 10 mg per kg a day; can build to 20–30 mg per kg a day; therapeutic blood level range appears to be 4–12 mg per L | Drowsiness, nausea, rash, vertigo, irritability Monitor: CBC and LFTs for possible blood dyscrasias and hepatotoxicity; blood levels are necessary |

(continued on next page)

TABLE 20-4 *(continued)*
**COMMON PSYCHOACTIVE DRUGS IN CHILDHOOD AND ADOLESCENCE**

| Drugs | Indications | Dosage | Adverse Reactions and Monitoring |
|---|---|---|---|
| **Benzodiazepines**—have been insufficiently studied in childhood and adolescence | Sometimes effective in parasomnias: sleepwalking disorder or sleep terror disorder; can be tried in generalized anxiety disorder | Parasomnias: diazepam (Valium) 2–10 mg before bedtime | Can cause drowsiness, ataxia, tremor, dyscontrol; can be abused |
| | Clonazepam (Klonopin) can be tried in all anxiety disorders, especially panic disorder | | |
| | Alprazolam (Xanax) can be tried in separation anxiety disorder | | |
| **Fenfluramine** (Pondimin)—an amphetamine congener | Well-studied in autistic disorder; generally ineffective, but some patients show improvement | Gradually increases to 1.0–1.5 mg per kg a day in divided doses | Weight loss, drowsiness, irritability, loose bowel movements |
| **Propranolol** (Inderal)—a β-adrenergic blocker | Aggression in MR, PDD, and cognitive disorder; awaits controlled studies | Effective dosage in children and adolescents is not yet established; range is probably 40–320 mg a day | Bradycardia, hypotension, nausea, hypoglycemia, depression; avoid in asthma |
| **Clonidine** (Catapres) and guanfacine (Tenex)—presynaptic α-adrenergic blocking agents | Some success in ADHD; clonidine in Tourette's disorder | Clonidine—0.1–0.3 mg a day; 3–5.5 μg per kg a day Guanfacine—up to 3 mg a day | Orthostatic hypotension, sedation, dry mouth |
| **Cyproheptadine** (Periactin) | Anorexia nervosa | Dosages up to 8 mg four times a day | Antihistaminic side effects, including sedation and dryness of the mouth |
| **Naltrexone** (ReVia) | Self-injurious behaviors in MR and PDD; currently being studied in PDD | 0.5–2.0 mg per kg a day | Sleepiness, aggressivity Monitor LFTs, as hepatotoxicity has been reported in adults at high dosages |
| **Desmopressin** (DDAVP) | Nocturnal enuresis | 20–40 μg intranasally | Headache, hyponatremic seizures (rare) |

Table by Richard Perry, M.D.

TABLE 20–5
**DSM-IV DIAGNOSTIC CRITERIA FOR AUTISTIC DISORDER**

A. A total of six (or more) items from (1), (2), and (3), with at least two from (1), and one each from (2) and (3):
(1) qualitative impairment in social interaction, as manifested by at least two of the following:
(a) marked impairment in the use of multiple nonverbal behaviors such as eye-to-eye gaze, facial expression, body postures, and gestures to regulate social interaction
(b) failure to develop peer relationships appropriate to developmental level
(c) a lack of spontaneous seeking to share enjoyment, interests, or achievements with other people (e.g., by a lack of showing, bringing, or pointing out objects of interest)
(d) lack of social or emotional reciprocity
(2) qualitative impairments in communication as manifested by at least one of the following:
(a) delay in, or total lack of, the development of spoken language (not accompanied by an attempt to compensate through alternative modes of communication such as gesture or mime)
(b) in individuals with adequate speech, marked impairment in the ability to initiate or sustain a conversation with others
(c) stereotyped and repetitive use of language or idiosyncratic language
(d) lack of varied, spontaneous make-believe play or social imitative play appropriate to developmental level
(3) restricted repetitive and stereotyped patterns of behavior, interests, and activities, as manifested by at least one of the following:
(a) encompassing preoccupation with one or more stereotyped and restricted patterns of interest that is abnormal either in intensity or focus
(b) apparently inflexible adherence to specific, nonfunctional routines or rituals
(c) stereotyped and repetitive motor mannerisms (e.g., hand or finger flapping or twisting, or complex whole-body movements)
(d) persistent preoccupation with parts of objects
B. Delays or abnormal functioning in at least one of the following areas, with onset prior to age 3 years: (1) social interaction, (2) language as used in social communication, or (3) symbolic or imaginative play.
C. The disturbance is not better accounted for by Rett's disorder or childhood disintegrative disorder.

Used with permission, APA.

TABLE 20–6
**DSM-IV DIAGNOSTIC CRITERIA FOR RETT'S DISORDER**

A. All of the following:
(1) apparently normal prenatal and perinatal development
(2) apparently normal psychomotor development through the first 5 months after birth
(3) normal head circumference at birth
B. Onset of all of the following after the period of normal development:
(1) deceleration of head growth between ages 5 and 48 months
(2) loss of previously acquired purposeful hand skills between ages 5 and 30 months with the subsequent development of stereotyped hand movements (e.g., hand-wringing or hand washing)
(3) loss of social engagement early in the course (although often social interaction develops later)
(4) appearance of poorly coordinated gait or trunk movements
(5) severely impaired expressive and receptive language development with severe psychomotor retardation and restricted patterns of interest that is abnormal either in intensity or focus
(6) apparently inflexible adherence to specific, nonfunctional routines or rituals
(7) stereotyped and repetitive motor mannerisms (e.g., hand or finger flapping or twisting, or complex whole-body movements)
(8) persistent preoccupation with parts of objects
C. The disturbance causes clinically significant impairment in social, occupational, or other important areas of functioning.
D. There is no clinically significant general delay in language (e.g., single words used by age 2 years, communicative phrases used by age 3 years).
E. There is no clinically significant delay in cognitive development or in the development of age-appropriate self-help skills, adaptive behavior (other than in social interaction), and curiosity about the environment in childhood.
F. Criteria are not met for another specific pervasive developmental disorder or schizophrenia.

Used with permission, APA.

TABLE 20–7
**DSM-IV DIAGNOSTIC CRITERIA FOR ASPERGER'S DISORDER**

A. Qualitative impairment in social interaction, as manifested by at least two of the following:
 (1) marked impairment in the use of multiple nonverbal behaviors such as eye-to-eye gaze, facial expression, body postures, and gestures to regulate social interaction
 (2) failure to develop peer relationships appropriate to developmental level
 (3) a lack of spontaneous seeking to share enjoyment, interests, or achievements with other people (e.g., by a lack of showing, bringing, or pointing out objects of interest to other people)
 (4) lack of social or emotional reciprocity
B. Restricted repetitive and stereotyped patterns of behavior, interests, and activities, as manifested by at least one of the following:
 (1) encompassing preoccupation with one or more stereotyped and restricted patterns of interest that is abnormal either in intensity or in focus
 (2) apparently inflexible adherence to specific, nonfunctional routines or rituals
 (3) stereotyped and repetitive motor mannerisms (e.g., hand or finger flapping or twisting, or complex whole-body movements)
 (4) persistent preoccupation with parts of objects
C. The disturbance causes clinically significant impairment in social, occupational, or other important areas in functioning.
D. There is no clinically significant general delay in language (e.g., single words used by age 2 years, communicative phrases used by age 3 years).
E. There is no clinically significant delay in cognitive development or in the development of age-appropriate self-help skills, adaptive behavior (other than in social interaction), and curiosity about the environment in childhood.
F. Criteria are not met for another specific-pervasive developmental disorder or schizophrenia.

Used with permission, APA.


TABLE 20–8
**DSM-IV DIAGNOSTIC CRITERIA FOR CHILDHOOD DISINTEGRATIVE DISORDER**

A. Apparently normal development for at least the first 2 years after birth as manifested by the presence of age-appropriate verbal and nonverbal communication, social relationships, play, and adaptive behavior.
B. Clinically significant loss of previously acquired skills (before age 10 years) in at least two of the following areas:
 (1) expressive or receptive language
 (2) social skills or adaptive behavior
 (3) bowel or bladder control
 (4) play
 (5) motor skills
C. Abnormalities of functioning in at least two of the following areas:
 (1) qualitative impairment in social interaction (e.g., impairment in nonverbal behaviors, failure to develop peer relationships, lack of social or emotional reciprocity)
 (2) qualitative impairments in communication (e.g., delay or lack of spoken language, inability to initiate or sustain a conversation, stereotyped and repetitive use of language, lack of varied make-believe play)
 (3) restricted, repetitive, and stereotyped patterns of behavior, interests, and activities, including motor stereotypies and mannerisms
D. The disturbance is not better accounted for by another specific pervasive developmental disorder or by schizophrenia.

Used with permission, APA.


Concordance in monozygotic (MZ) twins is higher than in dizygotic (DZ) twins; at least 2% of siblings are afflicted, and language and learning problems are increased in families of autistic children. Associated genetic disorders include tuberous sclerosis and fragile X syndrome. Prenatal and perinatal insults are increased, but these may be insufficient without genetic predisposition. No site of organic damage is specific to autistic disorder. Cortical, cerebellar, brain stem, and immunological abnormalities have been implicated in subgroups because of findings from electroencephalogram (EEG), computed tomography (CT), magnetic resonance imaging (MRI), autopsy, and positron emission tomography (PET) studies. Subgroups have abnormal levels of neurotransmitters or their metabolites in blood or cerebrospinal fluid (CSF).

**2. Asperger's disorder.**   Cause is unknown, but family studies suggest a relation to autistic disorder.

**3. Rett's disorder.**   Probably has genetic basis, since it is only seen in girls; case reports indicate complete concordance in MZ twins.

**4. Childhood disintegrative disorder.**   Cause is unknown, but this disorder is associated with other neurological conditions, e.g., seizure disorders, tuberous sclerosis, metabolic disorders.

## C. Treatment

**1. Special education.**   Paramount. There is some evidence that early intensive special educational intervention is most beneficial. Thus, early diagnosis is important.

**2. Pharmacological.**   See Table 20–4.

  a. In nonsedating dosages, haloperidol in controlled studies reduced withdrawal, stereotypies, and hyperactivity. In a long-term study, dyskinesia occurred in 27% of children. It resolved after cessation of drug.

  b. Opioid antagonists, e.g., naltrexone (ReVia), are being explored. The major rationale is to reduce interpersonal withdrawal by blocking endogenous opioids as one does in addicts by blocking exogenous opioids.

  c. Lithium, β-adrenergic receptor antagonists (β-blockers), and antiepileptic drugs may be useful.

  d. Risperidone (Risperdal) has been beneficial in anecdotal reports.

  e. Fenfluramine (Pondimin) is effective in a few autistic children.

  f. Anticonvulsants are used in Rett's disorder to control seizures.

**3. Psychological.**   Individual psychotherapy is generally useless given the language and other cognitive impairments. Family support and counseling is crucial; parents should be told that autistic disorder does not result from faulty upbringing. Parents often require strategies for dealing with the child and siblings. Associations and self-help groups exist for parents of children with autistic disorder.

## V. Learning disorders, motor skills disorder, and communication disorders

Learning disorders (**reading disorder, mathematics disorder, disorder of written expression**, and **learning disorder not otherwise specified [NOS]**), motor skills disorder (**developmental coordination disorder**), and communication disorders (**expressive language disorder, mixed receptive-expressive language disorder, phonological disorder, stuttering**, and **learning disorder NOS**) share many characteristics and comorbidity. The prevalence of learning and motor skills disorders in general is about 5% and specifically ranges from 1% (for stuttering) to 3% (for the other communication disorders). The male-to-female ratio is 2:1 in all the disorders with the exceptions of written expression (unknown) and mathematics (possibly higher prevalence in girls than in boys).

TABLE 20–9
**DSM-IV DIAGNOSTIC CRITERIA FOR READING DISORDER, MATHEMATICS DISORDER, OR DISORDER OF WRITTEN EXPRESSION**

A. Reading achievement, mathematical ability, or writing skills, as measured by individually administered standardized tests (or functional assessments of writing skills), are substantially below those expected given the person's chronological age, measured intelligence, and age-appropriate education.
B. The disturbance in criterion A significantly interferes with academic achievement or activities of daily living that require reading skills, mathematical ability, or the composition of written texts (e.g., writing grammatically correct sentences and organized paragraphs).
C. If a sensory deficit is present, the difficulties are in excess of those usually associated with it.

Used with permission, APA.


TABLE 20–10
**DSM-IV DIAGNOSTIC CRITERIA FOR DEVELOPMENTAL COORDINATION DISORDER**

A. Performance in daily activities that require motor coordination is substantially below that expected given the person's chronological age and measured intelligence. This may be manifested by marked delays in achieving motor milestones (e.g., walking, crawling, sitting), dropping things, "clumsiness," poor performance in sports, or poor handwriting.
B. The disturbance in criterion A significantly interferes with academic achievement or activities of daily living.
C. The disturbance is not due to a general medical condition (e.g., cerebral palsy, hemiplegia, or muscular dystrophy) and does not meet criteria for a pervasive developmental disorder.
D. If mental retardation is present, the motor difficulties are in excess of those usually associated with it.

Used with permission, APA.


TABLE 20–11
**DSM-IV DIAGNOSTIC CRITERIA FOR EXPRESSIVE LANGUAGE DISORDER**

A. The scores obtained from standardized individually administered measures of expressive language development are substantially below those obtained from standardized measures of both nonverbal intellectual capacity and receptive language development. The disturbance may be manifest clinically by symptoms that include having a markedly limited vocabulary, making errors in tense, or having difficulty recalling words or producing sentences with developmentally appropriate length or complexity.
B. The difficulties with expressive language interfere with academic or occupational achievement or with social communication.
C. Criteria are not met for mixed receptive-expressive language disorder or a pervasive developmental disorder.
D. If mental retardation, a speech-motor or sensory deficit, or environmental deprivation is present, the language difficulties are in excess of those usually associated with these problems.

Used with permission, APA.


A. **Diagnosis, signs and symptoms.**   The criteria for the disorders are similar.

   1. **Learning disorders.**   See Table 20–9.
   2. **Motor skills disorder.**   See Table 20–10.
   3. **Communication disorders.**   See Tables 20–11 through 20–14.

B. **General considerations.**   Learning, developmental coordination, and communication disorders often coexist with one another and with attention-deficit and disruptive behavior disorders. Family incidence is increased.

   Little is known about neurobiology. In reading disorder, a few studies (CT scan, MRI, and autopsy) demonstrate a lack of normal hemispheric asymmetries in parietal or temporal lobes. Left-handedness and ambilaterality are increased in communication disorders (with the possible exception of

TABLE 20–12
**DSM-IV DIAGNOSTIC CRITERIA FOR MIXED RECEPTIVE-EXPRESSIVE LANGUAGE DISORDER**

A. The scores obtained from a battery of standardized individually administered measures of both receptive and expressive language development are substantially below those obtained from standardized measures of nonverbal intellectual capacity. Symptoms include those for expressive language disorder as well as difficulty understanding words, sentences, or specific types of words, such as spatial terms.
B. The difficulties with receptive and expressive language significantly interfere with academic or occupational achievement or with social communication.
C. Criteria are not met for a pervasive developmental disorder.
D. If mental retardation, a speech-motor or sensory deficit, or environmental deprivation is present, the language difficulties are in excess of those usually associated with these problems.

Used with permission, APA.·

TABLE 20–13
**DSM-IV DIAGNOSTIC CRITERIA FOR PHONOLOGICAL DISORDER**

A. Failure to use developmentally expected speech sounds that are appropriate for age and dialect (e.g., errors in sound production, use, representation, or organization such as, but not limited to, substitutions of one sound for another (use of /t/ for target /k/ sound) or omissions of sounds such as final consonants).
B. The difficulties in speech sound production interfere with academic or occupational achievement or with social communication.
C. If mental retardation, a speech-motor or sensory deficit or environmental deprivation is present, the speech difficulties are in excess of those usually associated with these problems.

Used with permission, APA.

TABLE 20–14
**DSM-IV DIAGNOSTIC CRITERIA FOR STUTTERING**

A. Disturbance in the normal fluency and time patterning of speech (inappropriate for the individual's age), characterized by frequent occurrences of one or more of the following:
(1) sound and syllable repetitions
(2) sound prolongations
(3) interjections
(4) broken words (e.g., pauses within a word)
(5) audible or silent blocking (filled or unfilled pauses in speech)
(6) circumlocutions (word substitutions to avoid problematic words)
(7) words produced with an excess of physical tension
(8) monosyllabic whole-word repetitions (e.g., "I-I-I see him")
B. The disturbance in fluency interferes with academic or occupational achievement or with social communication.
C. If a speech-motor or sensory deficit is present, the speech difficulties are in excess of those usually associated with these problems.

Used with permission, APA.

phonological disorder). Hearing impairment must be ruled out in communication disorders.

### C. Treatment

1. **Remediation.** Remediation for learning disabilities is usually provided in school and depends on severity. Most cases require no intervention or tutoring. Resource rooms or special class placement may be necessary. Speech therapy is often required with communication disorders. No intervention or tutoring is required in milder cases.

2. **Psychological.** Lowered self-esteem, school failure, and dropping-out are common with the disorders. Therefore, psychoeducation is crucial, and school counseling or individual, group, or family therapy may be indicated.

TABLE 20–15
**DSM-IV DIAGNOSTIC CRITERIA FOR ATTENTION-DEFICIT/HYPERACTIVITY DISORDER**

A.  Either (1) or (2):
  (1)  six (or more) of the following symptoms of **inattention** have persisted for at least 6 months to a degree that is maladaptive and inconsistent with developmental level:
  *Inattention*
  (a)  often fails to give close attention to details or makes careless mistakes in schoolwork, work, or other activities
  (b)  often has difficulty sustaining attention in tasks or play activities
  (c)  often does not seem to listen when spoken to directly
  (d)  often does not follow through on instructions and fails to finish schoolwork, chores, or duties in the workplace (not due to oppositional behavior or failure to understand instructions)
  (e)  often has difficulty organizing tasks and activities
  (f)  often avoids, dislikes, or is reluctant to engage in tasks that require sustained mental effort (such as schoolwork or homework)
  (g)  often loses things necessary for tasks or activities (e.g., toys, school assignments, pencils, books, or tools)
  (h)  is often easily distracted by extraneous stimuli
  (i)  is often forgetful in daily activities
  (2)  six (or more) of the following symptoms of **hyperactivity-impulsivity** have persisted for at least 6 months to a degree that is maladaptive and inconsistent with developmental level:
  *Hyperactivity*
  (a)  often fidgets with hands or feet or squirms in seat
  (b)  often leaves seat in classroom or in other situations in which remaining seated is expected
  (c)  often runs about or climbs excessively in situations in which it is inappropriate (in adolescents or adults, may be limited to subjective feelings of restlessness)
  (d)  often has difficulty playing or engaging in leisure activities quietly
  (e)  is often ``on the go'' or often acts as if ``driven by a motor''
  (f)  often talks excessively
  *Impulsivity*
  (g)  often blurts out answers before questions have been completed
  (h)  often has difficulty awaiting turn
  (i)  often interrupts or intrudes on others (e.g., butts into conversations or games)
B.  Some hyperactive-impulsive or inattentive symptoms that caused impairment were present before age 7 years.
C.  Some impairment from the symptoms is present in two or more settings (e.g., at school (or work) and at home).
D.  There must be clear evidence of clinically significant impairment in social, academic, or occupational functioning.
E.  The symptoms do not occur exclusively during the course of a pervasive developmental disorder, schizophrenia, or other psychotic disorder and are not better accounted for by another mental disorder (e.g., mood disorder, anxiety disorder, dissociative disorder, or a personality disorder).

*Code* based on type:
  **Attention-deficit/hyperactivity disorder, combined type:** if both criteria A1 and A2 are met for the past 6 months
  **Attention-deficit/hyperactivity disorder, predominantly inattentive type:** if criterion A1 is met but criterion A2 is not met for the past 6 months
  **Attention-deficit/hyperactivity disorder, predominantly hyperactive-impulsive type:** if criterion A2 is met but criterion A1 is not met for the past 6 months

**Coding note:** For individuals (especially adolescents and adults) who currently have symptoms that no longer meet full criteria, ``in partial remission'' should be specified.

Used with permission, APA.

  **3. Pharmacological.**   Only for associated psychiatric disorder, such as ADHD. No evidence that medication directly benefits children with learning, motor skills, or communications disorders.

## VI. Attention-deficit and disruptive behavior disorders

### A. Attention-deficit/hyperactivity disorder (ADHD).   Prevalence is probably 3–5%. The male-to-female ratio is 3–5:1.

  **1. Diagnosis, signs, and symptoms.**   See Table 20–15.

2. **General considerations.** ADHD, particularly the predominantly hyperactive-impulsive type, often coexists with conduct disorders or oppositional defiant disorder. ADHD also coexists with learning and communication disorders.

ADHD is thought to reflect subtle, yet unclear, neurological impairments. It is associated with perinatal trauma and early malnutrition. The incidence is increased in male relatives, and concordance is greater in MZ than in DZ twins. ADHD children are often temperamentally difficult. In neurotransmitter systems, the clearest evidence is of noradrenergic dysfunction. Nonfocal (soft) neurological signs are common. Cerebral blood flow (CBF) studies show frontal hypoperfusion; thus, frontal lobe dysfunction is suspected, allowing for disinhibition. ADHD is probably not related to sugar intake; few patients (perhaps 5%) are affected by food additives. 20–25% of persons with ADHD continue to show symptoms into adolescence, some into adulthood. Some, especially those with concomitant conduct disorder, become delinquent or later develop antisocial personality disorder.

3. **Treatment**
   a. **Pharmacological**—see Table 20–4.
      i.   Stimulants reduce symptoms in about 75%; they improve self-esteem by improving the patient's rapport with parents and teachers. Stimulants decrease hyperactivity. Plasma levels are not useful.
           (a) Dextroamphetamine (Dexedrine) is approved by the Food and Drug Administration (FDA) for ages 3 years and over.
           (b) Methylphenidate (Ritalin) is FDA-approved for ages 6 years and older. The sustained-release preparation does not have proven usefulness.
           (c) Pemoline (Cylert) is given in doses of 18.75–37.5 mg a day. It has a delayed onset of action.
      ii.  Clonidine (Catapres) and guanfacine (Tenex) are reported to reduce arousal in children with the disorder.
      iii. Antidepressants if stimulants fail; may be best in ADHD plus symptoms of depression or anxiety. Imipramine (Tofranil) and desipramine (Norpramin) have shown some efficacy in studies, but there are reports of four children dying suddenly while taking desipramine.
      iv.  Antipsychotics or lithium if other medications fail but only with severe symptoms and aggression (concomitant disruptive behavior disorder).
   b. **Psychological**—multimodality treatment is necessary for child and family. May include medication, individual psychotherapy, family therapy, and special education (especially with coexisting specific developmental disorder). These interventions are crucial in moderate or severe cases, given the risk of delinquency.

B. **Conduct disorder.** Prevalence ranges from 5–15% in studies. Accounts for many inpatient admissions in urban areas. The male-to-female ratio is 4–12:1.

TABLE 20–16
**DSM-IV DIAGNOSTIC CRITERIA FOR CONDUCT DISORDER**

A. A repetitive and persistent pattern of behavior in which the basic rights of others or major age-appropriate societal norms or rules are violated, as manifested by the presence of three (or more) of the following criteria in the past 12 months, with at least one criterion present in the past 6 months:

**Aggression to people and animals**
   (1) often bullies, threatens, or intimidates others
   (2) often initiates physical fights
   (3) has used a weapon that can cause serious physical harm to others (e.g., a bat, brick, broken bottle, knife, gun)
   (4) has been physically cruel to people
   (5) has been physically cruel to animals
   (6) has stolen while confronting a victim (e.g., mugging, purse snatching, extortion, armed robbery)
   (7) has forced someone into sexual activity

**Destruction of property**
   (8) has deliberately engaged in fire setting with the intention of causing serious damage
   (9) has deliberately destroyed others' property (other than by fire setting)

**Deceitfulness or theft**
   (10) has broken into someone else's house, building, or car
   (11) often lies to obtain goods or favors or to avoid obligations (i.e., "cons" others)
   (12) has stolen items of nontrivial value without confronting a victim (e.g., shoplifting, but without breaking and entering; forgery)

**Serious violations of rules**
   (13) often stays out at night despite parental prohibitions, beginning before age 13 years
   (14) has run away from home overnight at least twice while living in parental or parental surrogate home (or once without returning for a lengthy period)
   (15) is often truant from school, beginning before age 13 years

B. The disturbance in behavior causes clinically significant impairment in social, academic, or occupational functioning.

C. If the individual is age 18 years or older, criteria are not met for Antisocial Personality Disorder.

*Specify* type based on age at onset:
   **Childhood-onset type:** onset of at least one criterion characteristic of Conduct Disorder prior to age 10 years
   **Adolescent-onset type:** absence of any criteria characteristic of Conduct Disorder prior to age 10 years

*Specify* severity:
   **Mild:** few if any conduct problems in excess of those required to make the diagnosis **and** conduct problems cause only minor harm to others
   **Moderate:** number of conduct problems and effect on others are intermediate between "mild" and "severe"
   **Severe:** many conduct problems in excess of those required to make the diagnosis **or** conduct problems cause considerable harm to others

Used with permission, APA.

1. **Diagnosis, signs, and symptoms.** See Table 20–16.
2. **General considerations.** Conduct disorder is associated with family instability, including victimization by physical or sexual abuse. Propensity for violence correlates with child abuse, family violence, alcoholism, and signs of severe psychopathology, e.g., paranoia and cognitive or subtle neurological deficits. It is crucial to explore for these signs; findings can guide treatment.

   Conduct disorder often coexists with ADHD and learning or communication disorders. Suicidal thoughts and acts and alcohol and drug abuse correlate with conduct disorder.

   Some children with conduct disorder have low plasma dopamine β-hydroxylase levels. Abnormal serotonin levels have been implicated.

TABLE 20–17
**DSM-IV DIAGNOSTIC CRITERIA FOR OPPOSITIONAL DEFIANT DISORDER**

A. A pattern of negativistic, hostile, and defiant behavior lasting at least 6 months, during which four (or more) of the following are present:
  (1) often loses temper
  (2) often argues with adults
  (3) often actively defies or refuses to comply with adults' requests or rules
  (4) often deliberately annoys people
  (5) often blames others for his or her mistakes or misbehavior
  (6) is often touchy or easily annoyed by others
  (7) is often angry and resentful
  (8) is often spiteful or vindictive
  **Note:** Consider a criterion met only if the behavior occurs more frequently than is typically observed in individuals of comparable age and developmental level.
B. The disturbance in behavior causes clinically significant impairment in social, academic, or occupational functioning.
C. The behaviors do not occur exclusively during the course of a psychotic or mood disorder.
D. Criteria are not met for conduct disorder, and, if the individual is age 18 years or older, criteria are not met for antisocial personality disorder.

Used with permission, APA.

### 3. Treatment

a. **Pharmacological**—see Table 20–4. Lithium or haloperidol is of proven efficacy in many aggressive children with conduct disorder. Carbamazepine has shown success. β-Adrenergic receptor antagonists deserve study.

b. **Psychological**—multimodality as in ADHD. May include medication, individual or family therapy, tutoring, or special class placement (for cognitive or conduct problems). It is crucial to discover and fortify any interests or talents to build resistance to the lure of crime. If environment is noxious or if conduct disorder is severe, placement away from home may be indicated.

### C. Oppositional defiant disorder

**1. Diagnosis, signs and symptoms.** See Table 20–17.

**2. General considerations.** Oppositional defiant disorder can coexist with many disorders, including ADHD and anxiety disorders. It appears to result from parent-child struggles over autonomy; therefore, occurrence increases in families with overly rigid parents and temperamentally active, moody, and intense children.

### 3. Treatment

a. **Pharmacological**—drugs used for conduct disorder may be necessary, but only after careful weighing of benefits and risks and failure of other interventions.

b. **Psychological**—individual or family therapy is the intervention of choice. Behavior modification can be helpful.

## VII. Feeding and eating disorders of infancy or early childhood

**A. Pica.** The repeated ingestion of a nonnutritive substance, inappropriate to developmental level, for at least 1 month in infants who do not meet criteria for autistic disorder, schizophrenia, or Kleine-Levin syndrome. Prevalence is unclear; studies report 10–32%. It is associated with MR, neglect, and nutritional deficiency, e.g., iron or zinc. Lead or other poisonings can result.

TABLE 20–18
**DSM-IV DIAGNOSTIC CRITERIA FOR TOURETTE'S DISORDER**

A. Both multiple motor and one or more vocal tics have been present at some time during the illness, although not necessarily concurrently. (A tic is a sudden, rapid, recurrent, nonrhythmic, stereotyped motor movement or vocalization.)
B. The tics occur many times a day (usually in bouts) nearly every day or intermittently throughout a period of more than 1 year, and during this period there was never a tic-free period of more than 3 consecutive months.
C. The disturbance causes marked distress or significant impairment in social, occupational, or other important areas of functioning.
D. The onset is before age 18 years.
E. The disturbance is not due to the direct physiological effects of a substance (e.g., stimulants) or a general medical condition (e.g., Huntington's disease or postviral encephalitis).

Used with permission, APA.

It usually stops in early childhood. Treatment involves testing for lead intoxication and treating if necessary. Since cravings for dirt and ice may relate to iron and zinc deficiencies, such deficiencies should be ruled out. Parent guidance may be necessary. Infrequently, aversive conditioning is necessary.

**B. Rumination disorder.**   Repeated regurgitation, for at least 1 month, following a period of normal eating (in the absence of gastrointestinal [GI] illness) that is not due to anorexia nervosa or bulimia nervosa. Swallowed food is brought back into the mouth, ejected or rechewed, and swallowed. There is no distress. The condition is rare, with onset between 3 and 12 months of age. Immature, ungiving mothers who further reject because of the disorder may be associated with rumination. Little is known of outcome, but it ranges from spontaneous remissions, to malnutrition, to failure to thrive, to death. GI problems, e.g., pyloric stenosis, must be ruled out. Treatment involves parental guidance and behavioral techniques, which may include aversive behavior therapy when the disorder is severe.

**C. Feeding and eating disorder of infancy or early childhood.**   New category for children who persistently eat inadequately for at least 1 month in the absence of a general medical condition or another causal mental condition that results in failure to gain weight and the loss of significant weight. Onset is before 6 years of age. Because many children with the disorder are temperamentally difficult or developmentally delayed, or their caregivers lack patience or are neglectful, counseling of the caregivers is often crucial.

**VIII. Tic disorders**

**A. Tourette's disorder.**   (Also known as Gilles de la Tourette's syndrome.) Prevalence is about 4–5 per 10,000; mean age of onset is 7 years of age. The male-to-female ratio is 3:1.

   **1. Diagnosis, signs, and symptoms.**   See Table 20–18. Motor and vocal tics can be simple or complex. Simple tics generally are the first to appear.
   **Examples:**
   **Simple motor tics**—eyeblinking, head jerking, facial grimacing.
   **Simple vocal tics**—coughing, grunting, sniffing.

**Complex motor tics**—hitting self, jumping.
**Complex vocal tic**—coprolalia (use of vulgar words), palilalia (repeating own words), echolalia (repeating other's words).

2. **General considerations.** There is evidence of genetic transmission—increased tic disorders in families; significantly greater concordance in MZ twins than in DZ twins. Evidence of neurobiological substrate—EEG abnormalities in about 50% of patients; implication of dopamine abnormality; abnormal levels of homovanillic acid (dopamine metabolite) in CSF: stimulants, which are dopamine agonists, can worsen tics or precipitate their occurrence; dopamine antagonists generally improve tics. Tourette's disorder and other tic disorders must be differentiated from a multitude of other disorders and diseases, e.g., dyskinesias, Sydenham's chorea, Huntington's disease. Associated with Tourette's disorder: ADHD, learning problems, and obsessive-compulsive symptoms, of which there is increased incidence in first-degree relatives. Social ostracism is frequent. If the condition is untreated, the course is usually chronic with periods of lessening interspersed with exacerbation of tics.

3. **Treatment**
    a. **Pharmacological**—see Table 20–4.
        i. **Haloperidol**—leads to improvement, often marked, in about 85% of patients; sometimes requires dosages that are sedating.
        ii. **Pimozide (Orap)**—strongly antidopaminergic, as haloperidol is; there is a small potential for slowing cardiac conduction.
        iii. **Clonidine**—an $\alpha_2$-adrenergic agonist; not as effective as haloperidol or pimozide, but there is no risk of tardive dyskinesia. There is little evidence implicating a noradrenergic mechanism in Tourette's disorder.
    b. **Psychological**—counseling or therapy is often necessary for child, family, or both. The nature of Tourette's disorder, coping with it, and ostracism must be addressed. Group therapy may reduce social isolation.

B. **Chronic motor or vocal tic disorder.** Similar to Tourette's disorder, and diagnostic criteria are the same except that there are either single or multiple motor tics or vocal tics, not both. The prevalence is much greater than that of Tourette's disorder, but its severity and social impairment generally are less than with Tourette's disorder. Genetically, chronic motor or vocal tic disorder and Tourette's disorder frequently occur in the same families. The neurobiology appears to be the same, and the treatment is identical to that of Tourette's disorder.

C. **Transient tic disorder.** Prevalence is unclear; nonrigorous surveys report that 5–24% of school children have some sort of tic. The male-to-female ratio is 3:1.

1. **Diagnosis, signs, and symptoms.** See Table 20–19.
2. **General considerations.** In most cases, the tics are psychogenic, increasing during stress and tending to remit spontaneously. In a few cases, chronic motor or vocal tic disorder or Tourette's disorder eventually develops.

TABLE 20–19
**DSM-IV DIAGNOSTIC CRITERIA FOR TRANSIENT TIC DISORDER**

A. Single or multiple motor and/or vocal tics (i.e., sudden, rapid, recurrent, nonrhythmic, stereotyped motor movements or vocalizations).
B. The tics occur many times a day, nearly every day for at least 4 weeks, but for no longer than 12 consecutive months.
C. The disturbance causes marked distress or significant impairment in social, occupational, or other important areas of functioning.
D. The onset is before age 18 years.
E. The disturbance is not due to the direct physiological effects of a substance (e.g., stimulants) or a general medical condition (e.g., Huntington's disease or postviral encephalitis).
F. Criteria have never been met for Tourette's disorder or chronic motor or vocal tic disorder.

*Specify* if:
**Single episode** or **recurrent**

Used with permission, APA.

TABLE 20–20
**DSM-IV DIAGNOSTIC CRITERIA FOR ENCOPRESIS**

A. Repeated passage of feces into inappropriate places (e.g., clothing or floor) whether involuntary or intentional.
B. At least one such event a month for at least 3 months.
C. Chronological age is at least 4 years (or equivalent developmental level).
D. The behavior is not due exclusively to the direct physiological effects of a substance (e.g., laxatives) or a general medical condition except through a mechanism involving constipation.

*Code* as follows:
**With constipation and overflow incontinence**
**Without constipation and overflow incontinence**

Used with permission, APA.

**3. Treatment.** In mild cases, treatment may not be needed. In severe cases, behavioral techniques or psychotherapy is indicated. Medication used for other tic disorders is tried only in severe cases.

## IX. Elimination disorders

**A. Encopresis.** Prevalence is about 1% of 5-year-old children; encopresis is more common in boys than in girls.

**1. Diagnosis, signs, and symptoms.** See Table 20–20.

**2. General considerations.** Rule out physical disorder, such as aganglionic megacolon (Hirschsprung's disease). Inadequate toilet training can result in child-parent power struggles and functional encopresis. Some children appear to have ineffective GI motility, which contributes. Some fear using the toilet. Those with constipation and overflow incontinence can get impacted, have pain on defecating, and develop anal fissures. Leakage is continuous. Those without constipation and overflow often have oppositional defiant or conduct disorders. Encopresis often has precipitants, e.g., birth of a sibling or parental separation. Encopresis usually brings embarrassment and social ostracism. When encopresis is deliberate, associated psychopathology is usually severe. About 25% of patients also have enuresis. Encopresis can last for years but usually resolves.

**3. Treatment.** The child may require individual psychotherapy to address the meaning of the encopresis as well as any embarrassment or

TABLE 20–21
**DSM-IV DIAGNOSTIC CRITERIA FOR ENURESIS**

A. Repeated voiding of urine into bed or clothes (whether involuntary or intentional).
B. The behavior is clinically significant as manifested by either a frequency of twice a week for at least 3 consecutive months or the presence of clinically significant distress or impairment in social, academic (occupational), or other important areas of functioning.
C. Chronological age is at least 5 years (or equivalent developmental level).
D. The behavior is not due exclusively to the direct physiological effect of a substance (e.g., a diuretic) or a general medical condition (e.g., diabetes, spina bifida, a seizure disorder).

*Specify* type:
 **Nocturnal only**
 **Diurnal only**
 **Nocturnal and diurnal**

Used with permission, APA.

ostracism. Behavioral techniques often are helpful. Parental guidance and family therapy often is needed. Conditions, such as impaction and anal fissures, require consultation with a pediatrician.

**B. Enuresis (not due to a general medical condition).** Prevalence: Age 5—7% of boys, 3% of girls; age 10—3% of boys, 2% of girls; age 18—1% of boys, rare in girls. The diurnal subtype is the least prevalent and is more common in girls than in boys.

   1. **Diagnosis, signs, and symptoms.** See Table 20–21.
   2. **General considerations.** Enuresis tends to run in families; concordance is greater in MZ than in DZ twins. In some patients, bladders tend to be small, requiring frequent voiding. It does not seem to be related to a specific stage of sleep, as do sleepwalking or sleep terror disorders. Many patients have no coexisting mental disorder, and impairment reflects only the conflict with caregivers, loss of self-esteem, and social ostracism, if any. Enuresis is likely to coexist with other disorders and can be precipitated by such events as sibling birth or parental separation. Spontaneous remissions are frequent at ages 6–8 and puberty.
   3. **Treatment**
      a. **Pharmacological**—rarely used, given the rate of spontaneous remissions, success of behavioral approaches, and tolerance to drug. Imipramine often is effective in reducing or even eliminating wetting, but tolerance can develop after about 6 weeks. The mode of action is unclear; effects on bladder or sleep cycle are considered. Desmopressin has shown success.
      b. **Psychological**
         i. **Behavioral approaches**—record dry nights on a calendar and reward dry nights with a star and 5–7 consecutive dry nights with a gift. A bell (or buzzer) and pad apparatus is a successful treatment but is cumbersome.
         ii. **Psychotherapy**—not recommended unless psychopathology or other problems coexist, such as reduced self-esteem. The exploration of conflicts underlying enuresis has met with little success. Parental guidance related to the management of the disorder often is necessary.

TABLE 20–22
**DSM-IV DIAGNOSTIC CRITERIA FOR SEPARATION ANXIETY DISORDER**

A. Developmentally inappropriate and excessive anxiety concerning separation from home or from those to whom the individual is attached, as evidenced by three (or more) of the following:
   (1) recurrent excessive distress when separation from home or major attachment figures occurs or is anticipated
   (2) persistent and excessive worry about losing, or about possible harm befalling, major attachment figures
   (3) persistent and excessive worry that an untoward event will lead to separation from a major attachment figure (e.g., getting lost or being kidnapped)
   (4) persistent reluctance or refusal to go to school or elsewhere because of fear of separation
   (5) persistently and excessively fearful or reluctance to be alone or without major attachment figures at home or without significant adults in other settings
   (6) persistent reluctance or refusal to go to sleep without being near a major attchment figure or to sleep away from home
   (7) repeated nightmares involving the theme of separation
   (8) repeated complaints of physical symptoms (such as headaches, stomachaches, nausea, or vomiting) when separation from major attachment figures occurs or is anticipated
B. The duration of the disturbance is at least 4 weeks.
C. The onset is before age 18 years.
D. The disturbance causes clinically significant distress or impairment in social, academic (occupational), or other important areas of functioning.
E. The disturbance does not occur exclusively during the course of a pervasive developmental disorder, schizophrenia, or other psychotic disorder and, in adolescents and adults, is not better accounted for by panic disorder with agoraphobia.

*Specify* if:
   **Early onset:** if onset occurs before age 6 years

Used with permission, APA.

## X. Other disorders of infancy, childhood, or adolescence

### A. Separation anxiety disorder.
Prevalence is unknown. The male-to-female ratio is 1:1. Onset is from preschool to adolescence; some children evidence the most severe form of disorder when onset is about age 11.

1. **Diagnosis, signs, and symptoms.** See Table 20–22.
2. **General considerations.** Separation anxiety disorder clusters in families, but genetic transmission is unclear. Some data link affected children with parents who have a history of that disorder as well as current panic disorder, agoraphobia, or depression. Neurobiological data are lacking. Social debilitation is a risk in severe cases.
3. **Treatment**
   **a. Pharmacological**—see Table 20–4.
      **i. Antidepressants**—tricyclic and tetracyclic drugs, e.g., imipramine, are of use.
      **ii. Anxiolytics**—little researched in childhood anxiety disorders, with little evidence of efficacy.
      **iii. Antipsychotics**—not useful in anxiety disorders. The risk of side effects outweighs potential benefits.
      **iv. Antihistamines**—diphenhydramine (Benadryl) is sometimes used to relieve childhood anxiety. Usefulness is limited, and the child can have a paradoxical reaction.
   **b. Psychological**—multimodal treatment is recommended.
      **i. Individual psychotherapy**—inseparability from parents can result from rageful destructive feelings toward parents, which are repressed and projected onto the environment and then experienced as constant threats to the child and parents' well-being.

The feelings are relieved only by avoiding separation. Other theories include overly strong attachment bond and insecure mother-infant security system.

    **ii. Family therapy or parent guidance**—if parents are fostering separation anxiety.

    **iii. Behavior modification**—may be helpful to achieve separation from parents and return to school.

**B. Selective mutism.** Rare, more common in girls.

Diagnostically, a child who both speaks and comprehends refuses to talk for at least 1 month (but this period is not limited to the first month of school) in social situations. Begins between age 4 and 8, usually resolves in weeks to months. Associated with parental overprotection, parental ambivalence, communication disorders, shyness, and oppositional behavior. Treatment can include individual psychotherapy and parent counseling. Serotonin-specific reuptake inhibitors (SSRIs) may be helpful.

**C. Reactive attachment disorder of infancy or early childhood.** Prevalence and sex ratio are unknown. Often diagnosed and treated pediatrically.

Diagnostically, grossly inadequate caretaking (persistent disregard of physical or emotional needs or repeated change of caretaker) results in markedly disturbed social relatedness in a child who is younger than 5 years. Inhibited type is characterized by failure to initiate or respond to interactions accompanied by apathy, passivity, and lack of visual tracking. Disinhibited type is characterized by indiscriminate and shallow sociability. These failure-to-thrive children are apathetic, passive, and do not track visually. The disturbance is not due to MR or autistic disorder.

    **1. General considerations.** Physically, head circumference is generally normal; weight, very low; height, somewhat short. Pituitary functioning is normal. Associated with low socioeconomic status and mothers who are depressed, isolated, and have experienced abuse. Course—the earlier the intervention, the more reversible the disorder. Affectionless character can develop. Death can occur.

    **2. Treatment.** If the caregiver is unavailable, removal of child may be necessary and permanent. Severe malnourishment and other medical problems may require hospitalization of child. Some homes become adequate following parent education, the provision of a homemaker or financial aid, or treatment of mental disorders in family members.

**D. Stereotypic movement disorder.** Diagnostically, there are repetitive, seemingly nonfunctional behaviors for at least 4 weeks, e.g., hand shaking, rocking, head banging, nail biting, nose picking, hair pulling, that markedly interfere with normal activities or cause physical injury. The disorder is common in MR. It is not diagnosed for behaviors associated with obsessive-compulsive disorder, PDDs, or trichotillomania. Increased dopamine activity seems to increase stereotypic movements. Pervasive developmental disorder or tic disorder must be absent. Common in MR and blindness. Treatment varies. If movements increase with frustration, boredom, or tension, these conditions are addressed. Self-abusive behaviors may require medications, such as haloperidol, lithium, or opioid antagonists (which are currently under study) (Table 20–4).

## XI. Other disorders relevant to children and adolescents

**A. Schizophrenia with childhood onset.** Several studies confirm that some children have delusions or hallucinations (auditory or visual). Nevertheless, few children or young adolescents are schizophrenic, and delusions, hallucinations, and thought disorders are difficult to diagnose in children. Some children diagnosed as schizophrenic are diagnosed with mood disorder when followed to adolescence. Treat with antipsychotic medications (although studies are lacking). Psychotherapy, family therapy, and special schooling may be necessary. See Chapter 7.

**B. Mood disorders.** Some prepubertal children meet the criteria for major depressive disorder. The efficacy of antidepressant medication has yet to be demonstrated in child depressives. Prepubertal children and adolescents with mania, hypomania, or maniclike symptoms have been successfully treated with lithium. See Chapter 9.

**C. Other disorders.** Some children meet criteria for anxiety disorders, including generalized anxiety disorder, specific phobia, social phobia, obsessive-compulsive disorder, posttraumatic stress disorder, and panic disorders (see Chapter 10). Clomipramine (Anafranil) and SSRIs appear to benefit children with obsessive-compulsive disorder. Posttraumatic stress disorder can result from physical or sexual abuse.

Substance-related, gender identity, eating, somatoform, sleep, and adjustment disorders can also be diagnosed during childhood and adolescence.

## XII. Other childhood issues

**A. Child abuse and neglect.** An estimated 1 million children are abused or neglected annually in the United States, resulting in 2,000–4,000 deaths per year. The abused are apt to be of low birth weight or born prematurely (50% of all abused children), handicapped, (e.g., MR, cerebral palsy), or troubled (e.g., defiant, hyperactive). The abusing parent is usually the mother, who likely was abused herself. Abusing parents often are impulsive, substance abusers, depressed, antisocial, or narcissistic.

150,000–200,000 new cases of sexual abuse are reported each year. 2–8% of allegations appear to be false, and many other allegations cannot be substantiated. In 8 of 10 sexually abused children, the perpetrator, usually male, is known to the child. In 50%, the offender is a parent, parent surrogate, or relative.

**B. Suicide.** Serious attempts and completed suicides are rare in children younger than 13 years. Suicidal ideation, threats, and less serious gestures are much more frequent and often a precipitant to hospitalization. Suicidal children tend to be depressed (and sometimes preoccupied with death); however, angry, impulsive children, as well as children suffering recent emotional trauma, can be suicidal.

Suicidal behavior is increasing in adolescents and, as with children, often necessitates hospitalization. It correlates with depression, aggressive behavior, and alcohol abuse. Girls have more suicidal ideation and make more suicidal gestures or attempts. Serious attempts and successful suicides correlate with being male and the availability of alcohol, illicit drugs, or medications, which lower impulse control and can be used to overdose.

Parents often are unaware of their children's suicidal thoughts and behavior, thus necessitating direct questioning of children and adolescents about suicide. See Chapter 19.

C. **Firesetting.** Associated with other destruction of property, stealing, lying, self-destructive tendencies, and cruelty to animals. The male-to-female ratio is 9:1.

D. **Obesity.** Present in 5–20% of children and adolescents. A small percentage present with an obesity-hypoventilation syndrome similar to adult Pickwickian syndrome. These children can have dyspnea and sleep characterized by snoring, stridor, perhaps apnea, and hypoxia with oxygen desaturation. Death can result. Other conditions, such as hypothyroidism or Prader-Willi syndrome, should be ruled out. See Chapter 17.

E. **Acquired immune deficiency syndrome (AIDS).** AIDS has presented child and adolescent psychiatrists with a multitude of difficult problems. For example, the care of young patients from lower socioeconomic groups, already grossly inadequate because of insufficient resources, is further burdened by HIV-related illness or the death of parents and relatives. Young psychiatric patients with concomitant nonsymptomatic positive serology who need residential treatment are rejected for fear of the disease's transmission. In adolescence, AIDS has further complicated sexuality and the problem of substance abuse. See Chapter 4.

---

*For a more detailed discussion of this topic, see Fletcher JM, Taylor HG, Levin HS, Satz P: Neuropsychological and Intellectual Assessment of Children, Sec 9.6, p 581; Wadden TA: Obesity, Sec 26.3, p 1481; Cantwell DP, Baker L: Borderline Intellecutual Functioning and Academic Problem, Sec 28.4, p 1631; Child Psychiatry, Chap 33, pp 2151–2168; Young JG, Kaplan D, Padcualvaca DM, Brasic JM: Psychiatric Examination of the Infant, Child, and Adolescent, Chap 34, p 2169; Bregman JD, Harris JC: Mental Retardation, Chap 35, p 2207; Learning Disorders, Motor Skills Disorder, and Communication Disorders, Chap 36, pp 2243–2276; Campbell M, Shay J: Pervasive Developmental Disorders, Chap 37, p 2277; Arnold LE, Jensen PS: Attention-Deficit Disorders, Chap 38, p 2295; Vitiello B, Jensen PS: Disruptive Behavior Disorders, Chap 39, p 2311; Garfinkel PE: Feeding and Eating Disorders of Infancy and Early Childhood, Chap 40, p 2321; Hanna GL: Tic Disorders, Chap 41, p 2325; Mikkelsen EJ: Elimination Disorders; Other Disorders of Infancy, Childhood, and Adolescence, Chap 43, pp 2345–2366; Carlson GA, Abbott SF: Mood Disorders and Suicide, Chap 44, p 2367; Szatmari P: Schizophrenia with Childhood Onset, Chap 45, p 2393; Child Psychiatry: Psychiatric Treatment, Chap 46, pp 2399–2446; Child Psychiatry: Special Areas of Interest, Chap 47, pp 2447–2494, in CTP/VI.*

# 21

## Geriatric Psychiatry

### I. Introduction

Geriatric psychiatry is the branch of medicine concerned with the prevention, diagnosis, and treatment of physical and psychological disorders in the elderly and with the promotion of longevity and mental health.

### II. Epidemiology

Because Americans are living longer than in the past, the number and the relative percentage of elderly persons in the general population are markedly increased. According to the 1990 United States census, the oldest old—people at least 85 years old—are the fastest-growing group of the elderly population. Although the oldest old constitute only 1.2% of the total population, they have increased 232% since 1960. People at least 85 years old now constitute 10% of those 65 and older. Since 1960, the elderly population has grown 89%; the total population has increased 39%. There are 39 men for every 100 women 85 years or older.

### III. Medical background

The leading causes of death in the elderly are heart disease, cancer, stroke, Alzheimer's disease, and pneumonia. Central nervous system (CNS) changes and psychopathology are also frequent concomitants of the other major causes of geriatric demise.

Morbidity is common in aging. More than one half of persons age 65 and over report arthritic and related symptoms. Benign prostatic hyperplasia is present in three quarters of men over age 75. Urinary incontinence is believed to occur in as many as one fifth of the elderly, frequently in association with dementia. These common disorders result in behavior modification. Arthritis, for example, may restrict activity and alter lifestyle. The cognizant elderly, like other adults, are profoundly embarrassed by urinary difficulties and will restrict activities and hide or deny their disability in order to maintain self-esteem.

Cardiovascular disease is a prominent cause of morbidity and mortality in the elderly. Hypertension may be present in 40% of the elderly, many of whom are receiving diuretics or antihypertensive medications. Hypertension itself can result in CNS effects ranging from headaches to stroke, and pharmacotherapy for this condition can result in mood and cognitive disorders either indirectly, e.g., electrolyte disturbances due to diuretic treatment, or more directly, e.g., neurotransmitter changes associated with β-adrenergic receptor antagonists.

Sensory changes also accompany the aging process. One third of the aged have some degree of auditory disability. In one study, nearly one half of persons 75–85 years of age had lens cataract formation, and more than 70% had glaucoma. Difficulties with convergence, accommodation, and macular degeneration also are sources of visual disability in the aged. These sensory changes frequently interact with psychopathological disabilities, serving to magnify psychopathological deficit and color symptoms.

## IV. Clinical syndromes

### A. Depression

1. **Signs and symptoms.** The frequency of depression appears to increase with age, although the relapse rate, i.e., time between depressive episodes, appears to decrease. The frequency of suicide also increases markedly with age. Yet, there is good evidence that certain features of depression, namely obsessions and phobia, decrease with age.

   Epidemiological studies of depression in the elderly are confounded by confusion between depression and dementia. Family members of dementia patients commonly seek treatment for patients with the chief complaint of depression in the absence of any true mood disorder. The psychiatrist must recognize that paucity of speech, slowing of gait, flattening of affect, and decreased interest in and involvement with social and personal activities, which all indicate depression in a young patient, indicate early dementia in the elderly patient in the absence of clear-cut dysphoria. Cognitive assessment, which will reveal deficits in the dementia patient, will further clarify the diagnosis of dementia when applicable.

   Depression may coexist with dementia and is a common concomitant of the early stages of Alzheimer's disease (Global Deterioration Scale stages 3–5). When depression occurs in the context of Alzheimer's disease, the most common symptom is tearfulness, which is frequently accompanied by early signs of the characteristic sleep disturbance, suspiciousness, anxieties, and agitation, which form the behavioral syndrome of Alzheimer's disease. Other symptoms, reminiscent of depression in other contexts, may occur in the depressive syndrome of Alzheimer's disease, including somatic complaints and obsessive behaviors. Pervasive dysphoria, however, is relatively rare, and Alzheimer's disease patients with depression rarely, if ever, manifest suicidal behavior. Manneristic statements such as, "I wish I were dead," are common in Alzheimer's disease; however, such statements are not accompanied by suicidal plans, gestures, or actions.

   In contrast to psychosis, depression apparently never occurs in the advanced stages of Alzheimer's disease, although it is commonly the earliest manifestation of the disease and may precede the cognitive symptoms by many months or years.

   Depression is also a common concomitant of infarction or other brain insult, with or without coexisting dementia. Pathology affecting the frontal brain regions is believed to be particularly associated with affective symptoms. Depression associated with cerebral infarction is characteristically associated with emotional incontinence, i.e., sudden episodes of tearfulness without a pervasive, consistent, or affective dysphoria.

In addition to dementia and overt brain trauma, depression in the elderly is commonly the result of physical pathology with diverse etiology. For example, electrolyte disturbances from diuretics alone or in combination with other medications can result in a mood disorder, much as vitamin $B_{12}$ deficiency due to malabsorption can occur after gastrointestinal surgery.

**2. Treatment.** Primary (idiopathic) depressive disorders in the elderly are serious and, in many cases, even life-threatening conditions. Treatment modalities that should be given primary consideration include tricyclic antidepressants (TCAs), serotonin-specific reuptake inhibitors (SSRIs), bupropion (Wellbutrin), electroconvulsive therapy (ECT), and monoamine oxidase inhibitors (MAOIs).

**a. Antidepressants**—an increasingly diverse category of compounds, all of which are potentially useful in the elderly. All antidepressant drugs are equally effective in treating depression, making side effects the dominant consideration in selecting a drug.

  **i. Tricyclic drugs**—when used by elderly patients, the secondary amine agents desipramine (Norpramin) and nortriptyline (Aventyl, Pamelor) are preferred because of their low propensity to cause anticholinergic, orthostatic, and sedative side effects. Nortriptyline is less likely than are other tricyclic agents to cause orthostatic hypotension in patients with congestive heart failure. Because of the quinidinelike effect of all tricyclics, a pretreatment electroencephalogram (EEG) is essential to determine if the patient has a preexisting cardiac conduction defect.

  **ii. MAOIs**—useful in treating depression because monoamine oxidase (MAO) decreases in the aging brain and may account for diminished catecholamines and a resultant depression. MAOIs should be used with caution in elderly patients. Orthostatic hypotension is common and severe with MAOIs. Patients need to adhere to a tyramine-free diet to avoid hypertensive crises. The potential for serious drug interaction involving certain analgesics, such as meperidine (Demerol) and sympathomimetics, also requires that patients understand what food and drugs they may use. Tranylcypromine (Parnate) and phenelzine (Nardil) should be used cautiously in patients prone to hypertension.

  **iii. Bupropion**—generally well tolerated; it is nonsedating and does not produce orthostasis; it should be given in three divided doses.

  **iv. SSRIs**—in general, the SSRIs—such as fluoxetine (Prozac), sertraline (Zoloft), and paroxetine (Paxil)—are safe and well tolerated by elderly patients. As a group, the drugs may cause nausea and other gastrointestinal symptoms, nervousness, agitation, headache, and insomnia, most often to mild degrees. Fluoxetine is the drug most likely to cause nervousness, insomnia, and loss of appetite, particularly early in treatment. Sertraline is the drug most likely to produce nausea and diarrhea. Paroxetine causes some anticholinergic effects. SSRIs do not cause the characteristic side effects of the tricyclic agents. The absence of orthostatic

TABLE 21–1
**GERIATRIC DOSAGES OF DRUGS COMMONLY USED TO TREAT BIPOLAR I DISORDER**

| Generic Name | Trade Name | Geriatric Dosage Range (mg a day) |
|---|---|---|
| Lithium carbonate | Eskalith, Lithotabs, Lithonate, Lithobid | 75–900 |
| Carbamazepine | Tegretol | 200–1,200 |
| Valproate (valproic acid) | Depakene, Depakote | 250–1,000 |
| Clonazepam (a benzodiazepine) | Klonopin | 0.5–1.5 |

hypotension is a clinically significant factor in the use of SSRIs by the elderly.

**b. ECT**—may be the treatment of choice for depression in the elderly, particularly if cardiac factors limit or preclude the use of antidepressant medications or if refusal to eat presents an immediate, perhaps even life-threatening, problem. The risk of ECT is very low and is often less than that of pharmacotherapy. Any risks of treatment must be weighed against the risks of depression, including the patient's mental status and any suicidal risk.

**B. Bipolar disorder.** The relapse rate of mania and bipolar disorder increases with age. The mean length of morbid episodes is at least as long in aged patients as in younger adults. The great majority of cases of bipolar illness begin before age 50; onset after age 65 is considered unusual. When a manic episode occurs for the first time after the age of 65, an overt pathophysiological (organic) etiology should be strongly suspected. Possible etiologies include medication side effects or concomitant dementia.

The use of lithium in elderly patients is more hazardous than in young patients because age-related morbidity and physiological changes are common. Lithium is excreted by the kidneys, and decreased renal clearance or renal disease can increase the risk of toxicity. Thiazide diuretics decrease renal clearance of lithium; consequently, the concomitant use of these medications can necessitate adjustment in lithium dosage. Other medications may also interfere with lithium clearance. Lithium may cause CNS effects to which the elderly may be more sensitive. Because of these factors, more frequent serum monitoring of lithium concentrations is recommended in the elderly. Drugs used to treat elderly patients with bipolar disorder are listed in Table 21–1.

**C. Schizophrenia, paranoid states, and other late-life psychoses**

**1. Signs and symptoms.** Initial admissions to psychiatric hospitals for schizophrenia peak from 25 to 34 years of age and are relatively uncommon after age 65. Paranoid psychoses of diverse causes, however, are common in aged persons, including many elderly patients without any premorbid history of significant psychopathology. Sensory deficits appear to predispose to paranoid psychoses in some elderly patients. In others, cerebrovascular events and dementia are associated with the onset of paranoid symptoms. Medications or other pathophysiological causes should be carefully explored in all cases. Recent findings indicate that paranoid and delusional psychoses sometimes precede dementia of the Alzheimer's type. In other instances, these states may be associated with cerebrovascular factors, which are not always evident from clinical or neuroimaging findings. Neurotransmitter changes associated with aging may also predispose the elderly to psychosis. More specifically, in the elderly decrements in various neurotransmitter systems have been convincingly demonstrated. For example, decrements in dopaminergic functioning are associated with age-related cell loss in the substantia nigra, with or without overt parkinsonian symptoms. Age-related changes in noradrenergic functioning also are associated with physical evidence of cellular loss in the locus ceruleus. Similarly, age-related cholinergic neurotransmitter system changes are associated with decreased choline acetyltransferase enzyme activity. Collectively, these and other CNS neurochemical changes result in a resetting of the CNS neurotransmitter balance; these changes often predispose to psychosis in the elderly.

**2. Treatment.**  The changes in neurotransmitter systems in the elderly appear to be important to both the causes and the treatment of psychosis. In general, psychosis in the elderly frequently responds to much lower doses of medication than psychosis in young patients. The elderly also are more sensitive to many of the adverse effects of antipsychotic medications than younger adults.

Specifically, the elderly are very sensitive to extrapyramidal side effects. Elderly patients have been known to stop speaking, ambulating, and swallowing as a result of doses of medication that would be unlikely to produce significant problems in other patients. Partly as a result of age-related autonomic changes, the elderly also are highly susceptible to the orthostatic side effects of antipsychotics. Falling may be associated with extrapyramidal side effects, orthostatic side effects, and sedating effects of typical antipsychotics. These side effects frequently act in conjunction with other medications, arthritis, peripheral vascular disease, arrhythmias, transient ischemic attacks (TIAs), idiopathic parkinsonism, and other age-associated pathologies to further increase the risk of falling. Hip fracture resulting from falls, partly associated with medication, is a major cause of morbidity in the elderly and can be a proximal or distal factor associated with demise. Consequently, the potentially deleterious, and even life-threatening, side effects of antipsychotics in the elderly must be minimized.

Cholinergic neurotransmitter changes also are believed to predispose the elderly to anticholinergic side effects. It should be noted, however, that the antipsychotic with the highest anticholinergic potency, thioridazine (Mellaril), is roughly equivalent in anticholinergic potency to desipramine, the least anticholinergic antidepressant of the commonly used tricyclics and their derivatives. Furthermore, doses of antipsychotics prescribed in elderly patients are frequently much lower than those used in the treatment of younger adult patients. Consequently, in practice, anticholinergic side effects of antipsychotics in elderly patients are not as serious a concern as extrapyramidal, orthostatic, and sedating effects.

Clinical experience also indicates that the therapeutic effects of antipsychotic medications in the elderly may not become evident on a given dosage of medication for 4 weeks or longer. Because of these therapeutic factors and risks, the dictum in treating psychosis in the elderly is "start low and go slow." As in younger patients, side effect profiles should help determine the choice of medication; however, there is no consensus regarding the antipsychotic of choice for the elderly or even whether high-potency or low-potency antipsychotics are more desirable. Among the low-potency antipsychotics, thioridazine is frequently prescribed for the elderly, and a typical starting dosage is 10 mg 1–3 times daily; among the high-potency antipsychotics, haloperidol (Haldol) is frequently prescribed, and a typical starting dosage is 0.25 mg or 0.5 mg 1–3 times daily.

**D. Age-associated cognitive decline, Alzheimer's disease, and other dementing disorders.** Changes in cognition are among the most frequent and the most important (in terms of morbidity, mortality, and impact on family members and society in general) age-related medical conditions.

**1. Alzheimer's disease.** Cognitive changes in normal aging and in progressive Alzheimer's disease occur in a continuum. Barry Reisberg and associates describe seven major clinically distinguishable stages from normality to most severe Alzheimer's disease in the Global Deterioration Scale. These stages and their implications are summarized below.

**Stage 1: Normal**—no objective or subjective evidence of cognitive decrement.

Current epidemiological data indicate that only a minority of elderly persons fall within this category, perhaps 20% of persons over age 65.

**Stage 2: Normal for age**—subjective complaints of cognitive decrement.

Most persons over age 65 have subjective symptoms of not remembering the names and locations of objects as well as they did in the previous 5–10 years.

These symptoms can be troubling to aged persons. In Europe, such symptoms appear to be the leading reason why persons take medications of all forms. In the United States, elderly persons commonly take lecithin, multivitamins, and various nostrums for these complaints.

Present prognostic data do not indicate that these symptoms of age-associated memory impairment are the precursor of further decline in most elderly persons. Although medications and nostrums are frequently taken, there remains no convincing evidence of their efficacy.

**Stage 3: Compatible with incipient Alzheimer's disease**—subtle evidence of objective decrement in complex occupational or social tasks.

Subtle deficits may become evident in various ways. For example, the patient may become hopelessly lost when traveling to an unfamiliar location; decreased performance in a demanding occupation may be noted by coworkers; patients may display overt word- and name-finding deficits; concentration deficits may be evident to family members or on clinical testing; and an overt tendency to forget what has just been said and to repeat oneself may be manifest.

The prognosis associated with these subtle, but identifiable, symptoms varies. In some cases, these symptoms are the result of brain insults, such as small strokes, which may not be evident from the clinical history, neurological examination, or neuroimaging findings. In other cases, symptoms are due to subtle, and perhaps not clearly identifiable, psychiatric, medical, and neurological disorders of diverse causes. In other cases, the symptoms represent the earliest symptoms of Alzheimer's disease and may last as long as 7 years. The diagnosis of Alzheimer's disease in this stage, however, can be made with confidence only in retrospect.

Anxiety is a frequent psychiatric concomitant of the cognitive losses at stage 3. Given the frequently benign prognosis, the inability to diagnose with confidence at this stage, and the prolonged duration of these symptoms when they do represent the earliest signs of Alzheimer's disease, the most effective treatment for the anxiety is that the patient withdraw from anxiety-provoking activities. For example, withdrawal from a job that is beyond the patient's cognitive capacities can eliminate daily stress and humiliation. It can also eliminate, at least temporarily, the patient's problems, since patients at this stage do not have difficulty with routine tasks of daily living.

**Stage 4: Mild Alzheimer's disease**—clearly manifested deficits on a careful clinical interview.

Deficits manifest in concentration, memory, orientation, or functional capacity. Concentration deficit may be large enough that not only does the patient display a deficit on the standard subtraction of serial 7s task, but he or she has difficulty subtracting serial 4s from 40. Recent memory may suffer such that some major events of the previous week are not recalled. Detailed questioning may reveal that the spouse's knowledge of the patient's past is superior to the patient's own recall of his or her personal history. The patient may mistake the date by 10 days or more. The spouse (or other family members) may note that the patient no longer is able to balance a checkbook, no longer remembers to pay the rent or other bills properly, has difficulty preparing meals, or displays similar deficits in the ability to manage complex occupational and social tasks.

Alzheimer's disease can be diagnosed with confidence in this stage. It is possible to follow patients through the course of this stage, the mean duration of which has been estimated to be 2 years. Symptoms may plateau in this stage, and some patients may not manifest a further overt decline for 4 years or longer.

The most prominent psychiatric features of stage 4 are the patient's decreased interest in personal and social activities, accompanied by a flattening of affect. Depressive symptoms also may be noted, but are generally mild enough that no specific treatment is indicated. Depressive symptoms sometimes are severe enough to warrant treatment, frequently with a low dose of an antidepressant. Patients are still capable of living alone if assistance is provided with such complex, but essential, activities as paying the rent and managing the patient's bank account.

**Stage 5: Moderate Alzheimer's disease**—deficits large enough to prevent patients from surviving without assistance.

Patients at this stage can no longer recall major relevant aspects of their lives, e.g., they may not recall the name of the president, their correct current address, or the name of the school they attended. Patients at this stage frequently do not recall the current year and have enough difficulty in concentration and calculation as to err in subtracting serial 2s from 20. In addition to their inability to manage complex activities of daily living, patients generally have difficulty choosing the proper clothing to wear for the season and the occasion.

The duration of this stage is approximately 1½ years, although, as with the previous stage, some patients may plateau with these symptoms for many years.

Although generally more overt, the psychiatric symptoms at stage 5 are in many ways similar to those noted in stage 4. Consequently, the patient's denial and flattening of affect tend to be more evident. Depressive symptoms may occur. Anger and some of the more overt behavioral symptoms of Alzheimer's disease also are common. Depending on the nature and magnitude of the psychiatric symptoms, treatment with an antidepressant or an antipsychotic medication may be indicated. When the latter is used, the dictum previously stated for the treatment of psychosis in the elderly applies: "start low and go slow."

Patients who are living alone at this stage require at least part-time assistance for continued community survival. When additional community assistance is not feasible or available, institutionalization may be required. Patients who are residing with a spouse frequently resist additional assistance as an invasion of their home.

**Stage 6: Moderately severe Alzheimer's disease**—deficits large enough to necessitate assistance with basic activities of daily living.

Patients at this stage may occasionally forget the name of the spouse on whom they depend for survival. They frequently do not know their address but can generally recall some important aspects of their domicile, such as the street or the town. Patients have generally forgotten the schools they attended but recall some aspects of their early lives, such as their birthplace, former occupation, or one or both of their parents' names. Patients generally still can state their correct personal name. They may have difficulty counting backward from 10 by 1s.

Over the course of stage 6, which lasts approximately 2½ years, deficits in dressing and bathing increase progressively. In the latter part of this stage, toileting and continence become compromised.

Emotional and behavioral problems become most manifest and disturbing. Agitation, anger, sleep disturbances, physical violence, and negativity are examples of symptoms that commonly require treatment at this point in the illness. Although low doses of antipsychotics may be useful, high doses are frequently necessary for many patients, and a satisfactory response is sometimes difficult to obtain.

Patients require full-time assistance in community settings. If the patient lives with his or her spouse, the spouse will generally require at least part-time additional management assistance.

**Stage 7: Severe Alzheimer's disease**—deficits that necessitate continuous assistance with activities of daily living.

Speech activity is severely circumscribed early in this stage and is eventually lost. Ambulation and other motor capacities are also lost.

Most patients survive until this stage, when they commonly succumb at approximately the time ambulatory ability is lost. Although some patients survive in this stage for 6 years or longer, most patients succumb approximately 2–3 years after stage 7 begins. Pneumonia appears to be the most common proximate cause of death.

Although agitation can be a problem for some patients, psychotropic medication can frequently be discontinued successfully. Nursing homes may be better equipped than spouses for the management of patients. Many devoted spouses, however, prefer to continue to care for their partner, in which case, round-the-clock home health care assistance may be a necessary adjunct as management of incontinence and other basic life activities, such as bathing and feeding, become major concerns. Psychiatrists should be prepared to counsel family members regarding such issues as institutionalization and the continued meaning of life.

2. **Vascular dementia.** This is the second major cause of dementia in the elderly. It occurs most frequently in conjunction with Alzheimer's disease. Classic pathological studies have indicated that approximately 50% of dementia cases coming to autopsy are associated with Alzheimer's disease alone, 25% with Alzheimer's disease in association with cerebrovascular factors, and 15% with vascular dementia in the absence of neuropathological evidence of Alzheimer's disease.

Vascular dementia is believed to be the result of cerebral infarctions of varying size in multiple brain regions. Conditions associated with cerebral infarction, such as cardiac arrhythmias and hypertension, predispose to vascular dementia.

Clinically, vascular dementia is believed to follow a more stepwise course than the relatively gradual course of Alzheimer's disease. The time course of decline of vascular dementia is at least as rapid as that of Alzheimer's disease. In mixed cases, the presence of cerebral infarction appears to increase morbidity. Consequently, the rate of dementia and the time of death are relatively rapid in vascular dementia and in mixed dementia compared with Alzheimer's disease.

The clinical presentation of vascular dementia is more diverse than that of Alzheimer's disease. Speech disturbance or gait disturbance, for example, may occur at varying points in the evolution of vascular dementia pathology, whereas in Alzheimer's disease these deficits tend to occur at a specific point in the evolution of the dementia process.

Psychiatric disturbances occurring in vascular dementia include general dementia-related psychiatric conditions, such as the affective, psychotic, and agitation disturbances described at each stage of Alzheimer's disease. Emotional changes characteristic of stroke-related dementia also occur, e.g., emotional incontinence and other sudden, labile mood changes. Emotional incontinence generally is not treated with medication. The guidelines for the treatment of dementia-related psychiatric disturbances previously outlined for Alzheimer's disease apply for the treatment of affective, psychiatric, and other behavioral disturbances in vascular dementia.

The treatment for the underlying cause of vascular dementia is stroke prevention. These include the treatment of hypertension and cardiac arrhythmias and the use of platelet-deaggregating agents for the prevention of stroke. Among the latter, salicylates, such as aspirin, are perhaps the most effective.

3. **Other dementing disorders and differential diagnosis of dementia.** Other causes of dementia include Pick's disease, Creutzfeldt-Jakob disease, Huntington's disease, alcohol abuse, normal pressure hydrocephalus, and dementias secondary to diverse physiological disturbances.

a. **Pick's disease**—a degenerative dementia that is difficult to distinguish clinically from Alzheimer's disease. Neuropathologically, Pick's disease differs in that autopsy brain examination reveals so-called Pick bodies and not the characteristic neurofibrillary tangles, senile plaques, or granulovacuolar degeneration of Alzheimer's disease. Pick's disease also tends to affect the frontal region of the brain, whereas Alzheimer's disease is a much more diffuse cerebral process. Pick's disease has a somewhat younger age distribution than Alzheimer's disease, accounting for a significant percentage of dementia patients in the sixth decade of life. Clinically, Pick's disease appears to be marked by more frontal lobe features than Alzheimer's disease. Pick's disease has no known treatment.

b. **Creutzfeldt-Jakob disease**—a rare condition, occurring in approximately one person per million. Onset and course are variable and acute; subacute and chronic forms have been described. Frequently, Creutzfeldt-Jakob disease is distinguished from Alzheimer's disease by its course, which may be more rapid, or by the occurrence of focal and localized neural pathology. The latter includes cranial nerve signs, such as auditory deficits associated with 8th nerve involvement, and gait disturbance, associated with cerebellar involvement. Occasionally, Creutzfeldt-Jakob disease closely mimics the course of Alzheimer's disease.

c. **Huntington's disease**—may present with a dementia disturbance prior to the appearance of choreiform pathology and should be considered in the differential diagnosis of dementia.

d. **Alcohol-induced persisting dementia or amnestic disorder**—frequently distinguished from Alzheimer's disease by the presence of confabulation and by a memory deficit out of proportion to cognitive and functional disturbances in other areas.

e. **Normal pressure hydrocephalus**—marked by gait disturbance, urinary incontinence, and dilated cerebral ventricles out of proportion to the magnitude of cortical atrophy and dementia. Urinary incontinence, neuroradiological findings, and the relatively early appearance of gait disturbance assist in distinguishing this condition from Alzheimer's disease.

f. **Dementias secondary to diverse physiological disturbances**—the diagnosis of dementia, which may be secondary to more than 50

TABLE 21-2
**FUNCTIONAL STAGING AND PROGRESSION IN NORMAL AGING AND ALZHEIMER'S DISEASE**

| Functional Assessment Stage | Characteristics | Clinical Diagnosis | Estimated Duration in Alzheimer's Disease* |
|---|---|---|---|
| 1 | No decrement | Normal adult | |
| 2 | Subjective deficit in word finding | Normal aged adult | |
| 3 | Deficits noted in demanding employment settings | Compatible with incipient Alzheimer's disease | 7 years |
| 4 | Requires assistance in complex tasks, e.g., handling finances, planning dinner party | Mild Alzheimer's disease | 2 years |
| 5 | Requires assistance in choosing proper attire | Moderate Alzheimer's disease | 18 months |
| 6a | Requires assistance dressing | Moderately severe Alzheimer's disease | 5 months |
| 6b | Requires assistance bathing properly | | 5 months |
| 6c | Requires assistance with mechanics of toileting (such as flushing, wiping) | | 5 months |
| 6d | Urinary incontinence | | 4 months |
| 6e | Fecal incontinence | | 10 months |
| 7a | Speech ability limited to about a half-dozen words | Severe Alzheimer's disease | 12 months |
| 7b | Intelligible vocabulary limited to a single word | | 18 months |
| 7c | Ambulatory ability lost | | 12 months |
| 7d | Ability to sit up lost | | 12 months |
| 7e | Ability to smile lost | | 18 months |
| 7f | Ability to hold head up lost | | 12 months or longer |

Table by Barry Reisberg, MD. Table adapted from Reisberg B: Dementia: A systematic approach to identifying reversible causes. Geriatrics 41: 30, 1986.

possible primary etiologies, and the differentiation of these conditions from the major cause of dementia, Alzheimer's disease, is based on laboratory investigations and knowledge of the clinical course of Alzheimer's disease. The basic laboratory workup for dementia includes a complete blood count and differential, serum electrolytes and serum enzyme studies, serum $B_{12}$ and serum folate levels, thyroid levels, urinalysis, and a cerebral neuroimaging study. Positive findings from any of these studies must be interpreted by the clinician. They may indicate a primary etiology of dementia, which may be treatable; they may indicate added insult in the context of degenerative dementia; or they may be incidental. A knowledge of the clinical course of Alzheimer's disease can help the clinician in distinguishing these possibilities. A brief guide to the order and time course of the progression of functional loss in Alzheimer's disease can be found in Table 21–2. Table 21–3 shows differential diagnostic considerations when these functional changes occur prematurely in the evolution of the dementia process. Premature deficits should alert the clinician to possible increased morbidity or a possibly remediable underlying process.

TABLE 21–3
**DIFFERENTIAL DIAGNOSTIC CONSIDERATIONS OF FUNCTIONAL ASSESSMENT STAGE (FAST STAGE) NONORDINALITY**

| FAST Stage | FAST Characteristics | Differential Diagnostic Considerations: particularly if FAST stage occurs early (nonordinally) in the evolution of dementia |
|---|---|---|
| 1. | No functional decrement, either subjectively or objectively, manifest | |
| 2. | Complains of forgetting location of objects; subjective work difficulties | 2. Anxiety neurosis; depression |
| 3. | Decreased functioning in demanding employment settings evident to co-workers; difficulty in traveling to new locations | 3. Depression; subtle manifestations of medical pathology |
| 4. | Decreased ability to perform complex tasks, such as planning dinner for guests, handling finances, and marketing | 4. Depression; psychosis; focal cerebral process (e.g., Gerstmann's syndrome) |
| 5. | Requires assistance in choosing proper clothing; may require coaxing to bathe properly | 5. Depression |
| 6. | (a) Difficulty putting clothes on properly | 6. (a) Arthritis; sensory deficit; stroke; depression |
| | (b) Requires assistance bathing; may develop fear of bathing | (b) Arthritis; sensory deficit; stroke; depression |
| | (c) Inability to handle mechanics of toileting | (c) Arthritis; sensory deficit; stroke; depression |
| | (d) Urinary incontinence | (d) Urinary tract infection; other causes of urinary incontinence |
| | (e) Fecal incontinence | (e) Infection; malabsorption syndrome; other causes of fecal incontinence |
| 7. | (a) Ability to speak limited to 1–5 words | 7. (a) Stroke; other dementing disorder (e.g., diffuse space occupying lesions) |
| | (b) Intelligible vocabulary lost | (b) Stroke; other dementing disorder (e.g., diffuse space occupying lesions) |
| | (c) Ambulatory ability lost | (c) Parkinsonism; neuroleptic-induced or other secondary extrapyramidal syndrome; Creutzfeldt-Jakob disease: normal pressure hydrocephalus; hyponatremic dementia; stroke; hip fracture; arthritis; overmedication |
| | (d) Ability to sit up independently lost | (d) Arthritis; contractures |
| | (e) Ability to smile lost | (e) Stroke |
| | (f) Ability to hold head up lost | (f) Head trauma; metabolic abnormality; other medical abnormality; overmedication; encephalitis; other causes |

Table by Barry Reisberg, MD. Table adapted from Reisberg B: Dementia: A systematic approach to identifying reversible causes. Geriatrics 41: 30, 1986.

## V. Psychotherapy in the elderly

Fundamental psychological processes in the elderly do not differ from those of younger adults. However, the aging process and associated pathological changes do result in psychological issues that are relatively particular to this age group. Common issues in therapy include evolving and changing relationships of the elderly with their adult children. For example, in the presence of pathology, the elderly may have both a desire for independence and, in the present social context, unrealistic expectations with regard to their adult children. Adult children, in turn, may harbor continuing resentments toward their parents from childhood or, conversely, may experience an unrealistic guilt with regard to what they should be doing for their parents in the event of illness or other traumatic events.

Family therapy, consequently, can be of particular value in the elderly, sometimes in conjunction with group or individual psychotherapy. Other goals of individual therapy particular to the elderly include the maintenance of self-esteem despite physical, marital, and social change; the meaningful use of unaccustomed leisure time; and clarification of options in the context of more or less overwhelming physical and social change. In general, psychotherapy in the elderly is relatively situation- and problem-oriented and seeks solutions within the established personality framework, rather than overwhelming personality change. Many elderly persons, however, respond remarkably to seemingly overwhelming changes and personal tragedies, such as loss of personal health or a spouse, revealing unseen social strengths and adaptive capacities.

---

*For a more detailed discussion of this topic, see Caine ED, Grossman G, Lyness JM: Delirium, Dementia, Amnestic, and Other Cognitive Disorders and Mental Disorders Due to a General Medical Condition, Chap 12, p 705; Geriatric Psychiatry, Chap 49, pp 2507–2662, in CTP/VI.*

# 22

# Bereavement and Death

## I. Grief, mourning, and bereavement

Generally synonymous terms that describe a syndrome precipitated by the loss of a loved one. Attempts have been made to characterize the stages of grief, which are listed in Table 22–1. Characteristics of bereavement in parents and children are listed in Table 22–2.

Grief can occur for reasons other than the death of a loved one: (1) the loss of a loved one through separation, divorce, or incarceration; (2) the loss of an emotionally charged object or circumstance, e.g., loss of a prized possession or of a valued job or position; (3) the loss of a fantasized love object, e.g., death of intrauterine fetus, birth of a malformed infant; and (4) the loss resulting from narcissistic injury, e.g., amputation, mastectomy.

Grief differs from depression in a number of ways, which are described in Table 22–3. Risk factors for major depressive episodes after the death of a spouse are listed in Table 22–4. Complications of bereavement are listed in Table 22–5.

### A. Dos and don'ts of grief management and therapy

1. *Do* encourage ventilation of feelings. Allow person to talk about loved ones. Reminiscing about positive experiences can be helpful.
2. *Don't* tell bereaved not to cry or get angry.
3. *Do* try to have a small group of people who knew the deceased talk about him or her in the presence of the grieving person.
4. *Don't* prescribe antianxiety or antidepressant medication on a regular basis. If the person becomes acutely agitated, it is better to offer verbal comfort than a pill. However, small doses of medications (diazepam [Valium] 5 mg) may help in the short term.
5. *Do* note that frequent short visits are better than a few long visits.
6. *Do* be aware of delayed grief reaction, which occurs some time after the death and may be marked by behavioral changes, agitation, lability of mood, and substance abuse. Such reactions may occur close to the anniversary of a death, an anniversary reaction.
7. *Do* note that anticipatory grief reaction happens in advance of loss and can mitigate acute grief reaction at the actual time of loss. This can be a useful process if recognized when it is occurring.
8. *Do* be aware that the person grieving about a family member who died by suicide may not want to talk about his or her feelings of being stigmatized.

## II. Death and dying

The reactions of patients to being told by a physician that they have a terminal

TABLE 22–1
**GRIEF AND BEREAVEMENT**

| Stage | John Bowlby | Stage | C.M. Parkes |
|---|---|---|---|
| 1 | **Numbness or protest.** Characterized by distress, fear, and anger. Shock may last moments, days, or months | 1 | **Alarm.** A stressful state characterized by physiological changes, e.g., rise in blood pressure and heart rate; similar to Bowlby's first stage |
| 2 | **Yearning and searching for the lost figure.** World seems empty and meaningless, but self-esteem remains intact. Characterized by preoccupation with lost person, physical restlessness, weeping, and anger. May last several months or even years | 2 | **Numbness.** Person appears superficially affected by loss, but is actually protecting himself or herself from acute distress |
| 3 | **Disorganization and despair.** Restlessness and aimlessness. Increase in somatic preoccupation, withdrawal, introversion, and irritability. Repeated reliving of memories | 3 | **Pining (searching).** Person looks for or is reminded of the lost person. Similar to Bowlby's second stage |
| | | 4 | **Depression.** Person feels hopeless about future, cannot go on living, and withdraws from family and friends |
| 4 | **Reorganization.** With establishment of new patterns, objects, and goals, grief recedes and is replaced by cherished memories. Healthy identification with deceased occurs | 5 | **Recovery and reorganization.** Person realized that his or her life will continue with new adjustments and different goals |

TABLE 22–2
**BEREAVEMENT IN PARENTS AND CHILDREN**

| Loss of a Parent | Loss of a Child |
|---|---|
| Protest phase. Child has strong desire for the deceased parent | May be a more intense experience than the death of an adult |
| Despair phase. Child experiences hopelessness, withdrawal, and apathy | Feelings of guilt and helplessness may be overwhelming |
| Detachment phase. Child relinquishes emotional attachment to dead parent | Stages of shock, denial, anger, bargaining, and acceptance occur |
| Child may transfer need for a parent to one or more adults | Manifestations of grief may last a lifetime |
| | Up to 50% of marriages in which a child dies end in divorce |

illness that will lead to death vary. The reactions are described as a series of stages by thanatologist Elisabeth Kübler Ross (Table 22–6).

Be aware that stages do not always occur in sequence. There may be shifts from one stage to another. Moreover, children under 5 years of age do not appreciate death; they see it as a separation similar to sleep. Between 5 and 10 years of age, there is a growing awareness of death as something that occurs in others, particularly parents. After 10 years of age, death is conceptualized as something that can happen to the child.

## A. Dos and don'ts with the dying patient

1. *Don't* have a rigid attitude, e.g., "I always tell the patient." Let the patient be your guide. Most patients will want to know the diagnosis, whereas others will not. Determine what the patient already knows and

TABLE 22–3
**GRIEF VERSUS DEPRESSION**

| Grief | Depression |
|---|---|
| Normal identification with deceased. Little ambivalence toward deceased | Abnormal overidentification with deceased. Increased ambivalence and unconscious anger toward deceased |
| Crying, weight loss, decreased libido, withdrawal, insomnia, irritability, decreased concentration and attention | Similar |
| Suicidal ideas rare | Suicidal ideas common |
| Self-blame relates to how deceased was treated. No global feelings of worthlessness | Self-blame is global. Person thinks he or she is generally bad or worthless |
| Evokes empathy and sympathy | Usually evokes interpersonal annoyance or irritation |
| Symptoms abate with time. Self-limited. Usually clears within 6 months to 1 year | Symptoms do not abate and may worsen. May still be present after years |
| Vulnerable to physical illness | Vulnerable to physical illness |
| Responds to reassurance and social contacts | Does not respond to reassurance and pushes away social contacts |
| Not helped by antidepressant medication | Helped by antidepressant medication |

TABLE 22–4
**RISK FACTORS FOR MAJOR DEPRESSIVE EPISODE AFTER DEATH OF A SPOUSE**

History of depression: major depressive disorder, dysthymic disorder, depressive personality disorder, bipolar disorder

Under 30 years of age

Poor general health

Limited social support system

Unemployment

Poor adaptation to the loss

TABLE 22–5
**COMPLICATIONS OF BEREAVEMENT**

Disturbance in the process of grief
   Absent or delayed grief
   Exaggerated grief
   Prolonged grief

Increased vulnerability to adverse affects
   General medical morbidity
   Mortality
   Psychiatric disorders
     Anxiety disorders
     Substance use disorders
     Depressive disorders

Table adapted from and courtesy of Sidney Zisook, MD

TABLE 22–6
**DEATH AND DYING (REACTIONS OF DYING PATIENTS)**

**Elisabeth Kübler-Ross**

| | |
|---|---|
| Stage 1 | **Shock and denial.** Patient's initial reaction is shock, followed by denial that anything is wrong. Some patients never pass beyond this state and may go doctor shopping until they find one who supports their position |
| Stage 2 | **Anger.** Patients become frustrated, irritable, and angry that they are ill; they ask, ``Why me?'' Patients in this stage are difficult to manage because their anger is displaced onto doctors, hospital staff, and family. Sometimes anger is directed at themselves in the belief that illness has occurred as punishment for wrong doing |
| Stage 3 | **Bargaining.** Patient may attempt to negotiate with physicians, friends, or even god, that in return for a cure, he or she will fulfill one or many promises, e.g., give to charity, attend church regularly |
| Stage 4 | **Depression.** Patient shows clinical signs of depression; withdrawal, psychomotor retardation, sleep disturbances, hopelessness, and possibly suicidal ideation. The depression may be a reaction to the effects of illness on his or her life, e.g., loss of job, economic hardship, isolation from friends and family, or it may be in anticipation of the actual loss of life that will occur shortly |
| Stage 5 | **Acceptance.** Person realizes that death is inevitable and accepts its universality |

understands about the prognosis. Do not stifle hope or break through a patient's denial if that is the major defense, as long as the patient can obtain and accept necessary help. If the patient refuses to obtain help as a result of denial, gently and gradually help the patient to understand that help is necessary and available. Reassure the patient that he or she will be taken care of regardless of behavior.

2. *Do* stay with patient for a period of time after telling him or her the condition or diagnosis. There may be a period of shock. Encourage the patient to ask questions and provide truthful answers. Indicate that you will return to answer any questions that the patient or family may have.

3. *Do* make a return visit after a few hours, if possible, to check on the patient's reaction. If there is a measure of anxiety, 5 mg of diazepam (Valium) can be prescribed as needed for 24–48 hours.

4. *Do* advise family members of medical facts. Encourage them to visit and allow the patient to talk of his or her fears. Family members not only have to deal with the loss of a loved one but also are faced with their own personal mortality, which causes anxiety.

5. *Do* always check for the presence of living will or do not resuscitate (DNR) wishes of the patient or family. Try to anticipate their wishes regarding life-sustaining procedures.

6. *Do* alleviate pain and suffering. There is no reason for withholding narcotics for fear of dependence in a dying patient. Pain management should be vigorous.

*For more detailed discussion of this topic, see Zisook S: Death, Dying, and Bereavement, Sec 29.6, p 1713, in CTP/VI.*

# 23

# Psychotherapy

## I. General introduction

In psychiatry, a number of different theories or paradigms are used as models to explain human behavior. Each etiological theory has corresponding therapeutic techniques that are based on the different underlying explanatory models of behavior. Biological therapies, for instance, postulate a biological substrate for behavior, and the corresponding interventions involve biological treatments, such as psychopharmacology and electroconvulsive therapy (ECT). Other therapies view behavior from perspectives other than the biological; these corresponding treatments are generally called psychotherapies. Biological treatments are covered in Chapter 24.

Most psychiatrists believe that the different theories of behavior are not mutually exclusive, but rather, when taken together, provide a complex and integrated picture of a person's thoughts and actions from different perspectives. Certain clinical problems and patients may respond more to one therapy than to another; therefore, psychiatrists must be adept at using a number of different therapeutic techniques and interventions in order to treat patients skillfully. This chapter describes each of the psychotherapies in relation to the underlying theory with which it is associated.

## II. Psychoanalysis and psychoanalytic psychotherapy

These two forms of treatment are based on Sigmund Freud's theories of a dynamic unconscious and psychological conflict. The major goal of these forms of therapy is to help the patient develop insight into unconscious conflicts, which are based on unresolved childhood wishes and are manifested as symptoms, and to develop more consciously adult patterns of interacting and behaving.

**A. Psychoanalysis.** The most intensive and rigorous of this type of therapy. The patient is seen 3–5 times a week, generally for a minimum of several hundred hours over a number of years. The patient lies on a couch with the analyst seated behind, out of the patient's visual range. The patient attempts to say freely and without censure whatever comes to mind, to free associate, in order to follow as deeply as possible the train of thoughts to their earliest roots. This includes associating to dream material and to transference feelings that are evoked in the process. The analyst uses interpretation and clarification to help the patient work through and resolve conflicts that have been affecting the patient's life, often unconsciously. Psychoanalysis requires that the patient be stable, highly motivated, verbal, and psychologically minded. The patient also must be able to tolerate the stress generated by analysis without becoming overly regressed, distraught, or impulsive.

B. **Psychoanalytically oriented psychotherapy.** Based on the same principles and techniques as classic psychoanalysis but is less intense. There are two types: insight-oriented or expressive psychotherapy and supportive or relationship psychotherapy. Patients are seen 1–2 times a week and sit up facing the psychiatrist. The goal of resolution of unconscious psychological conflict is similar to that of psychoanalysis, but there is a greater emphasis on day-to-day reality issues and a lesser emphasis on the development of transference issues. Patients suitable for this therapy include those suitable for psychoanalysis, as well as those with a wider range of symptomatic and characterological problems. Patients with personality disorders also are suitable for this therapy.

In supportive psychotherapy, the essential element is support, rather than the development of insight. This type of therapy often is the treatment of choice for patients with serious ego vulnerabilities, particularly psychotic patients. Patients in a crisis situation, such as acute grief, also are suitable. This therapy can be long term, lasting many years, especially in the case of chronic patients. Support can take the form of limit-setting, increasing reality testing, reassurance, advice, and help with developing social skills (Table 23–1).

C. **Brief dynamic psychotherapy.** A short-term treatment, generally consisting of 10–40 sessions for a period of less than 1 year. The goal, based on Freudian theories, is to develop insight into underlying conflicts, which leads to psychological and behavior changes.

This therapy is more confrontational than the other insight-oriented therapies in that the therapist is very active in repeatedly directing the patient's associations and thoughts to conflictual areas. The number of hours is explicitly agreed on by the therapist and patient prior to the onset of therapy, and a specific, circumscribed area of conflict is chosen to be the focus of treatment. More extensive change is not attempted. Patients suitable for this therapy must be able to define a specific central problem to be addressed and must be highly motivated, psychologically minded, and able to tolerate the temporary increase in anxiety or sadness that this type of therapy can evoke. Patients who are not suitable include those with fragile ego structures, e.g., suicidal or psychotic patients, and those with poor impulse control, e.g., borderline patients, substance abusers, and antisocial personalities.

## III. Behavior therapy

The basic assumption of this therapy is that maladaptive behavior can change without insight into its underlying causes. Behavioral symptoms are taken at face value and not as symptoms of a deeper problem. Behavior therapy is based on the principles of learning theory, including operant and classic conditioning. Operant conditioning is based on the premise that behavior is shaped by its consequences; that is, if behavior is positively reinforced it will increase, if it is punished it will decrease, and if it elicits no response it will be extinguished. Classical conditioning is based on the premise that behavior is shaped by its being coupled with or uncoupled from anxiety-provoking stimuli. Just as Ivan Pavlov's dogs were conditioned to salivate at the sound of a bell once the bell had become associated with meat, a person can be conditioned to feel fear in

TABLE 23–1
**PSYCHOANALYSIS AND PSYCHOANALYTIC PSYCHOTHERAPY**

| Features | Psychoanalysis | Psychoanalytic Psychotherapy | |
|---|---|---|---|
| | | Insight-Oriented (Expressive) | Supportive (Relationship) |
| Basic Theory | Psychoanalytic Psychology | Psychoanalytic Psychology | Psychoanalytic Psychology |
| Frequency and duration | 4 to 5 times weekly, 2 to 5+ years. Sessions usually about 50 minutes. New modifications: shorter sessions | 1 to 3 times weekly, few sessions to several years. Sessions usually from 20 minutes to 50 minutes | Daily sessions to once every few months, one session to a lifelong process. Sessions may be brief, ranging from a few minutes to an hour |
| Activity of patient and therapist | Freely hovering attention by the analyst, free association by the patient. Interpretation of transference and resistance. Analyst assumes neutral role | Freely hovering attention by the therapist but with more focusing than in analysis. Less emphasis on free association, more on discussion by the patient. Analyst is more active | Expressive techniques generally avoided except for some cathartic effects. Therapist actively intervenes, advises, fosters discussion, selects focus. Therapist participates as a real person around current issues |
| Interpretive emphasis | Focus on resistance and transference to the analyst | Greater emphasis on interpersonal events and external events, less on transferences to the analyst than in analysis, but transference interpretation often effective. Transferences to persons other than the therapist often effectively interpreted | Interpretations of transferences by therapist generally avoided unless significantly interfering with the therapeutic relationship. Strong focus on external events. Clarification of interpersonal events |
| Transference | Transference neurosis fostered on foundation of the therapeutic alliance. Minimal reality orientation to external events | Transference neurosis discouraged; therapeutic alliance fostered. Considerably more reality oriented | Transference neurosis discouraged; real relationship and therapeutic alliance emphasized. Almost totally reality oriented |
| Regression | Fostered in the form of the transference neurosis | Generally discouraged except as necessary to gain access to fantasy material and other derivatives of the unconscious | Regression generally discouraged |
| Adjuncts | Couch. The use of psychotropic drugs is controversial; some psychoanalysts will not use drugs, others will. Will not see family members or do group psychotherapy | Couch less used. Mostly face-to-face therapy. Psychotropic drugs used as needed. May do combined group and individual therapy | Always face-to-face therapy. Couch contraindicated. Group methods, family therapy, or family contacts on a planned basis. Other therapists and agencies may be involved. Psychotropic drugs used frequently and as needed |

TABLE 23–1 *(continued)*
**PSYCHOANALYSIS AND PSYCHOANALYTIC PSYCHOTHERAPY**

| Features | Psychoanalysis | Psychoanalytic Psychotherapy | |
|---|---|---|---|
| | | Insight-Oriented (Expressive) | Supportive (Relationship) |
| Confidentiality | Absolute. May be compromised by third-party payers | Absolute. May be compromised by third-party payers | Absolute. May be compromised by third-party payers |
| Prerequisites | Relatively mature personality, favorable life situation, motivation for long undertaking, capacity to tolerate frustration, capacity for stable therapeutic alliance, psychological mindedness | Relatively mature personality, capacity for therapeutic alliance, some capacity to tolerate frustration, adequate motivation, and some degree of psychological mindedness | Some capacity for therapeutic alliance, personality capable of growth, reality situation not too unfavorable. Personality organization may range from psychotic to mature |
| Diagnostic indications | Neuroses, personality disorders, paraphilias, sexual disorders | Neuroses, personality disorders (especially borderline and narcissistic), paraphilias, sexual disorders, latent schizophrenia, cyclothymic disorder, psychosomatic disorders | Psychoses, adjustment disorders, impulse-control disorders, psychophysiological conditions, psychosomatic disorders |
| Goals | Reorganization of character structure, with diminution of pathologic defenses, integration of ultimate rejection of warded-off strivings and ideation. Understanding rather than symptom relief the objective, but symptom relief usually results. Correction of developmental lags in otherwise relatively mature personalities | Resolution of selected conflicts and limited removal of pathological defenses. Understanding the primary goal, usually with secondary relief of symptoms | Growth of the relatively immature personality through catalytic relationship with therapist counteracts the neurotogenic effects of prior significant relationships. Restoration of prior equilibrium, reduction of anxiety and fear in new situations. Help in tolerating unalterable situations |

neutral situations that have come to be associated with anxiety. Uncouple the anxiety from the situation, and avoidant and anxious behavior will decrease. Behavioral techniques include the following:

**A. Token economy.** A form of **positive reinforcement** used with inpatients. A patient is rewarded with various tokens (e.g., food, passes) for performing desired behaviors, e.g., dressing in street clothes, attending group therapy.

**B. Aversion therapy.** A form of conditioning in which an aversive stimulus, e.g., a shock or unpleasant smell, is paired with an undesired behavior. A less controversial form of aversion therapy involves the patient imagining something unpleasant coupled with the undesired behavior.

**C. Systematic desensitization.** A technique in which a patient with avoidant behavior linked to a specific stimulus, e.g., heights or airplane travel, is asked to construct a hierarchy of anxiety-provoking images in his or her imagination from the least to the most fearful, staying at each level of the hierarchy until anxiety diminishes. When this procedure is performed in real life rather than imagined, it is called graded exposure. These techniques work through a combination of positive reinforcement for confronting anxiety-provoking stimuli and the extinguishing of maladaptive behavior by the realization of an absence of negative consequences. Hierarchy construction often is associated with relaxation techniques, because it is felt that anxiety and relaxation are incompatible, thus leading to an uncoupling of the imagined images from anxiety (reciprocal inhibition).

**D. Flooding.**    A technique in which the patient is exposed immediately to the most anxiety-provoking stimulus, e.g., the top of a tall building if he or she is afraid of heights, instead of being exposed gradually or systematically to a hierarchy of feared situations. If this technique occurs in the imagination as opposed to real life, it is called implosion. Flooding is thought to be the most effective behavioral treatment of such disorders as phobias, if the patient can tolerate the anxiety associated with it.

Behavior therapy is believed to be most effective for clearly delineated, circumscribed maladaptive behaviors, e.g., phobias, compulsions, overeating, cigarette smoking, stuttering, and sexual dysfunctions. Treatment of conditions that can be strongly affected by psychological factors, such as hypertension, asthma, pain, and insomnia, may use behavioral techniques to induce relaxation and decrease aggravating stresses.

## IV. Cognitive therapy

Cognitive therapy is based on the theory that behavior is secondary to the way in which persons think about themselves and their roles in the world. Maladaptive behavior is secondary to ingrained, stereotyped thoughts, which can lead to cognitive distortions or errors in thinking. The theory is aimed at correcting these cognitive distortions and the self-defeating behaviors that result from them. Therapy is short-term, generally 15–20 sessions over 12 weeks, during which patients are made aware of their own distorted cognitions and the assumptions on which the questions are based. Homework is assigned: patients are asked to record what they are thinking in certain stressful situations (such as, ''I'm no good'' or ''No one cares about me'') and to ascertain the underlying, often relatively unconscious, assumptions that fuel the negative cognitions. This process has been called ''recognizing and correcting automatic thoughts.'' The cognitive model of depression includes the cognitive triad, which is a description of the thought distortions that occur when a person is depressed. The triad includes (1) a negative view of the self, (2) a negative interpretation of present and past experience, and (3) a negative expectation of the future.

Cognitive therapy has been most successfully applied to the treatment of mild to moderate, nonpsychotic depressions. It also has been effective as an adjunctive treatment with substance abusers and in increasing compliance with medication.

## V. Family therapy

Family therapy is based on the theory that a family is a system that attempts to maintain homeostasis, regardless of how maladaptive the system may be. This theory has been called a family systems orientation, and the techniques include focusing on the family rather than on the identified patient. The family therefore becomes the patient, as opposed to the individual family member who has been identified as sick. One of the major goals of a family therapist is to determine what homeostatic role, however pathological, the identified patient is serving in the particular family system. One example is the triangulated child—the child who is identified by the family as the patient is actually serving to maintain the family system by becoming involved in a marital conflict as a scapegoat, referee, or even surrogate spouse. The therapist's job is to help the family understand the triangulation process and address the deeper conflict that underlies the child's apparent disruptive behavior. Techniques include reframing and positive connotation (a relabeling of all negatively expressed feelings or behaviors as positive); for example, "this child is impossible" becomes "this child is desperately trying to distract and protect you from what he or she perceives is an unhappy marriage."

Other goals of family therapy include changing maladaptive rules that govern a family, increasing awareness of cross-generational dynamics, balancing individuation and cohesiveness, increasing one-on-one direct communication, and decreasing blaming and scapegoating.

## VI. Interpersonal therapy (IPT)

IPT is a short-term psychotherapy, lasting 12–16 weeks, developed specifically for the treatment of nonbipolar, nonpsychotic depression. Intrapsychic conflicts are not addressed. Emphasis is on current interpersonal relationships and on strategies to improve the patient's interpersonal life. Antidepressant medication is often used as an adjunct to IPT. The therapist is very active in helping to formulate the patient's predominant interpersonal problem areas, which define the treatment focus.

## VII. Group therapy

Group therapies are based on as many theories as are individual therapies. Groups range from those that emphasize support and an increase in social skills, to those that emphasize specific symptomatic relief, to those that work through unresolved intrapsychic conflicts. Focus may be on a person within the context of a group, on interactions that occur among persons in the group, or on the group as a whole. There can be resolution of both individual and interpersonal issues. Therapeutic factors include identification, universalization, acceptance, altruism, transference, reality testing, and ventilation. Groups provide a forum in which imagined fears and transference distortions can be immediately subjected to exploration and correction.

Groups tend to meet 1–2 times a week, usually for $1\frac{1}{2}$ hours. They may be homogeneous or heterogeneous, depending on diagnosis. Examples of homogeneous groups include those for weight-reduction and smoking-cessation, as well as groups whose members share the same medical or psychiatric problem, e.g., patients with acquired immunodeficiency syndrome (AIDS), posttraumatic stress disorder, or substance use disorders. Certain types of patients do not do well in certain types of groups. Psychotic patients who need structure and clear direction do not do well in insight-oriented groups. Paranoid patients, antisocial personalities, and substance abusers can benefit from group therapy but do not do well in heterogeneous insight-oriented groups. In general, acutely psychotic or suicidal patients do not do well in groups.

**A. Alcoholics Anonymous (AA).** An example of a large, highly structured, peer-run group that is organized around persons with a similar, central problem. AA emphasizes a sharing of experience, role models, ventilation of feelings, and strong sense of community and mutual support. Similar groups include Narcotics Anonymous (NA) and Sex Addicts Anonymous (SAA).

**B. Milieu therapy.** The multidisciplinary therapeutic approach used on inpatient psychiatric wards. The term "milieu therapy" reflects the idea that all activities on a ward are oriented toward increasing a patient's ability to cope in the world and to relate appropriately to others. Milieu therapy generally involves groups and may include art therapy, occupational therapy, activities of daily living groups, community meetings, group passes, and social events.

**C. Multiple family groups (MFGs).** Composed of families of schizophrenic patients. The groups discuss issues and problems related to having a schizophrenic person in the family and share suggestions and means of coping. MFGs are an important factor in decreasing relapse rates among schizophrenic patients whose families participate in the groups.

## VIII. Couples and marital therapy

As many as 50% of patients are estimated to enter psychotherapy primarily because of marital problems; another 25% experience marital problems along with their other presenting problems. Marital or couples therapy is an effective tool for helping each member of the couple to achieve self-knowledge while working on their problems. Couples and marital therapy encompasses a wide range of treatment techniques with the goal of increasing marital satisfaction or addressing marital impairment. As with family therapy, the relationship rather than either of the individuals is viewed as the patient.

For a more detailed discussion of this topic, see Theories of Personality and Psychopathology: Psychoanalysis, Chap 6, pp 431–486; Weiner MF, Mohl PC: Theories of Personality and Psychopathology: Other Psychodynamic Schools, Chap 7, p 487; Costa PT Jr, McCrae RR: Theories of Personality and Psychopathology: Approaches Derived from Philosophy and Psychology, Chap 8, p 507; Psychotherapies, Chap 31, pp 1767–1890; Kernberg PF: Individual Psychotherapy, Sec 46.1, p 2399; Licamele WL, Bernet W: Group Psychotherapy, Sec 46.2, p 2412; Sadavoy J, Lazarus LW: Individual Psychotherapy, Sec 49.7a, p 2593; Lansky MR: Family Therapy, Sec 49.7b, p 2598; Leszcz M: Group Therapy, Sec 49.7c, p 2599, in CTP/VI.

# 24

## Psychopharmacology and Other Biological Therapies

## I. Basic principles of psychopharmacology

Because the pharmacotherapy for mental disorders is one of the most rapidly evolving areas of clinical medicine, any practitioner who prescribes such drugs must remain current with the research literature. The key areas for regular update are the emergence of new agents, e.g., risperidone (Risperdal), tacrine (Cognex), venlafaxine (Effexor); new indications for existing agents, e.g., valproate (Depakene, Depakote); the clinical usefulness of plasma concentrations; and the identification and treatment of drug-related adverse effects.

Drug therapy and other biological treatments of mental disorders may be defined as attempts to modify or correct pathological behaviors, thoughts, or moods by chemical or other physical means. The relations between the physical state of the brain and its functional manifestations (behaviors, thoughts, and moods) are highly complex and imperfectly understood. However, the various parameters of normal and abnormal behavior—such as perception, affect, and cognition—may be profoundly affected by physical changes in the central nervous system (CNS), e.g., by cerebrovascular disease, epilepsy, and legal and illicit drugs.

**A. Classification of drugs.** The classic division of psychotherapeutic drugs is as follows: (1) anxiolytics and hypnotics, (2) antipsychotics, (3) antidepressants, and (4) antimanics.

These divisions are historically determined by their original clinical use. With most psychotropic drugs, however, clinical experience has shown that they have more than one clinical application. In actual practice, psychotropic drugs are used for purposes other than the primary approved indication. In addition, many compounds used for the treatment of endocrine, cardiovascular, and neurological conditions are now frequently used to augment existing treatment regimens.

It also is common clinical practice for drugs to be used in higher doses than approved by the Food and Drug Administration (FDA). The FDA's view is that it is generally appropriate for clinicians to prescribe within the guidelines of community norms.

Some combination drugs are used with the rationale that they may increase the patient's compliance by simplifying the drug regimen. A problem with combination drugs, however, is that the clinician has less flexibility in adjusting the dose of one of the components and thus minimizing side effects. The use of combination drugs also may cause two drugs to be administered when only one is actually effective.

**B. Pharmacokinetics.** The principal divisions of pharmacokinetics are drug absorption, distribution, metabolism, and excretion.

1. **Absorption.** Orally administered drugs must dissolve in the fluid of the gastrointestinal (GI) tract before the body can absorb them. The absorption depends on the drug's concentration and lipid solubility and the GI tract's local pH, motility, and surface area. Some antipsychotic drugs are available in depot forms that allow the drug to be administered only once every 1–4 weeks. Intravenous (IV) administration is the quickest route to achieve therapeutic blood levels, but it also carries the highest risk of sudden and life-threatening adverse effects.

2. **Distribution.** Drugs can be freely dissolved in the blood plasma, bound to dissolved plasma proteins (primarily albumin), and dissolved within the blood cells. The distribution of a drug to the brain is determined by the blood-brain barrier, the brain's regional blood flow, and the drug's affinity with its receptors in the brain. The volume of distribution can also vary with the patient's age, sex, and disease state.

3. **Metabolism and excretion.** The four major metabolic routes for drugs are oxidation, reduction, hydrolysis, and conjugation. The liver is the principal site of metabolism, and bile, feces, and urine are the major routes of excretion. Psychoactive drugs also are excreted in sweat, saliva, tears, and milk; therefore, mothers who are taking psychotherapeutic drugs should not nurse their children.

   A drug's **half-life** is defined as the amount of time it takes for one-half of a drug's peak plasma level to be metabolized and excreted from the body.

   **Clearance** is a measure of the amount of drug excreted per unit of time. If a disease process or another drug interferes with the clearance of a psychoactive drug, then the drug may reach toxic levels.

**C. Pharmacodynamics.** The major pharmacodynamic considerations include the receptor mechanism; the dose response curve; the therapeutic index; and the development of tolerance, dependence, and withdrawal phenomena.

The dose response curve plots the drug concentration against the effects of the drug. The **potency** of a drug refers to the relative dose required to achieve a certain effect. Haloperidol (Haldol), for example, is more potent than chlorpromazine (Thorazine) because generally only 5 mg of haloperidol are required to achieve the same therapeutic effect as 100 mg of chlorpromazine. Both haloperidol and chlorpromazine, however, are equal in their maximal efficacies, i.e., the maximum clinical response achievable by the administration of a drug.

The side effects of most drugs often are a direct result of their primary pharmacodynamic effects and are better conceptualized as adverse effects. The **therapeutic index** is a relative measure of a drug's toxicity or safety.

A person may become less responsive to a particular drug as it is administered over time, which is referred to as **tolerance**. Tolerance is associated with the appearance of physical dependence, which may be defined as the necessity to continue administering the drug in order to prevent the appearance of withdrawal symptoms.

**D. Clinical guidelines.** Optimal results with drug therapy are dependent on several factors. Drugs work best when used according to lessons that have been learned from clinical and research experience. Optimizing results of psychotropic drug therapy involve the five Ds: diagnosis, drug selection, dose, duration, and dialogue.

   **1. Diagnosis.** Careful diagnosis is the first step toward optimal drug treatment. Selection of an inappropriate medication based on a mistaken diagnosis may not only delay the ultimate resolution of the underlying disorder but also actually worsen the patient's clinical condition.

   **2. Drug selection.** Factors that determine drug selection include diagnosis, past history of drug response to a particular agent, and the overall medical status of the patient. By far the most important reasons to choose a drug are its relative side-effect profile and safety. Although all available drugs are equivalent in overall efficacy, they differ immensely in how well they are tolerated and how lethal they are in overdose. Drugs should not be selected because of their sedative effects.

   There once was a tendency to treat mental disorders with nonspecific sedation. This approach often reduced subjective distress or insomnia for a brief period, but did little to shorten the course of the underlying disorder. In addition, sedation itself can significantly impair cognition and psychomotor performance. Nonsedating antidepressants, such as fluoxetine (Prozac), or anxiolytics, such as buspirone (BuSpar), are preferable to sedating compounds.

   The Drug Enforcement Administration (DEA) has classified drugs according to abuse potential (Table 24–1), and clinicians are advised to be more cautious when prescribing Schedule II drugs than when prescribing less-controlled and uncontrolled substances.

   **3. Dose.** The two most common causes of treatment failure involving psychotropic drugs are underdosing and an inadequate therapeutic trial of a drug. It is well established that antidepressant drugs produce higher rates of improvement when taken at doses above the equivalent of 225 mg a day of imipramine (Tofranil). The development of adverse effects at higher dose levels tends to deter patient compliance, and physicians often are reluctant to encourage dose escalations in a patient complaining of these side effects. Once the decision has been made to treat a patient with medication, all effort should be made to achieve therapeutic dose levels.

   **4. Duration.** For most psychotropic drugs, 3 weeks is the minimum period of treatment needed to determine whether a drug will prove effective. Ideally, a therapeutic trial should continue for 4–6 weeks if clinical conditions permit. It is important to recognize that psychotropic drugs generally produce their effects with long-term administration. Some patients may respond more rapidly than others.

   **5. Dialogue.** Patients will generally have less trouble with adverse effects if they have been told to expect them. But clinicians should distinguish between probable or expected adverse effects and rare or unexpected adverse effects.

   Patients often feel that taking a psychotherapeutic drug means that they are really sick or not in control of their lives or that they may

TABLE 24–1
**CHARACTERISTICS OF DRUGS AT EACH DEA LEVEL**

| DEA Control Level (Schedule) | Characteristics of Drug at Each Control Level | Examples of Drugs at Each Control Level |
|---|---|---|
| I | High abuse potential<br>No accepted use in medical treatment in the United States at the present time and therefore, not for prescription use<br>Can be used for research | LSD, heroin, marijuana, peyote, PCP, mescaline, psilocybin, nicocodeine, nicomorphine, MDA, MDMA |
| II | High abuse potential<br>Severe physical dependence liability<br>Severe psychological dependence liability<br>No refills; no telephonic prescriptions | Amphetamine, methamphetamine, opium, morphine, codeine, hydromorphine, phenmetrazine, cocaine, amobarbital, secobarbital, pentobarbital, methylphenidate, dronabinol (tetrahydrocannibol), glutethimide |
| III | Abuse potential less than levels I and II<br>Moderate or low physical dependence liability<br>High psychological liability<br>Prescriptions must be rewritten after 6 months or 5 refills | Methyprylon, nalorphine, sulfonmethane, benzphetamine, phendimetrazine, clortermine, mazindol chlorphentermine, compounds containing codeine, opium, hydrocodone, dihydrocodeine, diethylpropion |
| IV | Low abuse potential<br>Limited physical dependence liability<br>Limited psychological dependence liability<br>Prescriptions must be rewritten after 6 months or 5 refills | Phenobarbital, benzodiazepines,[a] chloral hydrate, ethchlorvynol, ethinamate, meprobamate, paraldehyde |
| V | Lowest abuse potential of all controlled substances | Narcotic preparations containing limited amounts of nonnarcotic active medicinal ingredients |

[a] In New York State, benzodiazepines are treated as Schedule II substances, which require a triplicate prescription for a maximum of 1 month's supply.

become addicted to the drug and have to take it forever. A simplified approach to these concerns is to describe the psychiatric disorder partially as a disease or chemical imbalance analogous to diabetes as a disease of the pancreas. Psychiatrists should explain the difference between drugs of abuse that affect the normal brain and psychiatric drugs that are used to treat emotional disorders.

## E. Special considerations

**1. Children.** It is best to begin with a small dose and to increase the dose until clinical effects are observed. However, the clinician should not hesitate to use adult doses in children if the dose is effective and there are no side effects.

**2. Geriatric patients.** Psychiatrists should begin treating geriatric patients with a small dose, usually approximately one-half the usual dose. The dose should be raised in small amounts, more slowly than in middle-aged adults, until either a clinical benefit is achieved or unacceptable adverse effects appear. Although many geriatric patients require a small dose of medication, many others require the usual adult dosage.

3. **Pregnant and nursing women.** Avoid administering any drug to a woman who is pregnant (particularly during the first trimester) or who is nursing a child. This rule, however, occasionally needs to be broken when the mother's psychiatric disorder is severe. The two most teratogenic drugs in the psychopharmacopeia are lithium and anticonvulsants. Lithium administration during pregnancy is associated with a higher incidence of birth abnormalities, including Ebstein's anomaly, a serious abnormality in cardiac development.

4. **Medically ill patients.** Like children and geriatric patients, medically ill patients should receive the most conservative clinical practice, which is to begin with a small dose, increase it slowly, and watch for both clinical and adverse effects. Plasma drug levels may be a particularly helpful clinical test in these patients.

## II. Anxiolytics and hypnotics

The drugs of choice for the treatment of anxiety are the benzodiazepines and buspirone. These compounds offer a wide margin of safety compared with older anxiolytic and hypnotic drugs, such as chloral hydrate (Noctec), barbiturates, and meprobamate (Miltown). Antidepressant drugs, most notably the tricyclics, monoamine oxidase inhibitors (MAOIs), and serotonin-specific reuptake inhibitors (SSRIs) are also effective as antianxiety agents. They are commonly used to treat panic disorder, and occasionally to treat generalized anxiety disorder. Clomipramine (Anafranil) and SSRIs are used to treat obsessive-compulsive disorder.

A. **Benzodiazepines.** There are 15 benzodiazepines available for clinical use in the United States. They are widely prescribed, with at least 10% of the population using one of these drugs each year (Table 24–2).

Although best known for their role in treating anxiety, these compounds produce other pharmacological effects (Table 24–3).

Discontinuation of benzodiazepines can result in symptom recurrence, rebound, e.g., transient worsening of pretreatment symptoms, or withdrawal symptoms, e.g., emergence of new symptoms. Several factors contribute to the development of benzodiazepine withdrawal symptoms (Table 24–4). Drug type and duration of use are the most significant factors, but other considerations are also important. Some patients may need to take benzodiazepines for prolonged periods. This is particularly true for patients being treated for panic disorder. Concern about dependence should lead to caution when prescribing, but should not result in avoidance of benzodiazepine use when indicated. Some patients taking benzodiazepines for years do not develop withdrawal reactions, whereas others encounter difficulties after only a few weeks of use.

Apart from being subjectively distressing, withdrawal symptoms can lead to the perception that the symptoms are part of the underlying disorder and thus result in unnecessary continued use of the drug.

The most important distinction among the benzodiazepines is their elimination half-life—the relative rate of drug excretion.

Long half-life compounds tend to accumulate with repeated dosage. This increases the risk of excessive daytime sedation, difficulties with concentra-

TABLE 24–2
**BENZODIAZEPINES**

| Drug | Approximate Dose Equivalents[a] | Dose Forms | Benzodiazepines Rate of Absorption | Major Active Metabolites | Average Half-Life of Metabolites (hrs) | Short-Acting/ Long-Acting[b] | Usual Adult Dosage Range (mg per day) |
|---|---|---|---|---|---|---|---|
| Alprazolam (Xanax) | 0.25 | 0.25, 0.5, 1, 2 mg tablets | Medium | α-Hydroxyalprazolam, 4-hydroxyalprazolam | 12 | Short | 0.5–6 |
| Chlordiazepoxide (Librium) | 10 | 5, 10, 25 mg tablets; 5, 10, 25 mg capsules; 100 mg parenteral | Medium | Desmethylchlordiazepoxide, demoxopam, desmethyldiazepam, oxazepam | 100 | Long | 15–100 |
| Clonazepam (Klonopin) | 0.5 | 0.5, 1, 2 mg tablets | Rapid | None | 34 | Long | 0.5–10 |
| Clorazepate (Tranxene) | 7.5 | 3.75, 7.5, 11.25, 15, 22.5 mg tablets; 3.75, 7.5, 15 mg capsules | Rapid | Desmethyldiazepam, oxazepam | 100 | Long | 7.5–60 |
| Diazepam (Valium) | 5 | 2, 5, 10 mg tablets; 15 mg capsules (extended release); 5 mg/mL parenteral; 5 mg/5 mL, 5 mg/mL solution | Rapid | Desmethyldiazepam, oxazepam | 100 | Long | 2–60 |
| Estazolam (ProSom) | 0.33 | 1, 2 mg tablets | Rapid | 4-Hydroxy estazolam, 1-oxo estazolam | 17 | Short | 1–2 |
| Flurazepam (Dalmane) | 5 | 15, 30 mg capsules | Rapid | Desalkylflurazepam, N-l-hydroxyethylflurazepam | 100 | Long | 15–30 |
| Halazepam (Paxipam) | 20 | 20, 40 mg tablets | Medium | Desmethyldiazepam, oxazepam | 100 | Long | 60–160 |
| Lorazepam (Ativan) | 1 | 0.5, 1, 2 mg tablets; 2 mg/mL, 4 mg/mL parenteral | Medium | None | 15 | Short | 2–6 |
| Midazolam (Versed)[c] | 1.25–1.7 | 1 mg/mL, 5 mg/mL parenteral | N/A | l-Hydroxymethylmidazolam | 2.5 | Short | Parenteral form only; 7.5–45 |

| Oxazepam (Serax) | 15 | 15 mg tablets; 10, 15, 30 mg capsules | Slow | None | 8 | Short | 30–120 |
| Prazepam (Centrax) | 10 | 10 mg tablets; 5, 10, 20 mg | Slow | Desmethyldiazepam, oxazepam | 100 | Long | 20–60 |
| Quazepam (Doral) | 5 | 7.5, 15 mg tablets | Rapid | 2 oxoquazepam, N-desalkyl-2-oxoquazepam, and 3-hydroxy-2-oxoquazepam glucoronide | 100 | Long | 7.5–15 |
| Temazepam (Restoril) | 5 | 15, 30 mg capsules | Medium | None | 11 | Short | 15–30 |
| Triazolam (Halcion) | 0.1 | 0.125, 0.25 mg tablets | Rapid | None | 2 | Short | 0.125–0.25 |

[a]High-potency drugs have an approximage dose equivalent of under 1.0: 1.0–10, medium potency; over 10, low potency.
[b]Short-acting benzodiazepines have a half-life of under 25 hrs.
[c]Used only by anesthesiologists—no clinical use in psychiatry.

TABLE 24–3
**PHARMACOLOGICAL EFFECTS OF BENZODIAZEPINES**

| Effects | Clinical Applications/Consequences |
|---|---|
| *Therapeutic effects* | |
| Sedative | Insomnia, conscious sedation, alcohol withdrawal |
| Anxiolytic | Panic attacks, generalized anxiety |
| Anticonvulsant | Seizures |
| Muscle relaxant | Muscle tension, muscle spasm |
| Amnestic | Adjunct to chemotherapy or anesthesia |
| Antistress | Mild hypertension, irritable bowel syndrome, angina |
| *Adverse effects* | |
| Sedative | Daytime sleepiness, impaired concentration |
| Amnestic | Mild forgetfulness, anterograde memory impairment |
| Psychomotor | Accidents, falls |
| Behavioral | Depression, agitation |
| Decreased $CO_2$ response | Worsening of sleep apnea and other obstructive pulmonary disorders |
| Withdrawal syndrome | Dependence—anxiety, insomnia, excess sensitivity to light, excess sensitivity to sound, tachycardia, mild systolic hypertension, tremor, headache, sweating, abdominal distress, craving, seizures |

TABLE 24–4
**KEY FACTORS IN THE DEVELOPMENT OF BENZODIAZEPINE WITHDRAWAL SYMPTOMS**

| Factor | Explanation |
|---|---|
| Drug type | High-potency, short half-life compounds, e.g., alprazolam, triazolam, lorazepam |
| Duration of use | Risk increases with time |
| Dose level | Higher doses increase risk |
| Rate of discontinuation | Abrupt withdrawal instead of taper increases risk of severe symptoms, including seizures |
| Diagnosis | Panic disorder patients more prone to withdrawal |
| Personality | Patients with passive-dependent, histrionic, somatizing or asthenic traits are more likely to experience withdrawal |

tion and memory, and increased risk of falls. Rates of hip fractures due to falls are higher in elderly patients taking these drugs than in those taking more rapidly eliminated compounds.

The long half-life of these drugs is accounted for by a common long half-life metabolite, desmethyldiazepam. Its elimination half-life ranges from 50–120 hours.

Short half-life benzodiazepines have the advantage of producing less impairment with regular use. However, they appear to produce a more severe withdrawal syndrome.

Benzodiazepines differ in potency, i.e., the milligrams needed to achieve comparable clinical effects.

High-potency benzodiazepines appear to be effective in suppressing panic attacks.

Rate of absorption is another major consideration in benzodiazepine selection. With the exception of clorazepate (Tranxene), all benzodiazepines are rapidly and completely absorbed from the GI tract, although the presence of food somewhat delays the process. Subtle differences in absorption rate among these drugs may become clinically significant. Diazepam (Valium)

TABLE 24–5
**DRUGS AFFECTING THE RATE OF ELIMINATION OF OXIDIZED BENZODIAZEPINES**

| Increase Elimination Half-Life | Decrease Elimination Half-Life |
| --- | --- |
| Cimetidine | Chronic ethyl alcohol use |
| Propranolol | Rifampin |
| Oral contraceptives (estrogens) | |
| Chloramphenicol | |
| Propoxyphene | |
| Isoniazid | |
| Disulfiram | |
| Allopurinol | |
| Tricyclic antidepressants | |
| Acute ethyl alcohol use | |

and triazolam (Halcion), for example, have a rapid onset; chlordiazepoxide (Librium) and oxazepam (Serax) work more slowly. All intramuscularly (IM) injected benzodiazepines except lorazepam (Ativan) are poorly absorbed, resulting in unpredictable plasma levels. Drugs affecting the rate of elimination of benzodiazepines are presented in Table 24–5.

The five benzodiazepines used primarily as hypnotics are flurazepam (Dalmane), temazepam (Restoril), quazepam (Doral), estazolam (ProSom), and triazolam. Benzodiazepines shorten sleep latency and increase sleep continuity, making them useful for the treatment of insomnia. They also have a complex effect on sleep architecture.

The most clinically significant of the effects on sleep stages is the reduction of stages 3–4, also known as slow-wave sleep. Disorders such as sleepwalking and night terrors occur in these deep stages of sleep. Benzodiazepines also suppress rapid eye movement (REM)-related disorders, most notably violent behavior during REM (REM behavior disorder).

Zolpidem (Ambien) is a hypnotic medication that appears to bind to the GABA-benzodiazepine receptor complex. It is not a member of the benzodiazepine class, however, but is an imidazopyridine. The usual bedtime dose is 10 mg. It has a half-life of about 2–3 hours and is metabolized primarily by conjugation. Emesis and dysphoric reactions have been reported as adverse effects.

## B. Buspirone

1. **General introduction.** Buspirone is the first anxiolytic of the azaspirone class. It is pharmacologically unrelated to the benzodiazepines. In some early clinical trials it was found to be comparable to the benzodiazepines in anxiolytic efficacy.

2. **Clinical guidelines.** Buspirone is available in 5 and 10 mg tablets, with a recommended initial dosing schedule of 5 mg 3 times a day (TID). The maximum recommended daily dose is 60 mg. The therapeutic dose of buspirone is approximately 30 mg a day.

3. **Drug-drug interactions.** Concurrent administration of buspirone produces an increase in haloperidol serum levels. Combining buspirone with MAOIs can elevate blood pressure.

4. **Time course and improvement.** A major consideration in patient compliance with buspirone is the gradual onset of efficacy over a period of several days to weeks. Like antidepressants, buspirone is unlikely to

cause patients to notice significant improvement in symptoms before 7 days. Maximum therapeutic effects are generally experienced after 3–4 weeks of treatment. The observed lag period in onset of clinical efficacy argues against the utility of buspirone on an as-needed basis.

5. **Lack of sedation or interaction with CNS depressants.** The incidence of drowsiness reported by patients is no greater than with placebo. Alcohol and buspirone apparently do not enhance each other's effects.

6. **Lack of functional impairment.** Both short- and long-term buspirone treatment have failed to cause any adverse effect on psychomotor skills.

7. **Lack of potential for abuse or physical dependence.** Buspirone is not a DEA-controlled drug (see Table 24–1) and is not widely abused. The drug tends to produce dysphoria at doses above therapeutic levels. Single doses of 40 mg or more produce a highly unpleasant subjective sensation.

8. **Withdrawal.** Buspirone-treated patients experience no withdrawal syndrome, even with abrupt discontinuation. The finding implies that the likelihood of mistaking rebound anxiety or withdrawal symptoms for a return of the original anxiety symptoms is minimal.

9. **Adverse effects.** Six side effects occur with statistically significant incidence greater than that of placebo: (1) dizziness, (2) nausea, (3) headache, (4) nervousness, (5) lightheadedness, and (6) excitement.

10. **Overdose.** With doses as high as 375 mg a day, the most commonly observed symptoms are nausea, vomiting, dizziness, drowsiness, miosis, and gastric distress. No deaths have been reported either with deliberate or accidental overdose.

11. **Concurrent use with benzodiazepines.** Buspirone may be used concurrently with benzodiazepines in several circumstances: (1) treatment-resistant cases, (2) when severe insomnia merits the use of a benzodiazepine as a hypnotic, and (3) during a switching period, in which buspirone treatment is initiated before the benzodiazepine is discontinued. Buspirone will not prevent the benzodiazepine withdrawal syndrome.

## III. Antipsychotic drugs

**A. General information.** This group of drugs constitutes the major treatment for some of the most disturbed patients seen by psychiatrists. Antipsychotic drugs are mainly used to treat acute schizophrenic episodes and to prevent reemergence of psychotic symptoms in schizophrenic patients. These compounds also are useful for other psychiatric conditions, including mania, psychotic disorder due to a general medical condition, substance-induced psychotic disorder, and Tourette's disorder.

Standard antipsychotic drugs also have been called neuroleptics or major tranquilizers. The word "neuroleptic" refers to the effect of these drugs on motor activity rather than their clinical effects and is thus inappropriate. The term "major tranquilizer" is misleading because it suggests that these compounds are similar to benzodiazepines and other antianxiety drugs (the minor tranquilizers). Antipsychotic drugs are pharmacologically unrelated to the antianxiety agents, and their clinical effects do not result from nonspecific sedative action.

**B. Therapeutic effects.** These drugs achieve their major therapeutic effects when used in acute psychoses. Effects include reduction of the so-called positive symptoms, e.g., hallucinations, delusions, uncooperativeness, and thought disorder. Psychomotor activity (excitement or retardation) and information processing also are normalized. Positive symptoms of schizophrenia respond more consistently to antipsychotic drugs. Negative, or deficit, symptoms, e.g., affective flattening, apathy, anhedonia, blocking, poverty of speech, and social withdrawal, are less responsive to these drugs.

In general, negative schizophrenic symptoms persist over time, even during remissions, and have proved difficult to treat.

**C. Types of drugs.** In 1952, chlorpromazine was the first drug found to have a major effect on schizophrenic symptoms. Since then, other phenothiazine analogues have been developed along with several other compounds that are similar in their tricyclic structure. Compounds unrelated to the tricyclics also are available.

**D. Efficacy.** Despite the structural diversity of these drugs, no one compound is consistently superior to another. All antipsychotic compounds are equally effective when used at optimal doses. They differ in potency and in side effects. Some patients nevertheless respond better to one drug than another. There is no reliable way to predict this response.

Although some patients may show some immediate improvement in agitation or anxiety when started on an antipsychotic drug, these effects are mainly the result of nonspecific sedation. The actual impact of these drugs on psychotic symptoms develops with regular administration over a period of several weeks.

**E. Mechanism of action.** The mechanism of action of the typical antipsychotic drugs is probably more complex than is currently hypothesized. Their presumed mode of action involves the postsynaptic blockade of CNS dopamine (DA) type 2 ($D_2$) receptors.

**F. Potency.** A major distinction among these drugs is their efficacy at a given dose. Some drugs given at dosages that are less than 80 mg a day are called high-potency compounds. As a rule, the low-potency drugs produce more sedation, orthostatic hypotension, and anticholinergic effects than the high-potency drugs, which cause more frequent and severe extrapyramidal symptoms. The therapeutic dosages and relative potencies are listed in Table 24–6.

**G. Pharmacokinetics.** Several aspects of antipsychotic drug metabolism are clinically significant. Phenothiazines generally are well absorbed, but there may be significant differences among patients. Rates of metabolism also vary greatly. Because of the complexity of metabolites of phenothiazines, routine plasma level determinations are of limited clinical value. Liquid preparations generally are more completely absorbed than tablets or capsules. Because this route bypasses first-pass metabolism involving the liver, higher blood levels are obtained with IM administration than with oral (PO) adminis-

TABLE 24-6
**ANTIPSYCHOTICS: TYPICAL THERAPEUTIC DOSES**

| Drug | Chlorpromazine Equivalent (mg) | Relative Potency | Therapeutic Dose mg/day[a] |
|---|---|---|---|
| Chlorpromazine (Thorazine) | 100 | Low | 150–2000 |
| Triflupromazine (Vesprin) | 30 | Medium | 20–150 |
| Thioridazine (Mellaril) | 100 | Low | 100–800 |
| Mesoridazine (Serentil) | 50 | Medium | 10–400 |
| Perphenazine (Trilafon) | 10 | Medium | 8–64 |
| Trifluoperazine (Stelazine) | 3–5 | High | 5–60 |
| Fluphenazine (Prolixin) | 3–5 | High | 5–60 |
| Acetophenazine (Tindal) | 15 | Medium | 20–100 |
| Chlorprothixene (Taractan) | 75 | Low | 100–600 |
| Thiothixene (Navane) | 3–5 | High | 5–60 |
| Loxapine (Loxitane) | 10–15 | Medium | 30–250 |
| Haloperidol (Haldol) | 2–5 | High | 2–100 |
| Molindone (Moban) | 5–10 | Medium | 10–225 |
| Pimozide (Orap) | 1–2 | High | 2–20 |
| Clozapine (Clozaril) | 100 | Low | 150–600 |
| Risperidone (Risperdal) | 0.6 | High | 4–16 |

[a]Extreme range

tration. Because of generally long half-lives, antipsychotic drugs can be given once a day. Drugs that are lipophilic are difficult to dialyze in case of overdose.

**H. Adverse effects.** Antipsychotic drugs produce a broad range of side effects. These are a result of the multiple neurotransmitter systems affected by these drugs. Many patients who might benefit from the use of these drugs refuse to take them because of effects that can be distressing even to highly motivated patients, let alone those who are fearful and mistrustful. An important consideration in drug selection is avoidance of the most uncomfortable or dangerous adverse reactions—tardive dyskinesia and neuroleptic malignant syndrome.

1. **Obstructive jaundice.** Jaundice, which is rare, mainly occurs with chlorpromazine, about 1–5 weeks after start of treatment. (Symptoms include fever, nausea, right upper quadrant pain, malaise, and pruritus). Jaundice is not seen with nonphenothiazines. It may resolve spontaneously. If it occurs, consider discontinuing the chlorpromazine.

2. **Endocrine effects.** Side effects related to endocrine changes include weight gain, shift in glucose tolerance, false-positive pregnancy test, impotence or decreased sexual desire, amenorrhea, galactorrhea, and gynecomastia (due to increased prolactin level).

3. **Skin and eye effects.** Skin and eye effects include photosensitivity (use sunscreen), maculopapular rash, blue-gray metallic skin discoloration, deposits in anterior lens and posterior cornea, and pigmentary retinopathy with high doses of thioridazine (Mellaril). The anticholinergic activity of these drugs can precipitate narrow-angle glaucoma and blurred vision, particularly cycloplegia.

4. **Sedation.** Sedation is caused mainly by histamine type 1 ($H_1$) blockade and is seen most often with low-potency drugs, such as chlorproma-

zine. Some tolerance to sedation develops. If sedation remains a problem, reduce the dose or switch to a high-potency drug, such as haloperidol.

5. **Anticholinergic effects**
   a. Consist mainly of dry mouth, constipation, blurred near vision, delayed micturition, and glaucoma.
   b. Although mainly annoying, these effects are a major source of non-compliance.
   c. These adverse effects can lead to fecal impaction and urinary retention and can result in central atropinelike psychoses, a delirium related to anticholinergic toxicity.
   d. Management of anticholinergic side effects includes: neostigmine (Prostigmin) (15–30 mg 3 times a day) or bethanechol (Urecholine) (25 mg 2 times a day to 4 times a day) for urinary retention. Physostigmine (Antilirium) eye drops are not practical; reading glasses may help. Laxatives for constipation should be used judiciously.

6. **Orthostatic (postural) hypotension**
   a. Caused by $\alpha_1$-adrenergic blockade.
   b. Seen most often with aliphatic phenothiazines, mainly chlorpromazine, at high doses or when given IM. Can be caused by clozapine, when started at high dose.
   c. Do not treat with epinephrine, which is a $\beta$-adrenergic stimulant and thus may worsen orthostasis. Use metaraminol (Aramine) or norepinephrine (NE).

7. **Cardiac effects**
   a. Sudden death (rare).
   b. Electrocardiogram (EKG) changes (prolonged QT and PR intervals, ST depression, and blunted T waves).

8. **Hematological effects.**   Benign drop in white blood cell count (WBC), thrombocytopenia, pancytopenia, or agranulocytosis. Leukocyte count may decline slowly. Stabilizes at about 3,000; not usually symptomatic. Nevertheless, patient's blood count should be followed.

   Complete loss of granulocytes. Has an incidence of 1 in 500,000. Occurs abruptly—less than 8 weeks after start of treatment. Chlorpromazine most often is implicated. Symptoms include sudden sore throat and fever. Stop drug immediately and refer for medical treatment (usually antibiotics and reverse isolation).

9. **Neurological effects**
   a. **Pseudoparkinsonism**—the most common reversible drug-induced movement disorder (15% of patients). Its incidence increases with age. Like Parkinson's disease itself, this condition is characterized by dysfunction in tone (e.g., generalized rigidity), movement (e.g., bradykinesia, akinesia, tremor, festinating gait), and posture (e.g., flexed posture).

   Current theory holds that drug-induced parkinsonism and other extrapyramidal effects, such as tardive dyskinesia, are the result of nigrostriatal dopamine system blockade. Treatment consists primarily of antiparkinsonian medication.

Other interventions include a dose reduction of antipsychotic drug or the use of a phenothiazine with a relatively low liability for producing pseudoparkinsonism, e.g., thioridazine. See Chapter 25.

**b. Acute dystonic reactions**
  i. Experienced by at least 10% of patients.
  ii. Most common in young men.
  iii. Mechanism may involve excessive stimulation of hypersensitive DA receptors.
  iv. Attacks subside spontaneously in hours to days.
  v. Attacks are aborted spontaneously with anticholinergics or diazepam.

**c. Akathisia**
  i. Motor and mental restlessness.
  ii. Increasing doses of antipsychotic drugs may only increase restlessness.
  iii. Treated with anticholinergics, benzodiazepines, β-blockers.

**d. Neuroleptic malignant syndrome**
  i. Unexplained hyperthermia with increase in muscle tone and involuntary movements after initiating or increasing antipsychotic drugs.
  ii. Pulmonary complications and acute renal failure (secondary to dehydration) are common.
  iii. One-quarter of typical cases culminate in stupor, coma, and death.
  iv. Treat with dantrolene (Dantrium) (200 mg a day) or bromocriptine (Parlodel) (up to 60 mg a day).
  v. A medical emergency. Stop antipsychotic drug.

**e. Lethal catatonia.**
  i. Rare syndrome in patients on long-term treatment.
  ii. Prodrome of increasing mental and physical agitation lasting weeks to months.
  iii. May culminate in stupor, coma, and death.
  iv. Differentiate from neuroleptic malignant syndrome by absence of extrapyramidal rigidity, involuntary movements, and other clinical features listed in Table 24–7.

**f. Tardive dyskinesia**
  i. Symptoms include repetitive lip smacking, masticatory and tongue movements, and choreic movements of the trunk and limbs.
  ii. Occurs during or after discontinuation of long-term antipsychotic drug treatment. More common in women than in men.
  iii. Mechanism probably involves denervation hypersensitivity secondary to long-term dopaminergic blockade.
  iv. Irreversible in most patients.
  v. Anticholinergics do not prevent and may actually exacerbate the disease.
  vi. Treat by substituting responsible drug with a different antipsychotic and then slowly withdrawing the substitute drug.

TABLE 24-7
**CLINICAL DIFFERENCES BETWEEN LETHAL CATATONIA AND NEUROLEPTIC MALIGNANT SYNDROME**

| Stage | Lethal Catatonia | Neuroleptic Malignant Syndrome |
|---|---|---|
| | Prodrome lasting 2 weeks–2 months, consisting of behavioral and personality changes or frank schizophrenic symptoms<br>Possible acute onset with no prodrome | Period of prior antipsychotic drug exposure can be hours to months<br>Develops rapidly over a few hours to days<br>No prodromal phase has been described |
| Initial symptoms | Excitement, intense anxiety, and restlessness lasting a few days<br>Possible self-destructive or assaultive behavior<br>Hallucinatory experiences and delusional thinking usually present<br>Possible fever, tachycardia, and acrocyanosis<br>Sudden death may occur | Tremors and dyskinesias are early signs<br>Muscle hypertonicity described as lead pipe or plastic rigidity<br>Severe excitement and intense anxiety are not major features<br>Autonomic instability with tachycardia, labile hypertension, and possible diaphoresis<br>Fever may not be present initially<br>Acrocyanosis has not been described<br>May occur in nonpsychotic patients treated with antipsychotics<br>No deaths reported during early phase |
| Full syndrome | Continued increasing excitement with wild agitation and violent, destructive behavior, lasting 3–15 days, and possible choreiform movements<br>Mutism, rigidity, or stupor may alternate with excitement<br>Refusal of food and fluids<br>Increasing and fluctuating fever, rapid and weak pulse, profuse, clammy perspiration, hypotension | Appearance of most major symptoms (severe muscle rigidity, persistent autonomic instability, fever) usually occurs after 2–9 days<br>Possible agitation, confusion, and clouding of consciousness |
| Final stage | Cachexia, convulsions, delirium, coma, exhaustion<br>Death may occur | Severe complications, e.g., rhabdomyolysis with elevated creatine phosphokinase, myoglobinuria, renal failure, and intravascular thrombosis with pulmonary embolism and respiratory failure<br>Possible 20–30% mortality rate with full syndrome |
| Treatment | Antipsychotic drugs and other treatments to reduce severe psychotic symptoms | Immediate cessation of all dopamine-blocking antipsychotic drugs<br>Dopamine agonists (to reduce central hypodopaminergic state), calcium channel blockers (to reduce muscle rigidity), beta-adrenergic blockers (to reduce tachycardia), other supportive measures as needed<br>Consider using electroconvulsive therapy (ECT) |

Table adapted from Castillo E, Rubin RT, Holsboer-Trachsler E: Clinical differentiation between lethal catatonia and neuroleptic malignant syndrome. Am J Psychiatry *146:* 326, 1989. Used with permission.

**g. Rabbit syndrome**
  i.  Late-onset, drug-induced extrapyramidal symptoms.
  ii.  Rapid, fine rhythmic movements of the lips.
  iii. Unlike buccolingual movements of Tourette's disorder, rabbit syndrome improves with antiparkinsonian drugs.
**h. Seizures**—all antipsychotic drugs can lower the seizure threshold.

TABLE 24–8
**CONSIDERATIONS IN THE DRUG SELECTION**

| Factor | Comment |
| --- | --- |
| Diagnosis | The more clear-cut the diagnosis of schizophrenia, the more important an antipsychotic be used. |
| Past history of drug response | The success or failure of a particular drug in treating a past episode in the patient or biological family. |
| Medical status | Specific conditions, such as prostatic hypertropy, glaucoma, cardiac disease or constipation, argue against use of strongly anticholinergic drugs. In patients with parkinsonism, use low potency agents. |
| Severe depression | Because thioridazine and mesoridazine are more lethal in overdose, they should be avoided in potentially suicidal patients. |
| Cognitive disorder | Although used to treat behavioral disturbances associated with cognitive disorders, the more anticholinergic drugs can worsen mental status and cause delirium. |

I. **Drug selection.** Factors to be considered in drug selection include characteristics of both the patient and the pharmacological compound (Table 24–8).

The popularity of high-potency drugs, such as haloperidol, is largely the result of the low degree of both sedation and anticholinergic effects. Even though the risk of extrapyramidal symptoms is great, most clinicians prefer to treat them as they emerge.

1. **Phenothiazines**

a. **Aliphatic, e.g., chlorpromazine (Thorazine), triflupromazine (Vesprin)**—chlorpromazine is the most widely used of the low-potency drugs. Usually these drugs are associated with marked sedation, postural hypotension, and an intermediate profile with respect to frequency of extrapyramidal symptoms.

b. **Piperazine, e.g., perphenazine (Trilafon), trifluoperazine (Stelazine), fluphenazine (Prolixin), acetophenazine (Tindal)**—more potent than the aliphatics. One advantage of the piperazine drugs is the decreased likelihood of causing sedation and orthostatic hypotension. A disadvantage is a high incidence of extrapyramidal side effects.

i. **Perphenazine**—causes fewer extrapyramidal symptoms than other piperazines, but more sedation and cardiovascular effects. It seems to be the pharmacological middle of antipsychotic drugs.

ii. **Trifluoperazine**—associated with low sedative effects and moderate degrees of hypotension and anticholinergic activity. Apart from extrapyramidal effects, it is generally well tolerated.

iii. **Fluphenazine**—one of two antipsychotic drugs available in a long-acting injectable preparation. Fluphenazine comes in a decanoate form, which is generally administered as an IM injection every 2 weeks. In some cases, an injection can last up to 6 weeks. Fluphenazine decanoate is indicated over oral drugs in patients who do not comply with oral regimens or who have absorption problems. Fluphenazine also is available as an enanthate preparation, but this formulation is less frequently used because of its shorter duration and slower onset of action. All patients should take a trial dose of oral fluphenazine before being started on depot preparations.

c. **Piperidine, e.g., thioridazine, mesoridazine (Serentil)**

i. **Thioridazine**—the more commonly used of these two piperidines. It has the advantage of producing a low incidence of extrapyramidal symptoms; consequently, concurrent antiparkinsonian medication is rarely needed. Sedation, hypotension, and anticholinergic effects are similar to those of the aliphatics. Thioridazine has significant calcium antagonist channel activity, which is thought to cause inhibition of ejaculation in about 5% of male patients taking the drug, as well as more pronounced EKG changes than other phenothiazines have. In addition to an increased QR interval, thioridazine causes broadened, flattened, or clove T waves. Thioridazine has an absolute upper dosage limit of 800 mg a day. This restriction is based on the finding that pigmentary retinopathy occurs at doses of 1 g a day or over.

ii. **Mesoridazine**—similar to thioridazine in most side effects but does not cause retinal or ejaculatory disturbances. It is approximately 2–3 times as potent as thioridazine.

2. **Thioxanthenes**

a. **Thiothixene (Navane)**—has high extrapyramidal effects, but low sedative and low hypotensive effects. It is similar to trifluoperazine and haloperidol in properties.

b. **Chlorprothixene (Taractan)**—thioxanthene analogue of chlorpromazine, with similar sedative and hypotensive effects, but minimal extrapyramidal symptoms.

3. **Butyrophenones.** **Haloperidol (Haldol)** is rapidly absorbed from the GI tract—the highest plasma level is achieved in 2–5 hours, and the drug is slowly excreted. Half-life is 24–36 hours. IM haloperidol (5–20 mg every 2 hours) is considered by many to be the drug of choice in acutely agitated psychotics because of minimal sedation and hypotension. Extrapyramidal symptoms are common, but there are less anticholinergic and cardiovascular effects, liver damage, ocular damage, blood disorders, and phototoxicity than with chlorpromazine and other antipsychotics. A long-acting depot form is available.

4. **Dihydroindolines.** **Molindone (Moban)**, the only available dihydroindolone, is structurally unrelated to other antipsychotic drugs. It is as effective as other antipsychotic drugs and produces similar adverse effects. Nevertheless, studies suggest that molindone produces a generally lower incidence of anticholinergic effects, orthostatic hypotension, seizures, and weight gain than other antipsychotic agents. Despite this possibly favorable profile, it is not widely used.

5. **Diphenylbutylpiperidines.** **Pimozide (Orap)** is a highly potent and pure dopamine antagonist. It is approved for the treatment of Tourette's disorder, but is equally effective as standard antipsychotic drugs in the treatment of schizophrenia.

Compared with other high-potency compounds, pimozide appears to carry a greater risk of arrhythmias than standard anticonvulsant drugs do. Several reports suggest that pimozide is effective in treating mono-symptomatic hypochondriasis and the delusions of delusional disorder.

J. **Clinical use.** Because of the various adverse effects of antipsychotic drugs, patients usually undergo a complete blood count (CBC) and liver profile at the outset of treatment. An EKG is advised for older patients. In ambulatory patients, it is advisable to initiate antipsychotic drug treatment at low doses (the equivalent of 100 mg a day of chlorpromazine) and titrate the dosage upward as the patient's condition warrants and side effects permit. Two different antipsychotics should not be given concurrently; combined therapy does not enhance drug effectiveness and may increase the risk of side effects.

1. **Absorption.** Certain factors may interfere with the intestinal absorption of antipsychotic drugs and thus decrease the amount of active drug that reaches the CNS. Since absorption is delayed by food and decreased by antacids, patients should receive their medication between meals and about 2 hours after using antacids. Anticholinergic antiparkinsonism drugs also delay gastric emptying, resulting in increased degradation of antipsychotics in the stomach. One of the advantages of injectable forms of antipsychotic drugs is that they tend to provide higher plasma levels than oral preparations.

2. **Administration.** Patients may be given their medication in divided doses early in treatment. After several days, however, plasma levels of the drug become stable, and administration of the total daily dose at bedtime is advisable. Giving medication at bedtime may be necessary if sedating antipsychotic drugs, such as chlorpromazine or thioridazine, are used. One disadvantage of giving the total daily dose at bedtime is the increased risk of orthostatic hypotension if the patient gets out of bed during the night.

Antipsychotic drugs typically take days to weeks to provide maximal therapeutic effect. Improvement usually occurs in the third or fourth week of treatment, assuming doses are adequate. Unless side effects preclude continued use of the drug, a trial period of 6–8 weeks with the proper dosage is advisable.

Some patients react to initial doses of antipsychotic medication with dysphoria, usually leading to noncompliance. Anticholinergic medications are effective in reducing antipsychotic-induced dysphoria and, consequently, in improving compliance.

Because antipsychotic drugs are nonaddicting, some practitioners prefer to prescribe low doses of these compounds instead of antianxiety medications. This practice is not advisable in view of the potentially serious side effects of antipsychotic drug use.

In monitoring a patient's response to treatment, it is helpful to focus on specific target symptoms, such as auditory hallucinations or suspiciousness. Any reduction or lack of improvement in these symptoms can provide a frame of reference for the degree of success of the drug regimen.

TABLE 24–9
**ANTIPSYCHOTIC DRUG INTERACTIONS**

| Drug | Consequence |
| --- | --- |
| Tricyclic antidepressants | Increased concentrations of both |
| Anticholinergics | Anticholinergic toxicity, decreased absorption of antipsychotics |
| Antacids | Decreased absorption of antipsychotics |
| Cimetidine | Decreased absorption of antipsychotics |
| Food | Decreased absorption of antipsychotics |
| Buspirone | Elevation of haloperidol levels |
| Barbiturates | Increased metabolism of antipsychotics, excessive sedation |
| Phenytoin | Decreased phenytoin metabolism |
| Guanethidine | Reduced hypotensive effect |
| Clonidine | Reduced hypotensive effect |
| α-Methyldopa | Reduced hypotensive effect |
| Levodopa | Decreased effects of both |
| Succinylcholine | Prolonged muscle paralysis |
| Monoamine oxidase inhibitors | Hypotension |
| Halothane | Hypotension |
| Alcohol | Potentiation of CNS depression |
| Cigarettes | Decreased plasma levels of antipsychotics |
| Epinephrine | Hypotension |
| Propranolol | Increased plasma concentrations of both |
| Warfarin | Decreased plasma concentrations of warfarin |

Patients who have responded well to a specific drug during earlier treatment should receive the same drug during subsequent psychotic episodes. When a family member has been treated successfully with a specific drug and the patient has never been treated before, it is best to prescribe the same or a similar drug for the patient.

Other factors that influence the selection of a drug include the person's medical status and lifestyle and possible drug interactions (Table 24–9). For example, patients with conduction disturbances of the heart should not be treated with thioridazine because it produces nonspecific EKG changes that may confound the monitoring of the cardiac condition and may increase the risk of arrhythmias (see Table 24–9).

Dosage during the acute phase of a psychotic illness should be higher than maintenance doses. For example, the equivalent of 400 mg of chlorpromazine is considered the average effective dose in the treatment of acute schizophrenia; by comparison, the effective range for prevention of relapse is between 150 and 300 mg. Sometimes it is necessary to exceed the conventional dose by a wide margin, so that the patient receives 1,000 mg or even 1,600 mg of chlorpromazine. However, it is advisable to avoid routine megadoses, and when they are used the reasons should be scrupulously considered and treatment should be conducted in an inpatient setting.

It is always best to use the lowest effective dose, because this reduces the incidence and severity of side effects; however, there is a dose below which the antipsychotic drug does not exhibit clinical efficacy. The use of such homeopathic doses of medication is a disservice to the patient exposed to the risks of drug treatment without the possibility of its benefits.

TABLE 24–10
**OTHER DRUGS USED IN TREATMENT OF PSYCHOSIS**

| | |
|---|---|
| Reserpine | Acts as a presynaptic dopamine depleter. Slow onset, marginal efficacy, and risk of depression and suicide. No longer used in schizophrenia. |
| Lithium | Apart from reducing manic symptoms, lithium also has been reported to be useful in treating refractory schizophrenic patients when given in conjunction with antipsychotic drugs. |
| Carbamazepine | Some patients get worse with antipsychotic drugs. It is thought they may have atypical psychoses that respond to carbamazepine and other anticonvulsants. Manic psychosis also responds to carbamazepine. |
| Benzodiazepines | IM lorazepam is useful for acute agitation with psychosis of uncertain cause. There are reports of adjunctive use of benzodiazepines with antipsychotic drugs, producing an improvement in negative symptoms and reducing required dose levels of antipsychotic. |
| β-Adrenergic blockers | β-Adrenergic blockers may be effective in treating aggressive behavior or rage in schizophrenic patients. |

3. **Compliance.** Long-acting injectable (depot) antipsychotics are effective in preventing psychotic relapse and rehospitalization among schizophrenic patients. Patients who benefit most from long-acting preparations are those who are partially or completely noncompliant in taking medication. Noncompliance is a common problem with oral antipsychotic therapy; 40–50% of schizophrenic outpatients and nearly 40% of day hospital patients fail to take medication as prescribed. The usual dose of the most widely used long-acting antipsychotic, fluphenazine decanoate, is 12.5–50.0 mg every 2 weeks. The use of lower doses, such as 1.25–5.0 mg every 2 weeks, is associated with increased relapse rates. Rates of adverse effects are no higher among patients receiving fluphenazine decanoate than among patients taking standard oral antipsychotics.

Abrupt discontinuation of medication increases the risk of withdrawal symptoms, including sweating, nausea, diarrhea, tremor, restlessness, and insomnia. In differentiating the withdrawal syndrome from a return of psychotic symptoms, it is noted that withdrawal symptoms appear within several days of the last dose, then diminish by the second week, whereas relapse begins after several weeks and becomes progressively more severe.

Some other drugs that are used to treat psychotic conditions are listed in Table 24–10.

K. **Atypical antipsychotic drugs.** Two currently available antipsychotic drugs, clozapine (Clozaril) and risperidone, are considered atypical because they produce little or no extrapyramidal side effects. They also exhibit greater efficacy than standard antipsychotic agents in treating negative symptoms of schizophrenia. Despite these advantages of the atypical drugs, their use is restricted because of cost and, in the case of clozapine, risk of such serious side effects as agranulocytosis and seizures.

1. **Clozapine.** Clozapine differs from all other available antipsychotic drugs, which have their major effects as antagonists of DA receptors, particularly $D_2$ receptors. Clozapine has a high affinity for the serotonin

type 2 (5-hydroxytryptamine [5-HT$_2$]), $\alpha_1$- and $\alpha_1$-adrenergic, cholinergic (muscarinic), and histamine type 1(H$_1$) receptors. Moreover, clozapine's DA type 1 (D$_1$) antagonist activity is much greater than its D$_2$
antagonist activity. Clozapine is more effective in blocking dopaminergic activity in the basal ganglia; that observation may explain the lack
of extrapyramidal adverse effects with clozapine. There is no evidence
that clozapine actually alleviates persistent extrapyramidal symptoms
or reduces symptoms of tardive dyskinesia.

a. **Indications**—the major indication is the treatment of psychotic
   patients, usually affected with schizophrenia, who have not responded
   to traditional antipsychotic drugs or who cannot tolerate the adverse
   effects associated with those drugs. Clozapine has been shown to be
   as effective as standard antipsychotics in both the short-term and the
   long-term management of psychosis. Approximately 30% of patients
   who have not responded to standard antipsychotic treatments do
   respond to clozapine treatment. Low-dose clozapine (25–125 mg a
   day) has recently been used in the treatment of parkinsonism. Clozapine is also more effective than standard antipsychotic drugs in controlling aggressive and violent patients.

b. **Clinical guidelines**—a compliant patient who has been unsuccess-
   fully treated with two or three different antipsychotic drugs from
   different classes in sufficient doses (1,000 mg chlorpromazine equivalents), each for at least 2 months, is probably a candidate for
   treatment with clozapine. Some patients treated with standard antipsychotic drugs have intolerable adverse effects. Those patients are
   also candidates for treatment with clozapine. Clozapine may be
   of particular use in patients with coexisting Parkinson's disease
   and psychosis.

   The patient's preadministration history should include information
   on blood disorders, epilepsy, and any hepatic or renal diseases. Blood
   disorders and epilepsy are contraindications to clozapine therapy.
   Hepatic and renal diseases make it imperative that clozapine be administered at low dosages. Preadministration laboratory examination
   should include an electrocardiogram (EKG); several CBCs with WBCs,
   which can then be averaged; and liver and renal function tests. Clozapine is available in 25 and 100 mg tablets. 1 mg of clozapine is equivalent
   to approximately 2 mg of chlorpromazine. The initial dosage is usually
   25 mg 1 or 2 times daily, which can be raised gradually to 300 mg
   a day divided into 2 or 3 daily doses. The gradual increase in dosage is
   necessitated by the development of hypotension, syncope, and sedation,
   adverse effects to which patients develop tolerance with continued
   treatment. The usual effective treatment range is 400–500 mg a day,
   although dosages up to 600 mg a day are not unusual. After the
   decision to terminate the drug, clozapine treatment should be tapered
   whenever possible to avoid cholinergic rebound symptoms of diaphoresis, flushing, diarrhea, and hyperactivity.

   Weekly WBCs are indicated to monitor the patient for the development of agranulocytosis. Although careful monitoring is expensive,

early identification of agranulocytosis can prevent a fatal outcome. Agranulocytosis is not dose-dependent, and because it is not limited to the early treatment period, ongoing blood monitoring is necessary. If the WBC is less than 3,000 cells per $mm^3$ or the granulocyte count is less than 1,500 per $mm^3$, bone marrow should be aspirated to evaluate hematopoietic activity. Patients with agranulocytosis from clozapine should not be reexposed to the drug. Physicians can monitor the WBC through any laboratory. Proof of monitoring must be presented to the pharmacist weekly in order to obtain medication.

Blood levels of clozapine indicate that therapeutic effects occur when levels are above 350 ng per mL.

c. **Adverse effects**—the feature of clozapine that distinguishes it from standard antipsychotics is the absence of extrapyramidal adverse effects. Clozapine does not cause acute dystonia, parkinsonism, akathisia, rabbit syndrome, or akinesia. It also appears that clozapine does not cause tardive dyskinesia. Clozapine may pass into breast milk.

The two most serious adverse effects associated with clozapine use are agranulocytosis and seizures. Agranulocytosis is defined as a decrease in the number of white blood cells, with a specific decrease in the number of polymorphonuclear leukocytes, and a relative lymphopenia. The erythrocytes and platelet concentrations are unaffected. In the United States, from February 1, 1990 to March 31, 1994, there were 324 reported cases of clozapine-related agranulocytosis, which was 0.4% of treated patients. Of these, 12 patients died. Clozapine is also associated with the development of benign cases of leukocytosis, leukopenia, eosinophilia, and elevated erythrocyte sedimentation rates.

Clozapine is also associated with the development of dosage-dependent seizures. Approximately 14% of patients taking more than 600 mg a day of clozapine, 1.8% of patients taking 300–600 mg a day, and 0.6% of patients taking less than 300 mg a day have seizures. Those percentages are higher than those of standard antipsychotics. If seizures develop in a patient, clozapine should be temporarily stopped. Phenobarbital treatment can be initiated, and clozapine can be restarted at approximately 50% of the previous dosage, then very gradually raised again. Carbamazepine (Tegretol) should not be combined with clozapine because of its association with agranulocytosis.

The most common adverse effects associated with clozapine treatment are sedation, tachycardia, constipation, dizziness, hypotension, hyperthermia, and sialorrhea. Weight gain, fainting spells, myoclonus, periodic catalepsy, GI upset, and anticholinergic side effects have also been reported. The tachycardia is due to vagal inhibition and can be treated with peripherally acting β-adrenergic antagonists, such as atenolol (Tenormin, Tenoretic), although that treatment may aggravate the hypotensive effects of the clozapine. Hyperthermia of 1° to 2°F may develop, causing concern about infection because of agranulocytosis. Clozapine should be withheld in those cases, and, if the WBC is normal, clozapine can be reinstituted more slowly and at a lower dosage.

d. **Drug-drug interactions**—clozapine should not be used with any other drug that is also associated with agranulocytosis. Such drugs include carbamazepine, propylthiouracil, sulfonamides, and captopril (Capoten). CNS depressants, alcohol, or tricyclic antidepressants coadministered with clozapine may increase the risk of seizures, sedation, or cardiac effects. Lithium combined with clozapine may increase the risk of seizures, confusion, and movement disorders. Clozapine and cimetidine (Tagamet) may interact adversely. Concomitant use of clozapine and benzodiazepines is associated with orthostasis and syncope.

2. **Risperidone.** Risperidone is an antipsychotic drug with significant antagonist activity at the 5-HT$_2$ receptor and at the D$_2$ receptor. Research data indicate that it may be more effective than currently available dopamine receptor antagonists at treating both the positive and the negative symptoms of schizophrenia. The available research data also indicate that risperidone is associated with significantly fewer and less severe neurological adverse effects than are typical dopaminergic antagonist drugs.

a. **Clinical guidelines**—clinical trials have shown that risperidone is more effective than a placebo and may be superior to haloperidol in the treatment of schizophrenia and other psychotic disorders. The studies used dosages ranging of 2–16 mg a day of risperidone compared with a placebo and up to 20 mg a day of haloperidol. Dosages of 4, 6, and 8 mg a day of risperidone were the most effective and were reported to be more effective than haloperidol in reducing the negative symptoms of schizophrenia. Dosages of risperidone in that range were also reported to be associated with fewer extrapyramidal side effects than was haloperidol treatment. Additional studies of risperidone have shown that the drug is safe and generally well-tolerated, even with long-term treatment for periods of up to 12 months; longer periods of treatment are also likely to be safe and well-tolerated.

b. **Adverse effects**—at doses under 6 mg, extrapyramidal side-effects of risperidone are very low, but these symptoms increase significantly at higher doses. Some preliminary data suggest that higher doses of risperidone, e.g., 10–16 mg, have an antidyskinetic effect on buccolingual masticatory movements. In clinical trials, risperidone was associated with significantly less need for antiparkinsonian medication than haloperidol use.

In addition to extrapyramidal symptoms, risperidone use may be associated with anxiety, insomnia, somnolence, dizziness, constipation, nausea, dyspepsia, rhinitis, rash, and tachycardia. Dose-related side effects include sedation, fatigue, accommodation disturbances, orthostatic dizziness, palpitations or tachycardia, weight gain, diminished sexual desire, and erectile dysfunction. Rare side effects with long-term use include neuroleptic malignant syndrome, priapism,

TABLE 24–11
**CURRENTLY USED ANTIDEPRESSANT DRUGS**

| Drug/Class | Trade Name | Typical Therapeutic Dosage (mg/day) |
|---|---|---|
| **Tricyclics** | | |
| *Tertiary amines* | | |
| Amitriptyline | (Elavil) | 150–300 |
| Doxepin | (Sinequan) | 150–300 |
| Clomipramine[a] | (Anafranil) | 25–250 |
| Imipramine | (Tofranil) | 150–300 |
| Trimipramine | (Surmontil) | 150–300 |
| *Secondary amines* | | |
| Desipramine | (Norpramin) | 150–300 |
| Nortriptyline | (Pamelor) | 75–150 |
| Protriptyline | (Vivactil) | 15–30 |
| **Tetracyclics** | | |
| *Secondary amines* | | |
| Amoxapine | (Asendin) | 200–300 |
| Maprotiline | (Ludiomil) | 100–225 |
| **Monocyclic** | | |
| Bupropion | (Wellbutrin) | 300–450 |
| **Serotonin-specific reuptake inhibitors** | | |
| Fluoxetine[a] | (Prozac) | 20–60 |
| Sertraline | (Zoloft) | 50–200 |
| Paroxetine | (Paxil) | 20–50 |
| Fluvoxamine[a] | (Luvox) | 50–300 |
| **Serotonin-norepinephrine reuptake inhibitor** | | |
| Venlafaxine | (Effexor) | 75–300 |
| **Phenylpiperazines** | | |
| Trazodone | (Desyrel) | 300–600 |
| Nefazodone | (Serzone) | 300–500 |
| **Monamine oxidase inhibitors** | | |
| Tranylcypromine | (Parnate) | 20–60 |
| Phenelzine | (Nardil) | 30–90 |

[a]Approved for the treatment of obsessive-compulsive disorder.

thrombocytopenic purpura, and seizures in patients with concomitant hyponatremia.

## IV. Antidepressant drugs

**A. General introduction.**    Antidepressants are classified according to their chemical structure or mechanism of action (Table 24–11). Antidepressants produce synaptic changes with short-term administration (Tables 24–12 and 24–13) and changes in receptors with long-term administration (Table 24–14). For example, most antidepressant drugs produce a down-regulation of β-adrenergic and 5-HT$_2$ receptors.

A broad range of structurally diverse compounds produce improvement in depressive disorders. Controlled studies and clinical studies have demonstrated that:

TABLE 24–12
**SYNAPTIC CHANGES ASSOCIATED WITH SHORT-TERM ADMINISTRATION OF ANTIDEPRESSANTS**

Extracellular 5-HT and NE concentration
Rate of serotonergic neuronal firing
Rate of synthesis and release of 5-HT
5-HT turnover

TABLE 24–13
**ACUTE SYNAPTIC EFFECTS POSSIBLY LINKED TO THERAPEUTIC ACTIVITY**

Norepinephrine reuptake blockade
Serotonin reuptake blockade
Dopamine reuptake blockade
Serotonin type 1A receptor agonism
Serotonin type 2 monoamine oxidase
inhibition

TABLE 24–14
**RECEPTOR CHANGES ASSOCIATED WITH LONG-TERM ADMINISTRATION OF ANTIDEPRESSANTS**

β-Adrenergic receptor downregulation
$5\text{-HT}_2$ receptor downregulation
α-Adrenoceptor upregulation
$5\text{-HT}_{1A}$ receptor upregulation

1. Proper use of any antidepressant drug results in clinical improvement in at least 60–70% of depressed patients. By comparison, only 30% of placebo-treated patients improve in the same amount of time.
2. The onset of full antidepressant effects which may take several weeks. There is no reliable way of predicting who will respond to a particular drug or who will tolerate a particular side effect.
3. All antidepressants act on some aspect of the 5-HT or NE systems.
4. Generally, antidepressants have similar efficacy but are distinguished by their safety and side-effect profiles.
5. Many antidepressant side effects may be related to actions on various neurotransmitter systems.

**B. Drug selection.**   Important considerations in choosing an antidepressant drug are its relative sedative effect, anticholinergic effect, effect in seizure threshold, effects on cardiac function, and toxicity in overdose. Some drugs may produce unique side effects and may require special monitoring because of rare but potentially serious adverse reactions.

**C. Clinical use.**   Effective use of antidepressant drugs begins with accurate diagnosis. Diagnosis is important for several reasons. Depression may be mistaken for an anxiety disorder or another condition. Some subtypes, such as atypical depression, may respond better to some drugs. Drug selection involves choosing a drug that presents the fewest risks and best side-effect profile considering a patient's overall medical status. Once depression has been diagnosed and a drug chosen, it is crucial to use adequate doses of medication. In most cases, this involves at least the equivalent of 225 mg a day of imipramine.

There is no objective method of predicting whether a patient will respond more favorably to treatment with one type of drug than to another. The most reliable indication for choice of a specific drug is a history of positive response to that drug. Although not conclusively established as a clinical fact, there is some evidence that some depressive subtypes, such as with atypical features (atypical depression) and with seasonal pattern (seasonal affective disorder [SAD]), may respond better to MAOIs or bupropion (Wellbutrin). In cases of major depression, however, all drugs appear to be equally effective.

After a specific drug has been selected, the physician should have a clear treatment plan involving dosage, duration of the therapeutic trial, and alternative treatment strategies should the initial intervention fail. The physician should also assume an active role in communicating with the patient and family members.

Patients should have realistic expectations about therapeutic and adverse effects. Some depressed patients are reluctant to take medication, particularly if it is their first experience with acute depression. The lag of 2 to 3 weeks in onset of clinical effects, coupled with troublesome side effects, often leads to discouragement and noncompliance. For these reasons, it is helpful to explain the likely time course of improvement, common side effects, and contingency treatments, if necessary. Encouragement and information provided through frequent communication, can increase the likelihood of compliance and optimal therapeutic results.

With the exception of fluoxetine, to which most patients respond to a single fixed 20 mg dose throughout the course of treatment, all antidepressant treatment begins with a low test dose. The purpose of starting at lower doses is to determine drug tolerance and to minimize initial side effects. Dosage can be raised to about half the maximum recommended dose by the end of the first week, e.g., 150 mg of imipramine, 50 mg of nortriptyline. Patients stay on this dose until the end of the second treatment week. If there is no response at this point, the dose should be raised to the upper recommended limit.

Higher dosages, e.g., 300 mg a day of imipramine, are more effective than lower doses. Blood levels are subtherapeutic in up to 50% of patients treated with 200–225 mg a day of imipramine. Lack of clinical response after 4 weeks of treatment is an indication for plasma-level monitoring. Because inadequate dosage is the most common cause of treatment failure, treating physicians should not hesitate to escalate the dosage to the highest tolerated level.

Because of their generally long half-lives, tricyclics can be given in a single bedtime dose.

Most patients who ultimately benefit from antidepressant medication show signs of improvement by the end of the third treatment week. A significant subgroup of patients who are unresponsive after 4 weeks of treatment show a positive response, however, when the antidepressant trial is extended to a sixth week.

1. **Duration of use.**   There is no absolute rule on how long to continue antidepressant drug therapy after an acute depressive episode remits. Continuation therapy prevents relapse during the period of greatest risk

TABLE 24–15
**EVENTS ASSOCIATED WITH ANTIDEPRESSANT DISCONTINUATION**

Continued euthmia
Relapse of depression
Withdrawal syndrome
Conversion from depression to euthymia
Conversion to hypomania
Loss of response to the discontinued antidepressant in subsequent trials

(4–6 months following initial symptomatic recovery). Most experts recommend 6–9 months of therapy. During this period, a full therapeutic dose should be maintained.

The question of long-term maintenance therapy as a means of preventing future depressive episodes remains controversial. Some patients require long-term treatment, but there is little evidence that continuous antidepressant therapy prevents the onset of new episodes. Relapse or recurrence of depressive symptoms in patients treated successfully during an acute episode are about 30% at 1 year, 50% at 2 years, and 70% at 3 years.

2. **Treatment-resistant cases.** Some patients fail to improve even after all appropriate dose and duration criteria have been met. For them, several options are available.

One strategy is to switch to another, chemically unrelated drug. For instance, a patient who has not responded to imipramine might be switched to fluoxetine, trazodone (Desyrel), or one of the MAOIs. Before switching to another drug, however, many psychiatrists prefer to augment the existing drug with a second compound, e.g., lithium, thyroid hormones. Tricyclics also can be combined (with caution) with MAOIs.

When lithium is used in such combination therapy, its dosage is generally 600–900 mg a day, or serum concentrations between 0.6 and 0.8 mg per L. A typical combination of tricyclics with thyroid hormones involves 25–50 m$\mu$ a day of $T_3$ (L-triiodothyrone, liothyronine [Cytomel]) or 100 mg a day of $T_4$ ([L-thyroxine] [Levoxyl, Levothroid, Synthroid]).

In some treatment-refractory cases, psychostimulants, alone or in combination with antidepressants, help alleviate depressive symptoms. Psychostimulants, such as amphetamine (5–20 mg a day), may also be useful in patients who cannot tolerate antidepressant drugs.

An ever-present risk in treating depression with medication is the possibility that the patient will use the drugs to attempt suicide. Many of the antidepressant drugs, particularly the tricyclic and heterocyclic compounds (tetracyclics, trazodone), are lethal in overdose mainly because of their cardiac effects. When the risk of suicide is thought to be high and the patient is unable or unwilling to be hospitalized, SSRIs, venlafaxine, or nefazodone (Serzone) should be prescribed because of their relative safety in overdose.

Several outcomes are possible immediately following antidepressant discontinuation, including relapse, withdrawal, or hypomania (Table 24–15). Some patients, perhaps 10–15%, who discontinue medication after a good therapeutic response relapse after the drug is discontinued.

They often do not respond to the original drug when it is reinstated. Therefore, a patient who is both benefiting from and is tolerating an antidepressant well and who has a history of recurrent depressive episodes should be encouraged to remain on that drug. To avoid the risk of a withdrawal syndrome, when possible, drugs should be discontinued gradually.

**D. Adverse effects.** Available evidence shows that all currently available antidepressants are equally efficacious and possess a similar onset of action. Some, however, are appreciably more toxic when taken in overdose and are more likely to produce side effects. Most side effects are qualitatively similar among the drugs (Tables 24–16 and 24–17) but differ in frequency and severity. Some drugs produce idiosyncratic side effects.

**E. MAOIs.** The MAOIs have been available for several decades, but concern about potential interactions with tyramine-containing food and stimulant drugs have deterred many clinicians from routinely prescribing them. Nevertheless, they are highly effective in treating depression and often benefit patients who have not responded to treatment with other classes of drugs. Use of MAOIs has increased in recent years, mainly because of their effectiveness in treating panic disorder. Studies also suggest that MAOIs are more effective than tricyclics in the treatment of atypical depression, having a more pronounced effect on interpersonal sensitivity to rejection; the overall response rate in patients with atypical depression is 71% with MAOIs, 50% with tricyclics, and 28% with placebo.

The MAOIs currently available in the United States are irreversible and nonspecific inhibitors of both monoamine oxidase type A ($MAO_A$) and type B ($MAO_B$). These enzymes are responsible for degrading NE, 5-HT, and DA. The MAOIs include phenelzine (Nardil) and tranylcypromine (Parnate).

Hypertensive reactions may occur spontaneously but usually result from interactions between an MAOI and tyramine in food or interaction with sympathomimetic drugs. MAOIs should not be given to patients who cannot understand or comply with dietary and medication prescriptions. MAOIs should only be used as drugs of last resort in patients with asthma, who may need treatment with epinephrine during an attack.

MAOIs also may pose problems for patients undergoing procedures that require anesthesia or analgesia. They interact with narcotics to produce a potentially lethal syndrome characterized by agitation, fever, headache, seizures, and coma. They also may cause respiratory depression and coma. Meperidine (Demerol) has been implicated in fatal excitatory reactions. If analgesia is necessary, morphine may be used, but only if the dose is titrated and the patient closely monitored. Local anesthetics containing cocaine and epinephrine should be avoided.

Patients taking MAOIs should be given 50 mg tablets of chlorpromazine in the event that they feel symptoms of an hypertensive crisis. Should this happen, immediate medical attention is warranted.

In cases of MAOI-related emergencies, chlorpromazine, phentolamine (Regitine), or other $\alpha$-blocking agents are effective. Peripheral vasodilators also may prove useful.

TABLE 24–16
## SIDE EFFECTS OF ANTIDEPRESSANTS

*Anticholinergic*
- Dry mouth
- Constipation
- Loss of visual accommodation
- Urinary retention
- Paralytic ileus (absent bowel sounds)
- Precipitation of narrow angle glaucoma
- Memory disturbances
- Central anticholinergic toxicity
  —Confusion
  —Disorientation
  —Delirium
  —Auditory and visual hallucinations
  —Agitation
  —Hyperpyrexia
  —Concommitant anticholinergic symptoms

*Sedative*
- Fatigue
- Decreased energy
- Lassitude
- Hypersomnia

*Cardiovascular[a]*
Effects on heart rate, EKG, rhythm, and contractility
- Palpitations
- Mild tachycardia
- Delayed conduction (like quinidine, may be antiarrhythmic)
  —Prolonged PR, QRS, and QT intervals
  —Flattened T waves
- Clinical significance
  —Depends on underlying condition of cardiovascular system
  —At therapeutic levels, negligible effect on mechanical performance
- Overdose
  —QRS duration greater than 100 msec indicates severe toxicity
  —Aggravation of existing conduction defects
- Special cautions
  —Post-myocardial infarction when atroventricular (A-V) block develops
  —Coadministration of quinidine, lidocaine, phenytoin, thyroid medication

*Orthostatic hypotension*
- About 20% of patients experience up to a 25 mm Hg reduction in systolic pressure
- Clinical predictor: pretreatment change greater than 15 mm Hg
- Greatest risk: elderly and patients with congestive heart failure
- Unrelated to dose or plasma level

*Behavioral effects*
- Mania, excitement, agitation
- Central anticholinergic syndrome
- Nervousness

*Neurological effects*
- Tremor
- Paresthesias
- Peripheral neuropathy
- Parkinson's syndrome (with amoxapine)
- Generalized seizures
- Myoclonus

*Effects on sleep*
- Normalization of depressed sleep
  —REM suppression
  —Increased stage 4
  —Reduced nocturnal awakening
- Interference with sleep
- Night terrors
- Nightmares
- Nocturnal myoclonus

*Sexual disturbances*
- Decreased libido
- Erectile and ejaculation dysfunction

*Miscellaneous*
- Weight gain
- Sweating
- Skin rash
- Flushing
- Agranulocytosis, leukopenia, eosinophilia

*Withdrawal reactions*
- (Occur within first postdrug week, last for several days)
- GI symptoms
- Anxiety
- Agitation
- Shakiness

*Overdose*
- Myoclonic jerks
- Agitation, delirium, coma
- Metabolic acidosis
- Hyperpyrexia, neuromuscular irritability, seizures
- Ophthalmopegia with intact pupillary responses
- Paralytic ileus
- Cardiovascular manifestations (hypotension, QRS prolongation, arrhythmia)
- Respiratory depression

[a]Details of cardiovascular effects of individual antidepressants are listed in Table 24–17.

MAOI therapy should be discontinued 3 weeks prior to elective surgery. A major adverse effect of MAOIs is orthostatic hypotension. By comparison, the hypertensive reaction, which is the result of an interaction with certain foods or drugs, is rare. Almost all patients taking MAOIs experience postural hypotension. Other troublesome side effects include an inability to ejaculate or reach orgasm, paresthesias, anorexia, and pedal edema. Phenelzine use may result in severe weight gain.

Patients already on MAOIs should not be started on another type of antidepressant. Instead, a 2-week interval should separate the last dose of

TABLE 24–17
**CARDIOVASCULAR EFFECTS OF SOME ANTIDEPRESSANTS**

*Standard Tricyclics*
- Increased heart rate
- Slowed conduction as reflected by prolonged PR and QRS intervals
- Orthostatic hypotension a serious problem, particularly in patients with congestive heart failure (left ventricular function impaired)
- Less of a problem with nortriptyline than with other tricyclics

*Amoxapine*
- Slowed conduction at therapeutic dose
- Fatal in overdose because of heart block
- Orthostatic hypotension

*Maprotiline*
- Slowed conduction at therapeutic dose
- Fatalities in overdose due to heart block
- Orthostatic hypotension

*Trazodone*
- No effect on cardiac conduction at therapeutic doses
- No reported fatalities when taken alone in overdose
- Orthostatic hypotension
- Ventricular irritability (questionable)

*Fluoxetine*
- Clinically insignificant decrease in heart rate by 3 beats a minute
- No change in PR and QRS intervals
- One reported fatality when taken alone in overdose
- No known effect in blood pressure or ventricular function
- Minimal anticholinergic, histaminergic, and α-adrenergic effects

*Bupropion*
- Relatively free of cardiac side effects, with minimal effects in cardiac conduction
- No orthostatic hypotension

---

an MAOI and initiation of tricyclic, cyclic, or SSRI therapy. Patients already on a tricyclic can be started on an MAOI; those on fluoxetine should not be switched directly to an MAOI, but should be given a 5-week period without medication.

F. **Tricyclic antidepressants.**    The tricyclic antidepressant imipramine was discovered during clinical testing for antipsychotic drugs. Since then, many structurally related compounds, including tetracyclics, have been developed. The tertiary amines have two methyl groups on the terminal nitrogen atom of the side chain, whereas secondary amines have one methyl group.

The tricyclic and tetracyclic antidepressants inhibit the neuronal reuptake of both NE and 5-HT, thus increasing the amount of these neurotransmitters in the synapse. In general, tertiary amines are more potent blockers of 5-HT reuptake than secondary amines, which are more potent inhibitors of NE reuptake. These agents potently block many receptors, including cholinergic, histaminergic, and $\alpha_1$- and $\alpha_2$-adrenergic receptors.

As a group, the tertiary compounds produce significantly more sedation, dry mouth, constipation, and orthostatic hypotension than do secondary amine tricyclics (nortriptyline [Pamelor], desipramine [Norpramin], and protriptyline [Vivactil]). Although the increased side-effect profile of the tertiary compounds makes them troublesome to use in depression, they are often used for other conditions. Doxepin (Sinequan), trimipramine (Surmontil), and amitriptyline (Elavil), for example, are potent $H_1$- and $H_2$-receptor blockers, making them useful as antipruritic agents and in the treatment of gastric ulcer. They are also used to treat neurologically related pain.

From a clinical perspective, two of the secondary amine tricyclics—nortriptyline and desipramine—are better choices as first-line antidepressants than the tertiary compounds. They are markedly less sedating and have less anticholinergic activity, and are thus better tolerated by patients. Desipramine has the least anticholinergic effect of any tricyclic. Nortriptyline has been reported to produce less orthostatic hypotension in patients with congestive heart failure.

The tricyclics produce a broad spectrum of side effects, which are a frequent source of noncompliance. About one fourth of patients tolerate initial tricyclic therapy poorly.

The most subjectively distressing side effects are autonomic symptoms, such as dry mouth, constipation, and blurred vision; sweating and orthostatic hypotension; and behavioral and CNS symptoms, such as sedation, lethargy, agitation, and tremor. Other adverse effects that cause subjective distress include tachycardia, weight gain, and diminished sexual performance.

In morbidity and mortality, cardiovascular side effects cause the greatest concern. In addition to tachycardia, the tricyclics produce nonspecific ST-T changes, diminished T wave amplitude, increased PR-QT intervals, and prolongation of QRS complex. In fact, tricyclics produce quinidinelike effects and are considered type 1a antiarrhythmic drugs.

Although the cardiac effects of tricyclics present little risk to healthy patients, they can prove dangerous to patients with cardiac disease. The most serious risks are heart block and arrhythmias. It is standard practice to obtain an EKG in all patients before initiating tricyclic therapy.

Other side effects that need to be anticipated because of their potential severity are worsening of glaucoma; seizures; and triggering of mania, delirium, and agitation.

**G. Tetracyclics.**   Two antidepressants that are structurally and pharmacologically similar to the tricyclics are amoxapine (Asendin) and maprotiline (Ludiomil).

   **1. Amoxapine.**   Amoxapine is an analogue of loxapine, a potent antipsychotic drug. Amoxapine has clinically significant dopamine-blocking activity. Each 100 mg of amoxapine is equivalent to about 0.5–1.0 mg of haloperidol in antipsychotic activity. Thus, amoxapine appears to have full activity in depressive and psychotic symptoms. This combined effect can be put to therapeutic use in cases of severe depression involving psychotic symptoms. Amoxapine can obviate the need for a separate antipsychotic and antidepressant.

      Amoxapine has been shown to relieve symptoms rapidly in some patients, often at doses as low as 100 mg a day; the typical therapeutic dose range is 150–200 mg a day. Amoxapine has a short elimination half-life (8 hours) and should be taken in divided doses. Because it also blocks postsynaptic dopamine receptors, amoxapine's side-effect profile is characteristic of antipsychotic drugs; specifically, it can produce akathisia, dystonia, acute dyskinesia, and tardive dyskinesia. The overall incidence of amoxapine-induced extrapyramidal symptoms is low, but physicians should always be alert to their emergence during treatment.

Apart from its antipsychotic activity, amoxapine is similar to the NE-selective drugs, particularly maprotiline and desipramine, in side effects.

**2. Maprotiline (Ludiomil).** Maprotiline is the most selective inhibitor of NE reuptake. It is structurally and pharmacologically similar to desipramine, the second most selective NE blocker. The only significant structural difference between the two compounds is a bridge across the central ring of amoxapine; this molecular alteration accounts for maprotiline's being classified as a tetracyclic.

The major advantage of maprotiline is its mild to moderate degree of sedative and anticholinergic side effects. The most notable drawback of the drug is the increased incidence of seizures associated with its use. This higher incidence of seizures has been reported both at therapeutic doses and in overdose in patients without a history of seizure disorder. The risk of seizures is dose-related, a fact that warrants caution when the upper recommended dose of 225 mg a day is approached or exceeded. Caution should be also used when discontinuing benzodiazepines in patients who are receiving maprotiline, because the seizure threshold may be lowered.

Maprotiline has an elimination half-life of 43 hours. Its long half-life may require an extended period of observation following an overdose.

**H. Serotonin-norepinephrine reuptake inhibitors.** Like the tricyclics, venlafaxine (Effexor) inhibits both 5-HT and NE reuptake. In contrast to the tricyclics, it does not have any significant interactions with adrenergic, muscarinic, histaminergic, or serotonergic receptors. From a clinical perspective, this produces a side-effect profile that is much better tolerated than that of the tricyclics.

The most common side effect of venlafaxine is nausea. It is dose-related and tends to diminish with time. A rare side effect is systemic hypertension. It, too, is dose-related, but it tends to persist. At the lowest recommended starting dose—37.5 mg a day—the rate is 13%. All patients taking venlafaxine should have their blood pressure monitored during the first months of therapy and following dose increases. Blood pressure increases are not late-onset events. They occur early in treatment or follow upward dose adjustments.

The usual starting dose of venlafaxine is 37.5 mg twice a day in divided doses. An important distinction between the SSRIs, which have no clear dose-effect relations, and venlafaxine is that venlafaxine is more effective at higher doses. Nevertheless, most patients respond to a dose of 75 mg a day.

**I. Monocyclics.** Bupropion is a relatively pure NE reuptake inhibitor, with some dopamine reuptake blocking activity.

The side-effect profile of bupropion differs from that of standard antidepressants. A substantial proportion of patients experience some degree of increased restlessness, agitation, anxiety, and insomnia, especially at the start of the treatment (these effects can be treated by sedative-hypnotic drugs). These symptoms are severe enough to require discontinuation of bupropion in only 2% of patients.

The incidence of generalized seizures in patients taking bupropion has been reported to be approximately 0.4%, a rate that may exceed that of other

TABLE 24–18
**SEROTONIN-SPECIFIC REUPTAKE INHIBITORS**

|  | Fluoxetine | Sertraline | Paroxetine | Fluvoxamine |
|---|---|---|---|---|
| Half-life | | | | |
| *Parent* | 4–6 days | 1 day | 1 day | 15.6 hours |
| *Metabolite* | 4–16 days | 2–4 days | — | — |
| Effect of food on absorption | Yes | Yes | No | No |
| Plasma protein binding (%) | 95 | 99 | 95 | 80 |
| Cytochrome P$_{450}$ isoenzyme system inhibition | IID6 | IID6 | IID6 | IIIA4 |
| Available preparations | 10 mg, 20 mg capsules; 20 mg, 15 mg liquid | 50 mg, 100 mg tablets | 20 mg, 30 mg tablets | 50 mg, 100 mg tablets |

antidepressants. Therefore, bupropion is contraindicated in patients with a seizure disorder. Risk of seizure may be minimized if the total daily dosage is under 450 mg a day. Bupropion is available in 75 and 100 mg tablets. The total daily dosage is usually 200–225 mg a day. That dosage may be raised to 300–450 mg a day after 3 weeks. No single dose should exceed 150 mg.

Advantages of bupropion include the fact that it has no clinically significant effects on cardiac conduction or pulse rate and causes no significant orthostatic hypotension. It also produces few anticholinergic side effects, little or no weight gain, little or no daytime drowsiness, and no sexual side effects.

**J. SSRIs.** Since 1989, three SSRIs—fluoxetine, sertraline (Zoloft), and paroxetine (Paxil)—have been introduced for the treatment of depression in the United States, and an additional SSRI, fluvoxamine (Luvox), has been approved for the treatment of obsessive-compulsive disorder (Table 24–18). As a class, the SSRIs share a common mechanism of action of potently inhibiting the reuptake of 5-HT. They also have no significant interactions with adrenergic, histaminergic, muscarinic, or serotonergic receptors. Consequently, SSRIs cause considerably fewer side effects of the kind associated with the tricyclic and tetracyclic drugs, such as anticholinergic effects, weight gain, and sedation. SSRIs also show greater safety when taken in overdose.

SSRIs are widely used for disorders other than depression, most notably obsessive-compulsive disorder and eating disorders. Their broad spectrum of clinical effects reflects the widespread involvement of the 5-HT system in many biological functions.

The SSRIs are halogenated with either fluorine or chlorine, but otherwise are a structurally diverse class of antidepressants with distinct pharmacokinetic profiles.

The side-effect profile of the SSRIs can be considered to be a class effect, although minor between-drug pharmacological differences and patient sensitivities may result in persons experiencing some drugs as more tolerable than others. Commonly noted side effects include anxiety, insomnia, GI symptoms (such as nausea and diarrhea), headache, decreased appetite, and sexual dysfunction (delayed orgasm, decreased libido). Less common adverse effects include lethargy, fatigue, sweating, tremor, and extrapyramidal symptoms. Laboratory testing may reveal hyponatremia, elevated cholesterol, and prolonged bleeding time. Abrupt withdrawal of the SSRIs can result in a withdrawal syndrome.

Dose titration is not commonly required. The usual starting dose is the same as a full therapeutic dosage, except in patients with obsessive-compulsive disorder, anorexia nervosa, and bulimia nervosa, in which the dose may need to be increased. In general, the SSRIs are given once a day, usually in the morning to avoid insomnia.

1. **Fluoxetine.**   Fluoxetine has a half-life of up to 4–6 days and an active metabolite that has a half-life of up to 16 days. The major clinical significance of this long half-life lies in potential pharmacodynamic and pharmacokinetic interactions with other drugs after fluoxetine discontinuation. It is necessary, for example, to wait at least 5 weeks after the last fluoxetine dose before initiating MAOI therapy. The long half-life of fluoxetine, however, minimizes the risk of a withdrawal syndrome when treatment is stopped.

2. **Sertraline.**   Sertraline is the most selective of the SSRIs, although the relevance of this property is not established. Sertraline also possesses some dopamine reuptake blocking activity.

   Sertraline has a half-life of 1 day and a metabolite with some clinical activity that has a 2-day half-life. Compared to paroxetine and fluoxetine, sertraline has a much lower inhibitory effect on the cytochrome $P_{450}IID6$ isoenzyme. It is thus less likely to cause increased plasma levels of drugs that are coadministered with sertraline and also use that metabolic pathway. Some of these drugs include cimetidine, propranolol (Inderal), haloperidol, and phenytoin (Dilantin).

3. **Paroxetine.**   Paroxetine exhibits the greatest potency in 5-HT reuptake inhibition, but is not as selective as sertraline. The clinical significance of these distinctions is not known. Paroxetine has a half-life of 1 day and has no active metabolites.

   Clinical experiences indicate that when paroxetine is discontinued, the dose should be tapered gradually (over 1 month) in order to prevent a withdrawal syndrome.

4. **Fluvoxamine.**   Fluvoxamine is an SSRI that is not markedly different from other drugs of this class but that is approved only for the treatment of obsessive-compulsive disorder by the FDA. This fact has little to do with pharmacology; it mainly reflects marketing considerations. Other SSRIs, such as paroxetine and sertraline, are as effective as fluvoxamine in treating obsessive-compulsive disorder.

   Fluvoxamine has a half-life of about 15 hours, the shortest of the SSRIs. It has no active metabolites. Compared to the other SSRIs, whose plasma protein binding is 95% or higher, fluvoxamine, whose binding is approximately 80%, carries a lower risk of protein displacement drug interactions.

   Because fluvoxamine is a potent inhibitor of the cytochrome $P_{450}IIIA4$ enzyme, it exhibits pharmacokinetic interactions with alprazolam (Xanax), triazolam, terfenadine (Seldane), and astemizole (Hismanal). Increased concentration of terfenadine and astemizole are associated with ventricular tachycardia, and they should not be used in combination with fluvoxamine. In contrast to the other SSRIs, fluvoxamine is not a potent inhibitor of the $P_{450}IID6$ isoenzyme system.

Fluvoxamine should be started at 50 mg a day. The recommended dosage range is 100–300 mg a day. When using dosages above 100 mg a day, they should be divided into two doses.

**K. Phenylpiperazines.** Two phenylpiperazine agents, trazodone and nefazodone, are unique among the antidepressant drugs in that they are potent antagonists of the $5\text{-}HT_2$ receptor. They are, however, different in their profile of side-effects.

**1. Trazodone.** Trazodone is a highly specific 5-HT-reuptake blocker in vitro. Its therapeutic effects are due to its activity as a 5-HT -reuptake inhibitor and a $5\text{-}HT_2$ antagonist.

Cardiovascular effects of trazodone differ from those of the tricyclics. Generally, it produces a low incidence of cardiovascular effects owing to its lack of quinidinelike activity. However, trazodone has been shown to be arrhythmogenic, causing isolated premature ventricular contractions (PVCs), ventricular couplets, and short episodes (3–4 beats) of ventricular tachycardia.

It is suggested that trazodone be taken following a meal or light snack. When taken on an empty stomach, some patients (about 6%) experience dizziness.

Trazodone is safer than tricyclic antidepressants when taken alone in overdose. Taken with other CNS depressants or alcohol, however, the drug may have synergistic effects. It does not cause seizures in overdose.

About 1 in 800 male patients experience abnormal penile erections; most cases resolve spontaneously. If priapism develops, however, the patient should be directed to an emergency room, where intracorporeal epinephrine injections can be administered.

The most common side effects associated with trazodone use are sedation and orthostatic hypotension. Many clinicians use trazodone as a hypnotic agent in patients who fail to respond to benzodiazepines or when there is concern about drug abuse.

Trazodone has also been shown to be effective in treating agitation and aggression associated with organic mental disorders.

**2. Nefazodone.** Although an analogue of trazodone, nefazodone has a distinct combination of pharmacological effects and, as a consequence, a different side-effect profile. Like trazodone, nefazodone is a potent antagonist of postsynaptic $5\text{-}HT_{2A}$ receptors and an inhibitor of presynaptic 5-HT reuptake. Unlike trazodone, it also inhibits presynaptic NE reuptake. Other differences between nefazodone and trazodone include a markedly lower antagonism of $\alpha_1$-adrenergic receptors as well as a lack of affinity for $\alpha_2$- and $\beta$-adrenergic receptors. As a result of these differences, nefazodone is not associated with priapism or significant orthostatic hypotension. The incidence of orthostatic hypotension with nefazodone is under 3%.

As determined in clinical trials, nefazodone appears to produce a comparatively rapid reduction in anxiety symptoms associated with depression as well as early improvement in depression-related insomnia.

In terms of safety and tolerability, nefazodone causes no serious cardiovascular toxicity or EKG abnormalities. A small percentage of patients (under 2%) may develop sinus bradycardia. Nefazodone is not associated with significant weight change and does not cause either orgasmic dysfunction or decreased sexual desire. Even though nefazodone does not directly interact with muscarinic receptors, it is associated with mild anticholinergic side effects.

Nefazodone can inhibit the cytochrome $P_{450}$IIIA4 system and thus can elevate levels of drugs that also use that metabolic pathway. Two drugs that should not be used with nefazodone are terfenadine and astemizole. Plasma levels of the triazolo-benzodiazepines, e.g., alprazolam and triazolam, may also become elevated when coadministered with nefazodone. If benzodiazepines are used, lorazepam, oxazepam, or temazepam will not interact with nefazodone.

Nefazodone should be initiated at a dose of 100 mg twice a day. After 1 week, the dose can be increased to 150 mg twice a day. The therapeutic dose range is 300–600 mg a day and is similar for both young and elderly patients.

## V. Antimanic drugs

**A. Lithium.** Antipsychotic drugs are used in the treatment of mania to achieve rapid symptom control. Electroconvulsive therapy (ECT) can also dramatically improve acute manic symptoms. The mainstay of treatment for mania, however, is lithium. It not only helps to control acute episodes of mania, but it also reduces the risk of relapse. Several anticonvulsants and calcium channel antagonists can serve as alternatives to lithium.

**1. Administration.** Baseline thyroid function test, CBC, electrolytes, and blood urea nitrogen and creatinine (BUN/Cr) are required. If BUN/Cr are abnormal, progress to 2-hour creatinine clearance and then to 24-hour creatinine clearance. Follow with regular serum lithium levels and electrolytes (especially in patients also on diuretics). Monitor thyroid and renal status—lithium can cause renal insufficiency, hypothyroidism, and, rarely, hyperthyroidism.

Renal clearance parallels sodium clearance; sodium depletion can cause toxic lithium levels. The therapeutic index is low. Lithium can cause leukocytosis. Baseline EKG changes may include flattening, isoelectricity, or inversion of T waves. Lithium also has been reported to be arrhythmogenic, as well as causing various conduction defects (it is speculated that lithium substitutes for intracellular potassium). Lithium may have antipsychotic activity; often it is used with antipsychotics for treatment of acute mania with psychotic features; a direct antimanic effect may take up to 10–14 days.

**2. Lithium levels.** Draw a sample 8–12 hours after last dose, usually in the morning after a bedtime dose; one must measure the level at least

2 times a week while stabilizing the patient. Lithium's half-life is 22 hours, and it is excreted in urine (95%).

3. **Therapeutic range.** 0.6–1.2 mEq per L for maintenance; 1.0–1.5 mEq per L for acute mania. (Some patients may respond at lower levels, whereas others may require higher levels—the true therapeutic range may be wider, but a response at a level below 0.4 mEq per L is probably placebo).

B. **Other antimanic drugs.** Major new developments are the apparent usefulness of anticonvulsants and calcium antagonists. The $\alpha_2$-agonist clonidine (Catapres) has also been used.

1. **Anticonvulsants.** In general, anticonvulsants should be considered for use under the following circumstances: (1) inadequate response or intolerance to antipsychotics or lithium, (2) manic symptoms, (3) rapid cycling, (4) electroencephalogram (EEG) abnormalities, and (5) head trauma. The three most commonly used anticonvulsants are carbamazepine (Tegretol), valproate, and clonazepam (Klonopin).

a. **Carbamazepine**—structurally similar to the tricyclic antidepressants; FDA-approved for use in treating complex partial seizures, tonic clonic seizures, and paroxysmal pain syndromes, such as trigeminal neuralgia and phantom limb pain.

   i.   **Psychiatric uses:** (1) acute mania, (2) depression, (3) psychiatric symptoms secondary to seizure disorders, (4) acute exacerbations of schizophrenia (additive benefits with antipsychotics), (5) schizoaffective disorders, and (6) episodic dyscontrol syndromes.

   ii.  **Factors potentially predictive of antimanic response to carbamazepine:** (1) lithium nonresponders, (2) rapid cycling (more than four episodes a year), (3) more severely manic, depressed, anxious, or dysphoric patients, (4) more severely ill patients, (5) schizoaffective or psychotic features, (6) evidence of organic brain damage, and (7) subgroup with primarily manic episodes, no family history, or early onset.

   iii. **Pharmacology**—half-life—initially 3 days—12 hours or less at steady state; peak levels are reached 6 hours after intake.
        Metabolized almost exclusively by the liver (90%) through $P_{450}$ cytochrome system. Starting dose usually is 200 mg 2 times a day—increased by 200 mg every few days as needed.
        Therapeutic level is 8–12 µg/mL.

   iv.  **Drug interactions**
        (a) With all drugs also metabolized by $P_{450}$ system.
        (b) Phenytoin, phenobarbital, theophylline—decrease level of carbamazepine.
        (c) Erythromycin, lithium, verapamil (Calan, Isoptin), isoniazid, diltiazem, propoxyphene, cimetidine—increase level of carbamazepine.
        (d) Carbamazepine—decreases blood levels of clonazepam, haloperidol, tricyclic antidepressants, tetracycline, valproic acid, warfarin (Coumadin), ethosuximide (Zarontin), octa-

calcium phosphates; increases blood levels of clomipramine, digitalis.

v. **Preliminary workup**—physical examination, CBC with differential if WBC is less than 4,000; liver function tests (LFTs); renal function tests; for first month, weekly CBCs; afterwards, every 3 months.

vi. **Contraindications**—WBC is less than 3,000; hematocrit is less than 32%; red blood cells are fewer than 4,000,000/cu mm$^3$; platelets less than 100,000/mm$^3$; hemoglobin less than 11 g per 100 ml.

vii. **Common adverse effects:** (1) mild leukopenia, (2) nausea and vomiting, (3) rash (about 10%), (4) diplopia, (5) sedation, (6) dizziness, and (7) ataxia.

viii. **Rare adverse effects:** (1) Stevens-Johnson syndrome—exfoliative dermatitis, (2) hepatitis, (3) aplastic anemia, (4) agranulocytosis, and (5) thrombocytopenia.

ix. **Other important interactions and adverse effects:** (1) lithium and carbamazepine—neurotoxicity; (2) slows intracardiac conduction and may worsen preexisting cardiac conduction disease; (3) antidiuretic properties—stimulates antidiuretic hormone (ADH) receptor function; (4) suppresses circulating levels of $T_3$ and $T_4$.

b. **Valproate**—FDA approved for treating (1) absence seizures, (2) myoclonic seizures, (3) generalized tonic clonic seizures, and (4) manic episodes.

i. **Uses in psychiatry**—bipolar disorder and schizoaffective disorder.

ii. **Pharmacology**—half-life is about 8 hours; peak levels are reached 1–4 hours after intake; metabolized by liver.

iii. **Dosage**—starting dosage is about 250 mg 2 or 3 times a day; can increase every 2–3 days by 250 mg; usual dose range is 750–3,800 mg; therapeutic level is about 40–150 mg/L.

iv. **Common adverse effects**—nausea (5%), sedation (5%), hand tremor, weight gain; asymptomatic, transient, dose-dependent increase in LFTs.

v. **Rare adverse effects**—fatal hepatitis—showing an unclear relation to hepatic enzymes; seen in children on phenobarbital with mental retardation or seizure disorder; rare decrease in platelets or platelet dysfunction.

c. **Clonazepam**—FDA approved for treatment of (1) akinetic seizures, (2) myoclonic seizures, and (3) atypical absence seizures; also for infantile spasms.

i. **Psychiatric uses:** (1) acute mania—doses of about 2–16 mg a day, (2) panic attacks—doses of 3–6 mg a day, (3) drug withdrawal and detoxification from benzodiazepines, (4) Tourette's disorder, (5) unconfirmed antidepressant effects.

ii. **Mechanism of action**—unknown, but are hypothesized: (1) potentiates 5-HT synthesis, (2) potentiates γ-aminobutyric acid

(GABA)-ergic transmission, and (3) mimics neurotransmitter glycine.

 **iii. Pharmacology**—a 7-nitrobenzodiazepine derivative (in the same class as diazepam); half-life—79 hours; peak levels—1–3 hours after intake.

  Starting doses about 0.5 mg 2 times a day; can increase by 0.5 mg every 3 days to usual maximum of 3–6 mg a day (higher in acute mania); metabolized by the liver.

 **iv. Adverse effects:** (1) ataxia, (2) paradoxical behavior changes including disinhibition, and (3) drowsiness; less common—sexual dysfunction.

**d. Verapamil**

 **i. FDA-approved uses:** (1) angina pectoris, (2) hypertension, and (3) some supraventricular tachyarrhythmias.

 **ii. Nonpsychiatric uses (not FDA approved):** (1) migraines, (2) hypertrophic cardiomyopathies, (3) dysmenorrhea, (4) Raynaud's disease, (5) insulinomas, (6) cerebral vasospasm following intracerebral bleed, and (7) premature labor.

 **iii. Other possible uses in psychiatry**

  **(a) Depression**—no controlled studies.

  **(b) Anxiety**—anecdotal reports.

  **(c) Schizophrenia**—anecdotal reports.

 **iv. Pharmacology**—half-life of 5 hours; peak concentration—1–2 hours after intake; metabolized by liver; need to decrease dose by one-third in patients with liver dysfunction.

 **v. Dosage**—starting dosage is 80 mg 2 times a day. Can increase by 80 mg every other day to range of approximately 320–480 mg (maximum) or until therapeutic benefit is achieved.

 **vi. Adverse effects:** (1) hypotension, (2) bradycardia, (3) dizziness, (4) nausea, and (5) headache.

 **vii. Contraindications:** (1) severe liver dysfunction, (2) systolic blood pressure is less than 90 mm Hg, (3) sick sinus syndrome, and (4) 2°, 3° A-V block.

 **viii. Interactions**—decreased lithium level; studies show that verapamil may be additively cardiotoxic with lithium; increases carbamazepine levels.

## VI. Other drugs

 **A. b-Blockers.** β-Adrenergic receptor antagonists (β-blockers) have had many applications in other medical areas. The different agents have different degrees of action on $β_1$- and $β_2$-adrenergic receptors. They also have different degrees of lipid solubility that affect their centrally mediated effects, as well as side effects (most significantly, depression). Propranolol, the most widely studied β-blocker, blocks both β-1 and β-2 receptors and is highly lipid soluble. Always be cautious in prescribing β-blockers to patients with asthma or cardiac disease.

  **1. Pharmacology.** β-Adrenergic receptor antagonists act as sympatholytic drugs. In the CNS, the locus ceruleus contains the majority of noradrenergic and adrenergic neurons, which project widely throughout the brain. Within the brain, β-adrenergic receptors are located primarily postsynaptically and are blocked by the β-blockers.

2. **FDA-approved indications**
   a. Hypertension.
   b. Angina.
   c. Some tachyarrhythmias.
   d. Symptoms of thyrotoxicosis.
   e. Glaucoma.
   f. Prevention of migraine.

3. **Psychiatric uses (not FDA approved)**
   a. Performance anxiety—stage fright—best effects with peripherally acting (less lipophilic) β-blockers (atenolol [Tenormin], nadolol [Corgard]).
   b. Treatment of lithium-induced tremor.
   c. Neuroleptic-induced akathisia—usual dosages of about 20–80 mg a day of propranolol or equivalent.
   d. Ethanol withdrawal (plus benzodiazepine)—control tremor, improve vital signs.
   e. Impulsive violence in patients with organic mental syndrome.
   f. Generalized anxiety and panic disorders—autonomic symptoms only—dosages of 40–320 mg a day of propranolol or equivalent.

4. **Adverse effects.**   Hypotension, bradycardia, dizziness, depression, fatigue, nausea, and diarrhea.

B. **Clonidine.**   A centrally acting $\alpha_2$-agonist; causes decreased central adrenergic output; used for hypertension.

1. **Possible uses in psychiatry (not FDA approved)**
   a. **Opioid withdrawal**—suppresses autonomic symptoms; not effective in suppressing craving. Useful during withdrawal from methadone. Dosage is 0.1 mg 2 times a day or 3 times a day; taper with completion of withdrawal.
   b. **Tourette's disorder**—characterized by multiple motor and vocal tics developing in childhood. Clonidine—alternative to haloperidol; may take 2–3 months for response; start at 0.5 mg a day.
   c. **Mania**—for patients refractory to conventional treatments; dosage is 0.2–0.4 mg 2 times a day.
   d. **Anxiety disorders**—inconclusive results.
   e. **Neuroleptic-induced akathisia**—dosage is 0.2–0.8 mg a day.

2. **Pharmacology.**   Half-life is 9 hours. The drug is given 2 times a day; peak concentration is reached 1–3 hours after intake. Clonidine is very lipophilic—it readily crosses the blood-brain barrier. 50% is metabolized in liver, 50% is excreted unchanged by kidneys. Slow taper to prevent rebound hypertensive crisis.

3. **Adverse effects.**   Dry mouth, sedation, dizziness, nausea, impotence, fluid retention, synergistic effects with alcohol, vivid dreams and nightmares, insomnia, restlessness, depression, anxiety.

4. **Interactions.**   With tricyclic antidepressants—decreased antihypertensive effect.

## VII. ECT

ECT may be safer than tricyclic antidepressants for some patients. Usually reserved for patients who have failed other therapeutic attempts or for patients who are so acutely dangerous or suicidal that a course of pharmacotherapy might be too slow.

### A. Indications

1. Major depressive disorder (any type).
2. Bipolar disorder—depressed.
3. Bipolar disorder—manic (only after a medication failure or if patient is acutely dangerous).
4. Schizophrenia (this remains controversial)—nonchronic, acute, especially paranoid, catatonic, or with prominent affective symptoms.
5. Pregnancy—ECT often is the treatment of choice in suicidally depressed or psychotic pregnant patients who should not receive psychotropic drugs.

### B. Course.
ECT usually is given 3 times a week. Depressed patients usually require 6–10 treatments. Schizophrenic patients usually require 10–20 treatments. Each patient must be reassessed between treatments, and ECT should be stopped when there is no evidence of additional benefit from continuation.

1. Does not cure any illness but can induce remissions in an acute episode.
2. Should be followed by other treatments, e.g., medications and psychotherapy, after a course of ECT has been completed.
3. Also may be used prophylactically to prevent recurrence.

### C. Adverse effects

1. **Cardiac.**   PVCs (through vagal hyperactivity); sympathetically mediated ventricular arrhythmias; side effects of succinylcholine (Anectine)—hyperkalemia, direct cardiotoxicity of succinylcholine.
2. **Central nervous system.**   Transient memory impairment—retrograde and anterograde (usually resolves in 1–2 weeks); headaches; prolonged seizures (these can be treated initially with an increased dose of anesthetic; if this fails, then treat as if the case were status epilepticus); prolonged memory impairment—usually limited to events around the time of ECT, but may be worse, especially in patients with preexisting cognitive deficits; brain herniation—may occur as a result of increased intracranial pressure from seizures in a patient with an undiagnosed brain tumor.

### D. Medical workup.
CBC, urinalysis, serum chemistry profile, chest x-ray, spinal x-rays (to document preexisting fractures or other abnormalities), EKG, optional computed tomography (CT) scan of the head.

### E. Pertinent history

1. Hypertension—antihypertensive patients may require dosage adjustments to compensate for elevated blood pressure during a seizure. Nitroglycerin or propranolol often is given prophylactically in hypertensive patients.
2. Musculoskeletal injuries—require more muscle relaxants.
3. Taking reserpine or anticholinesterases—must stop for 1 week.
4. Lithium—some reports of increased cognitive impairment in patients treated with ECT while on lithium, so lithium is usually discontinued.

5. Tricyclic antidepressants—usually discontinued because of cardiovascular side effects.
6. Antipsychotics—usually continued because they decrease the seizure threshold and have few complicating effects.
7. MAOIs—no general consensus.
8. Drugs that raise the seizure threshold should be discontinued, e.g., anticonvulsants, benzodiazepines, lidocaine.

## F. Preparing the patient
1. Informed consent.
2. Alternative treatments.
3. Side effects.
4. Convalescent period (usually 1–3 weeks under close supervision until cognitive deficits resolve).

## G. Procedure.
No food after midnight; patient may have a liquid breakfast if ECT is scheduled for the afternoon. The area must be prepared for cardiopulmonary resuscitation and advanced cardiac life support. An anesthesiologist or anesthetist should be present. Someone adept at endotracheal intubation must be present. Requires suction, EKG monitoring, and usually EEG monitoring.

1. **Anticholinergics.** Atropine 0.5 mg IV until pulse increases by 10% (may also give IM a half hour before treatment). Decreases risk of arrhythmias and aspiration.

2. **Anesthesia.** Usually use barbiturates, and dosage should be adjusted to minimum effective amount because higher dosages will increase the seizure threshold and prolong the apneic period. Frequently used are:
   a. Thiopental (Pentothal) 100–300 mg—has longer half-life than methohexital and may cause a desired postictal sedation.
   b. Methohexital (Brevital) 30–160 mg—rapid, less cardiotoxic than thiopental.
   c. Ketamine (Ketalar) can be used if seizures are too brief or if no seizure occurs when device is on maximum setting.

3. **Muscle relaxants**
   a. Succinylcholine (Anectine) 40–80 mg—a competitive muscarinic agonist, which is displaced from the receptor slowly. Causes fasciculations initially and paralysis later. Half-life is increased by some antibiotics, quinidine, lithium, and phenelzine. A tourniquet applied to an extremity can be used to prevent distribution of muscle relaxant and allow the seizure to be observed in that extremity (especially if EEG monitoring is not available).
   b. Curare—a muscarinic antagonist, may be added if the patient complains of muscle pain. Curare will eliminate the fasciculations caused by succinylcholine.

4. **Types of electrical stimuli**
   a. Sine wave—delivers more energy and may cause more neurological and cognitive side effects.
   b. Brief pulse—requires longer duration of stimulation but delivers less actual energy to brain tissue.

TABLE 24–19
**BILATERAL VERSUS UNILATERAL NONDOMINANT**

|  | Bilateral | Unilateral |
|---|---|---|
| Clinical response | Probably equal | |
| Number of treatments needed | Maybe less | Maybe more |
| Amnesia | Greater | Less |
| Persistent cognitive deficits | More likely | Less likely |

## 5. Electrode placement.  See Table 24–19.

a. Bilateral—1–1.5 inches above midpoint between lateral canthus of the eye and upper tragus of the ear (estimate).

b. Nondominant unilateral—same as bilateral for first electrode on nondominant side. Second electrode is placed slightly lateral to vertex, leaving 4–5 inches between electrodes.

> **Note:** Always shave the area, remove debris and skin oil, and use an abrasive to improve skin adhesion. Also check electrode impedance to make sure it is as low as possible before administering stimulus. High impedance will require a larger stimulus and may cause skin burns.

## 6. Administering the stimulus

a. Check vital signs (temperature, cardiac rhythm, blood pressure, pulse).

b. Apply electrodes and make sure treatment bed is not grounded.

c. Clear patient's mouth, remove hearing aids.

d. Begin anesthesia (before muscle relaxants).

e. Muscle relaxants.

f. Ventilation.

g. Apply bite block.

h. Apply electrical stimulus.

i. Induce a seizure lasting 35–80 seconds (if direct EEG monitoring and the tourniquet test are not available, use seizure-induced tachycardia as a rough estimate).

> If three attempts are made during one period of anesthesia without an adequate seizure, stop and try again on the next scheduled day (usually 3 times a week) to avoid side effects of prolonged anesthesia and muscle relaxants.

## 7. Relative contraindications

a. Fever.

b. Significant arrhythmias.

c. Extreme hypertension.

d. Coronary ischemia.

## 8. Monitoring

a. **EKG**—expect sinus tachycardia, increased T wave amplitude during seizure (also increased blood pressure).

b. **EEG**—anesthetic effect (increased amplitude slow and fast waves), epileptic recruiting rhythm, tonic phase (high-frequency polyspike), clonic phase (repetitive polyspike and wave), termination period.

## VIII. Psychosurgery

Neurosurgical intervention to treat severe or incurable mental disorder. Frontothalamic tracts are severed. Reported to be useful in deteriorated schizophrenic patients or intractable obsessive-compulsive disorders. Not a recommended treatment and rarely used in the United States today.

---

*For a more detailed discussion of this topic, see Biological Therapies, Chap 32, pp 1895–2150; Popper CW: Pharmacotherapy, Sec 46.3, p 2418; Shader RI, Kennedy JS: Psychopharmacology, Sec 49.7d, p 2603; Hay DP: Electroconvulsive Therapy, Sec 49.7e, p 2616, in CTP/VI.*

# 25

# Medication-Induced Movement Disorders

## I. General introduction

The antipsychotic drugs are associated with a number of uncomfortable and potentially serious neurological adverse effects. They include (1) neuroleptic-induced parkinsonism, (2) neuroleptic-induced acute dystonia, (3) neuroleptic-induced acute akathisia, (4) neuroleptic-induced tardive dyskinesia, (5) neuroleptic malignant syndrome, and (6) medication-induced postural tremor.

## II. Neuroleptic-induced parkinsonism

**A. Diagnosis, signs, and symptoms.** Symptoms include muscle stiffness (lead-pipe rigidity), cogwheel rigidity, shuffling gait, stooped posture, and drooling. The pill-rolling tremor of idiopathic parkinsonism is rare, but a regular, coarse tremor similar to essential tremor may be present. A focal, perioral tremor, sometimes referred to as **rabbit syndrome,** is another parkinsonian effect seen with antipsychotics, although perioral tremor is more likely than other tremors to occur late in the course of treatment.

**B. Epidemiology.** Parkinsonian adverse effects occur in about 15% of patients who are treated with antipsychotics, usually within 5–90 days of the initiation of treatment. Women are affected about twice as often as men, and the disorder can occur at all ages, although it is most common after age 40.

**C. Etiology.** Caused by blockade of dopaminergic transmission in the nigrostriatal tract. All antipsychotics can cause the symptoms, especially high-potency drugs with low anticholinergic activity, e.g., trifluoperazine (Stelazine). Chlorpromazine (Thorazine) and thioridazine (Mellaril) are not likely to be involved.

**D. Differential diagnosis.** Includes idiopathic parkinsonism, other organic causes of parkinsonism, and depression, which can also be associated with parkinsonian symptoms.

**E. Treatment.** Can be treated with anticholinergic agents, amantadine (Symadine), or diphenhydramine (Benadryl) (Table 25–1). Anticholinergics should be withdrawn after 4–6 weeks to assess whether the patient has developed a tolerance for the parkinsonian effects; about half of patients with neuroleptic-induced parkinsonism need continued treatment. Even after the antipsychotics are withdrawn, parkinsonian symptoms may last up to 2 weeks and even up to 3 months in elderly patients. With such patients, the clinician may continue the anticholinergic drug after stopping the antipsychotic until the parkinsonian symptoms have completely resolved.

TABLE 25–1
**DRUG TREATMENT OF EXTRAPYRAMIDAL DISORDERS**

| Generic Name | Trade Name | Usual Daily Dosage | Indications |
|---|---|---|---|
| **Anticholinergic** | | | |
| Benztropine | Cogentin | PO 0.5–2 mg tid; IM or IV 1–2 mg | Acute dystonic reaction, |
| Biperiden | Akineton | PO 2–6 mg tid; IM or IV 2 mg | parkinsonsim, akinesia, |
| Procyclidine | Kemadrin | PO 2.5–5 mg bid–qid | akathisia, rabbit |
| Trihexyphenidyl | Artane, Tremin, Pipanol | PO 2–5 mg tid | syndrome |
| Ethopropazine | Parsidol | PO 50–100 mg bid–qid | |
| Orphenadrine | Norflex, Disipal | PO 50–100 mg bid–qid; IV 60 mg | |
| **Antihistaminergic** | | | |
| Diphenhydramine | Benadryl | PO 25 mg qid; IM or IV 25 mg | Acute dystonic reaction, parkinsonism, akinesia, rabbit syndrome |
| **Dopamine agonists** | | | |
| Amantadine | Symadine | PO 100–200 mg bid | Parkinsonism, akinesia, rabbit syndrome |
| **b-Adrenergic antagonists** | | | |
| Propranolol | Inderal | PO 20–40 mg tid | Akathisia, tremor |
| **a-Adrenergic antagonists** | | | |
| Clonidine | Catapres | PO 0.1 mg tid | Akathisia |
| **Benzodiazepines** | | | |
| Clonazepam | Klonopin | PO 1 mg bid | Akathisia, acute |
| Lorazepam | Ativan | PO 1 mg tid | dystonic reaction |

## III. Neuroleptic-induced acute dystonia

A. **Diagnosis, signs, and symptoms.**    Dystonic movements result from a slow, contained muscular contraction or spasm than can result in an involuntary movement. Dystonia can involve the neck (spasmodic torticollis or retrocollis), the jaw (forced opening resulting in a dislocation of the jaw or trismus), the tongue (protrusions, twisting), and the entire body (opisthotonos). Involvement of the eyes can result in an oculogyric crisis, characterized by the eyes' upward lateral movement. Other dystonias include blepharospasm and glossopharyngeal dystonia, resulting in dysarthria, dysphagia, and even trouble in breathing, which can cause cyanosis. Children are particularly likely to evidence opisthotonos, scoliosis, lordosis, and writing movement. Dystonia can be painful and frightening and often results in noncompliance with the drug treatment regimen.

B. **Epidemiology.**    About one tenth of all patients experience dystonia as an adverse effect of antipsychotics, usually in the first few hours or days of treatment. Dystonia is most common in young men (less than 40 years old) but can occur at any age in either sex.

C. **Etiology.**    Although it is most common with intramuscular (IM) doses of high-potency antipsychotics, dystonia can occur with any antipsychotic. It is least common with thioridazine and is uncommon with risperidone (Risperdal). The mechanism of action is thought to be the dopaminergic hyperactivity in the basal ganglia that occurs when the central nervous system levels of the antipsychotic drug begin to fall between doses.

**D. Differential diagnosis.** Includes seizures and tardive dyskinesia.

**E. Course and prognosis.** Dystonia can fluctuate spontaneously, responding to reassurance and resulting in the clinician's false impression that the movement is hysterical or completely under conscious control.

**F. Treatment.** Prophylaxis with anticholinergics or related drugs (see Table 25–1) usually prevents dystonia, although the risks of prophylactic treatment weigh against that benefit. Treatment with IM anticholinergics or intravenous (IV) or IM diphenhydramine (50 mg) almost always relieves the symptoms. Diazepam (10 mg IV), amobarbital (Amytal), caffeine sodium benzoate, and hypnosis have also been reported to be effective. Although tolerance for the adverse effect usually develops, it is sometimes prudent to change the antipsychotic if the patient is particularly concerned that the reaction may recur.

## IV. Neuroleptic-induced acute akathisia

**A. Diagnosis, signs, and symptoms.** Akathisia is a subjective feeling of muscular discomfort that can cause the patient to be agitated, pace relentlessly, alternately sit and stand in rapid succession, and feel generally dysphoric. The symptoms are primarily motor and cannot be controlled by the patient's will. Akathisia can appear at any time during treatment. Once akathisia is recognized and diagnosed, the antipsychotic dosage should be reduced to the minimal effective level.

**B. Treatment.** Treatment can be attempted with anticholinergics or amantadine, although those drugs are not particularly effective for akathisia. Drugs that may be more effective include propranolol (Inderal) (30–120 mg a day), benzodiazepines, and clonidine (Catapres). In some cases of akathisia, no treatment seems to be effective.

## V. Neuroleptic-induced tardive dyskinesia

**A. Diagnosis, signs, and symptoms.** Tardive dyskinesia is a delayed effect of antipsychotics; it rarely occurs until after 6 months of treatment. The disorder consists of abnormal, involuntary, irregular choreoathetoid movements of the muscles of the head, the limbs, and the trunk. The severity of the movements ranges from minimal—often missed by patients and their families—to grossly incapacitating. Perioral movements are the most common and include darting, twisting, and protruding movements of the tongue; chewing and lateral jaw movements; lip puckering; and facial grimacing. Finger movements and hand clenching are also common. Torticollis, retrocollis, trunk twisting, and pelvic thrusting occur in severe cases. Respiratory dyskinesia has also been reported. Dyskinesia is exacerbated by stress and disappears during sleep.

**B. Epidemiology.** About 10–20% of patients who are treated for more than a year develop tardive dyskinesia. About 15–20% of long-term hospital patients have tardive dyskinesia. Women are more likely to be affected than are men, and patients more than 50 years of age, patients with brain damage, children, and patients with mood disorders are also at high risk.

TABLE 25–2
**ABNORMAL INVOLUNTARY MOVEMENT SCALE (AIMS) EXAMINATION PROCEDURE**

| Patient Identification | Date |
|---|---|

Rated by

Either before or after completing the examination procedure, observe the patient unobtrusively at rest (e.g., in waiting room).

The chair to be used in this examination should be a hard, firm one without arms.

After observing the patient, rate him or her on a scale of 0 (none), 1 (minimal), 2 (mild), 3 (moderate), and 4 (severe) according to the severity of the symptoms.

Ask the patient whether there is anything in his or her mouth (e.g., gum, candy) and, if so, to remove it.

Ask the patient about the *current* condition of his or her teeth. Ask patient if he or she wears dentures. Do teeth or dentures bother patient *now*.

Ask patient whether he or she notices any movement in mouth, face, hands, or feet. If yes, ask patient to describe and indicate to what extent they *currently* bother patient or interfere with his or her activities.

0  1  2  3  4　Have patient sit in chair with hands on knees, legs slightly apart, and feet flat on floor. (Look at entire body for movements while in this position.)

0  1  2  3  4　Ask patient to sit with hands hanging unsupported. If male, between legs, if female and wearing a dress, hanging over knees. (Observe hands and other body areas.)

0  1  2  3  4　Ask patient to open mouth. (Observe tongue at rest within mouth.) Do this twice.

0  1  2  3  4　Ask patient to protrude tongue. (Observe abnormalities of tongue movement.) Do this twice.

0  1  2  3  4　Ask the patient to tap thumb, with each finger, as rapidly as possible for 10 to 15 seconds; separately with right hand then with left hand. (Observe facial and leg movements.)

0  1  2  3  4　Flex and extend patient's left and right arms. (One at a time.)

0  1  2  3  4　Ask patient to stand up. (Observe in profile. Observe all body areas again, hips included.)

0  1  2  3  4　*Ask patient to extend both arms outstretched in front with palms down. (Observe trunk, legs, and mouth.)

0  1  2  3  4　*Have patient walk a few paces, turn and walk back to chair. (Observe hands and gait.) Do this twice.

*Activated movements.

**C. Course and prognosis.** Between 5% and 40% of all cases of tardive dyskinesia eventually remit, and between 50% and 90% of all mild cases remit. However, tardive dyskinesia is less likely to remit in elderly patients than in young patients.

**D. Treatment.** The three basic approaches to tardive dyskinesia are prevention, diagnosis, and management. Prevention is best achieved by using antipsychotic medications only when clearly indicated and in the lowest effective dosages. The new antipsychotics (e.g., risperidone) are associated with less tardive dyskinesia than the old antipsychotics. Patients who are receiving antipsychotics should be examined regularly for the appearance of abnormal movements, preferably by using a standardized rating scale (Table 25–2).

Once tardive dyskinesia is recognized, the clinician should consider reducing the dosage of the antipsychotic or even stopping the medication altogether. Alternatively, the clinician may switch the patient to clozapine or to one of the new dopamine receptor antagonists, such as risperidone. In patients who cannot continue taking any antipsychotic medication, lithium, carbamazepine, or benzodiazepines may effectively reduce both the movement disorder symptoms and the psychotic symptoms.

## VI. Neuroleptic malignant syndrome

**A. Diagnosis, signs, and symptoms.** Neuroleptic malignant syndrome is a life-threatening complication that can occur anytime during the course of antipsychotic treatment. The motor and behavioral symptoms include muscular rigidity and dystonia, akinesia, mutism, obtundation, and agitation. The autonomic symptoms include hyperpyrexia (up to 107°F), sweating, and increased pulse and blood pressure. Laboratory findings include increased white blood cell count, creatinine phosphokinase, liver enzymes, plasma myoglobin, and myoglobinuria, occasionally associated with renal failure.

**B. Epidemiology.** Men are affected more frequently than are women, and young patients are affected more commonly than are elderly patients. The mortality rate can reach 20–30% or even higher when depot antipsychotic medications are involved.

**C. Pathophysiology.** Unknown.

**D. Course and prognosis.** The symptoms usually evolve over 24–72 hours, and the untreated syndrome lasts 10–14 days. The diagnosis is often missed in the early stages, and the withdrawal or agitation may mistakenly be considered to reflect increased psychosis.

**E. Treatment.** The first step in treatment is the immediate discontinuation of antipsychotic drugs; medical support to cool the patient; the monitoring of vital signs, electrolytes, fluid balance, and renal output; and the symptomatic treatment of fevers. Antiparkinsonian medications may reduce some of the muscle rigidity. Dantrolene (Dantrium), a skeletal muscle relaxant (0.8–2.5 mg/kg every 6 hours, up to a total dosage of 10 mg a day), may be useful in the treatment of the disorder. Once the patient can take oral medications, the dantrolene can be given in dosages of 100–200 mg a day. Bromocriptine (20–30 mg a day in four divided doses) or perhaps amantadine can be added to the regimen. Treatment should usually be continued for 5–10 days. When antipsychotic treatment is restarted, the clinician should consider switching to a low-potency drug or to clozapine, although neuroleptic malignant syndrome has also been reported to be associated with clozapine treatment.

## VII. Medication-induced postural tremor

**A. Diagnosis, signs and symptoms.** Tremor is a rhythmical alteration in movement that is usually faster than one beat a second.

**B. Epidemiology.** Typically, tremors decrease during periods of relaxation and sleep and increase with stress or anxiety.

**C. Etiology.** Whereas all the above diagnoses specifically include an association with a neuroleptic, a range of psychiatric medications can produce tremor—most notably lithium (Eskalith), antidepressants, and valproate (Depakene).

**D. Treatment.**
1. The lowest possible dosage of the psychiatric drug should be taken.
2. Patients should minimize their caffeine consumption.

TABLE 25-3
**DRUG-INDUCED CENTRAL HYPERTHERMIC SYNDROMES[a]**

| Condition (and Mechanism) | Common Drug Causes | Frequent Symptoms | Possible Treatment[b] | Clinical Course |
|---|---|---|---|---|
| **Hyperthermia** (↓ heat dissipation) (↑ heat production) | Atropine, lidocaine, meperidine NSAID toxicity, pheochromocytoma, thyrotoxicosis | Hyperthermia, diaphoresis, malaise | Acetaminophen per rectum (325 mg every 4 hours), diazepam oral or per rectum (5 mg every 8 hours) for febrile seizures | Benign, febrile, seizures in children |
| **Malignant hyperthermia** (↑ heat production) | NMJ blockers (succinylcholine), halothane (1:50,000) | Hyperthermia, **muscle rigidity, arrhythmias,** ischemic[c], hypotension, **rhabdomyolysis;** disseminated intravascular coagulation | Dantrolene sodium (1–2 mg/kg/min IV infusion)[d] | Familial, 10% mortality if untreated |
| **Tricyclic overdose** (↑ heat production) | Tricyclic antidepressants, cocaine | Hyperthermia, confusion, visual hallucinations, agitation, **hyperreflexia, muscle relaxation, anticholinergic effects** (dry skin, pupil dilation), arrhythmias | **Sodium bicarbonate** (1 mEq/kg IV bolus) if arrhythmias are present, physostigmine (1–3 mg IV) with cardiac monitoring | Fatalities have occurred if untreated |
| **Autonomic hyperreflexia** (↑ heat production) | CNS stimulants (amphetamines) | Hyperthermia excitement, **hyperreflexia** | Trimethaphan (0.3–7 mg/min IV infusion) | Reversible |
| **Lethal catatonia** (↓ heat dissipation) | Lead poisoning | Hyperthermia, intense anxiety, **destructive behavior, psychosis** | Lorazepam (1–2 mg iv every 4 hours), antipsychotics may be contraindicated | High mortality if untreated |
| **Neuroleptic malignant syndrome** (mixed: hypothalamic, ↓ heat dissipation, ↑ heat production) | Antipsychotics (neuroleptics), α-methyl DO, reserpine | Hyperthermia, **muscle rigidity, diaphoresis (60%), leukocytosis, delirium, rhabdomyolysis,** elevated CPK, autonomic deregulation, **extrapyramidal symptoms** | **Bromocriptine (2–10 mg every 8 hours po or ng tube),** lisuride (0.02–0.1 mg/hour IV infusion), Sinemet (carbidopa: levodopa (25/100) PO every 8 hours), dantrolene sodium (0.3–1 mg/kg IV every 6 hours) | Rapid onset, 20% mortality if untreated |

[a]Boldface indicates features that may be used to distinguish one syndrome from another. NSAID, nonsteroidal anti-inflammatory drugs; MAOI, monoamine oxidase inhibitors; NMJ, neuromuscular junction; CNS, central nervous system; DO, dopamine; CPK, creative phosphokinase; IV, intravenously; PO, orally; NG, nasogastric.
[b]Gastric lavage and supportive measures, including cooling, are required in most cases.
[c]Oxygen consumption increases by 7% for every 1 F up in body temperature.
[d]Has been associated with idiosyncratic hepatocellular injury, as well as severe hypotension in one case.

Table from Theoharides TC, Harris RS, Weckstein D: Neuroleptic . . . . .

3. The psychiatric drug should be taken at bedtime to minimize the amount of daytime tremor.
4. β-Adrenergic receptor antagonists, e.g., propanol (Inderal), can be given to treat drug-induced tremors.

## VIII. Hyperthermic syndromes

All of the medication-induced movement disorders may be associated with hyperthermia. Table 25–3 lists the various conditions associated with hyperthermia.

---

*For a more detailed discussion of this topic, see Wirshing WC: Neuropsychiatric Aspects of Movement Disorders, Sec 2.5, p 220; Schulz SC: Schizophrenia: Somatic Treatment, Sec 14.8, p 987; Grebb JA: Medication-Induced Movement Disorders, Sec 32.2, p 1909; Van Kammen DP, Marder SR: Dopamine Receptor Antagonists; Biological Therapies, Chap 32, pp 1895–2150; Popper CW: Pharmacotherapy, Sec 46.3, p 2418; Shader RI, Kennedy JS: Psychopharmacology, Sec 49.7d, p 2603, in CTP/VI.*

---

# 26
# Legal Issues

## I. General introduction

From a legal perspective, the clinical psychiatrist functions in two distinct contexts: (1) treating the patient and (2) performing certain legal evaluations.

Treating the patient involves a relationship of trust that places specific duties and responsibilities on the psychiatrist, such as the duties to maintain confidentiality and to obtain informed consent.

Legal evaluations include those for involuntary commitment, those related to various types of mental competence, and those in the criminal justice system.

A word of caution: laws and regulations can change rapidly as new legislation is passed or new cases are decided. It is strongly recommended that practitioners seek legal advice when there is uncertainty in psychiatric situations that raise legal issues.

## II. Legal issues in psychiatric practice

### A. Informed consent.
Proper informed consent requires that the patient be informed about the particular treatment, alternative treatments, and their potential risks and benefits; that the patient understands this information; and that the patient freely and knowingly gives consent. The psychiatrist should document the patient's consent, preferably with a signed form.

Exceptions to the rules of informed consent include:

1. **Emergencies.** Usually defined in terms of imminent physical danger to the patient or others.

2. **Therapeutic privilege.** Information that in the opinion of the psychiatrist would harm the patient or be antitherapeutic may be withheld.

### B. Confidentiality.
The therapeutic relationship gives rise to a legal and ethical duty of confidentiality, which requires the physician to hold secret all information given to him or her by a patient. Breach of confidentiality can result in an action for damages for defamation, invasion of privacy, or breach of contract.

Some exceptions to the duty of confidentiality include the requirements to report (1) contagious diseases, (2) gun and knife wounds, and (3) child abuse.

1. **The duty to warn.** The most important exception is the duty to warn, which requires psychotherapists to warn potential victims of their patient's expressed intention to harm the victim (Tarasoff I, 1974). In 1976 the Tarasoff II decision broadened the original ruling by requiring the therapist to take some action in the face of the threat of harm to another (the duty to protect).

2. **Release of information.** A patient must consent to disclosure of information in his or her record before the psychiatrist can release that

information. The actual physical record is the legal property of the psychiatrist or the institution; however, the patient has the legal right to his or her psychiatric records. The psychiatrist may claim therapeutic privilege as noted above, but disclosure must then be made to a representative of the patient, usually the patient's lawyer or advocate, according to the particular law of the state.

3. **Testimonial privilege.**   Protects the patient's right to privacy and belongs to the patient. The psychiatrist may not reveal information about patients against their will.

   Some exceptions to the doctrine of testimonial privilege are (1) hospitalization proceedings, (2) court-ordered examinations (military or civilian), (3) child custody hearings, and (4) malpractice claims.

C. **Laws governing hospitalization.**   1. The power of the state (society) to confine an individual (legally known as commitment) is based on two separate concepts: (1) The police power of the state to protect society for society's benefit. The issue here is the dangerousness of the individual. (2) The *parens patriae* power of the state, in which the needs of the individual are of concern. The issue here is the need for treatment.

   2. **Types of admissions procedures.**   Patients may be admitted to a psychiatric hospital in one of four ways:
      a. **Informal**—entry into and release from the hospital may be requested orally. The patient may leave at any time, even against medical advice.
      b. **Voluntary**—written application for admission with limitations placed on release (to allow for conversion into involuntary admission).
      c. **Involuntary**—if patients are a danger to themselves (suicidal) or to others (homicidal), they may be admitted to the hospital after a friend or relative applies for admission and two physicians confirm the need for hospitalization.
      d. **Emergency**—a temporary form of involuntary commitment for patients who are senile, confused, or unable to make their own decisions. In an emergency admission the patient cannot be hospitalized against his or her will for more than 15 days.

   3. **Criteria for commitment.**   Although specific criteria for commitment under the various categories differ across states, all require mental illness, dangerousness to self or others, need for care and treatment, or lack of judgment to care for themselves.

   4. **Procedural safeguards.**   Specific procedural safeguards for meeting the requirements of due process vary among states. These include (1) application requirements, (2) physician's evaluation, (3) patient's advocate, (4) judicial review, (5) limits on retention, and (6) notice of rights.

   5. **The right to treatment.**   The right of an involuntarily committed patient to active treatment has been enunciated by lower federal courts and enacted in some state statutes.

      The principle case, *Wyatt v. Stickney* (1972–1976), set the pattern of reform by requiring specific changes in the operations of institutions and their programs, including changes in the physical conditions, staffing, and quality of treatment provided.

The 1975 United States Supreme Court case of *Donaldson v. O'Connor* held that an involuntarily committed individual who is not dangerous and who can survive by himself or herself or with help must be released from the hospital.

6. **Right to refuse treatment.** One of the most controversial legal issues in the practice of psychiatry today is the right to refuse treatment. The issue arises when the patient's competence to make the necessary decisions is in question.

   a. **Status of the patient**—only involuntary patients may be treated against their will.

   b. **Who decides?** In the past, the treating psychiatrist had the prerogative simply to order treatment, e.g., medication, in the face of a patient's objection. Subsequently, procedures were developed to obtain a second or third opinion of psychiatrists in the facility (a so-called administrative review). That is still the extent of the process in many states.

7. **Involuntary outpatient commitment.** This procedure, which has been adopted in a number of states, permits the immediate hospitalization of an outpatient who does not comply with medical treatment. As such, it has been found to be a useful adjunct to hospitalization and treatment in the community.

## D. Malpractice

1. **Definition.** Literally denotes bad professional activity. Malpractice can be more broadly defined as occurrences in a professional practice that result in injury to the patient, which are the consequence of the psychiatrist's lack of care or skill. There need not be an intention to hurt the patient.

2. **Four Ds.** Four elements must be proved in a malpractice case:

   a. **Duty**—a standard of care; a requirement to exercise a particular degree of skill and care. The duty is predicated on the existence of a professional, i.e., therapist-patient, relationship. There is no duty to cure. The standard of care is usually a national standard rather than a local one.

   b. **Dereliction**—a failure to exercise this care, i.e., a breach of this duty. Dereliction may be due to carelessness, incompetence, inappropriate treatment, or failure to obtain the proper consent.

   c. **Direct causation**—a direct, or proximate, causal relationship between the dereliction of duty and the damage to the patient. Sometimes phrased as ''but for'' the dereliction of the duty, the damage would not have occurred.

   d. **Damages**—some specific damage or injury to the patient must be proved.

3. **Common causes of malpractice lawsuits in psychiatry**

   a. **Suicide**—the suicide of a psychiatric patient often raises the question of malpractice and is the most common basis of malpractice lawsuits in psychiatry. For that reason, careful documentation of the treatment of a suicidal patient is necessary.

**b. Improper somatic therapy**—the negligent administration of medications or electroconvulsive therapy is the second largest source of malpractice lawsuits in psychiatry. Tardive dyskinesia and fractures are the concerns.

**c. Negligent diagnosis**—although this is a relatively rare basis for a lawsuit, it may be used when there is a failure to properly assess a patient's dangerousness.

**d. Sexual activity with the patient**—an area of increasing concern, it is now a crime in a number of states. Sexual activity with a patient has been deemed unethical in the American Psychiatric Association (APA) ethical annotations and has been found to be a breach of contract as well as malpractice.

**e. Informed consent**—the alleged failure of the psychiatrist to obtain proper informed consent is often the basis of the malpractice lawsuit.

**4. Preventing liability**

a. Clinicians should provide only the care they are qualified to offer.

b. The decision-making process, the clinician's rationale for treatment, and an evaluation of the costs and benefits should all be documented.

c. Consultations help guard against liability because they provide a second opinion and allow the clinician to obtain information about the peer group's standard of practice.

## III. Legal issues in child and adolescent psychiatry

**A. Involuntary commitment of minors.** In a landmark decision, *Parham v. J.R.* (1979), the Supreme Court held that minors may be voluntarily committed to a psychiatric facility by their parents or guardians. The Court said parents should "retain a substantial if not dominant role" in the commitment decision.

However, although minors may be voluntarily committed to a psychiatric facility by their parents or guardians, such civil commitment of juveniles now requires various procedural safeguards. The Supreme Court held that civil commitment of juveniles requires the constitution's safeguards, including the right to counsel.

Once juveniles are committed, housing and treatment must be adequate. The Supreme Court has ruled that inadequate housing or lack of treatment for committed juveniles is unconstitutional.

**B. Consent of minors.** The principles of informed consent apply except that the issue of competence turns on the state's legal definition of minority for the particular issue involved.

An emancipated minor is usually one who is married or financially independent. For particular situations, usually related to contracts, the emancipated minor is treated as an adult.

**C. Custody.** The increasing divorce rate has led to a substantial increase in the number of cases of contested custody.

In cases of disputed custody, the almost universally accepted criterion is "the best interest of the child." In that context, the task of the psychiatrist is to provide an expert opinion and supporting data as to which party will best serve the interests of the child by being granted custody.

The mental disability of a parent can lead to the transfer of custody to the other parent or to a public agency. When the mental disability is chronic and the parent is incapacitated, a procedure for the termination of parental rights may result. That also is the case when evidence of child abuse is pervasive. In the Gault decision (1967), the Supreme Court held that a juvenile also has constitutional rights to due process and procedural safeguards, e.g., counsel, jury, trials.

## IV. Legal issues in psychiatry and civil law

**A. Mental competence.**  Psychiatrists often are called on to give an opinion about a person's psychological capacity or competence to perform certain civil, legal functions, e.g., to make a will, to manage one's financial affairs.

Competence is context related, i.e., the ability to perform a certain function for a particular legal purpose. It is especially important to emphasize that incompetence in one area does not imply incompetence in any or all other areas.

**B. Contracts.**  When a party to an otherwise legal contract is seriously mentally ill when the contract is made and the condition directly and adversely affects the person's ability to understand what he or she is doing (called "contractual capacity"), the law may void the contract.

The psychiatrist must evaluate the condition of the party seeking to void the contract at the time that the contract was supposedly entered into. The psychiatrist must then render an opinion as to whether the psychological condition of the party caused an incapacity to understand the important aspects or ramifications of the contract.

**C. Wills.**  The criteria concerning wills, called "testamentary capacity," are whether, when the will was made, the testator was capable of knowing without prompting (1) the nature of the act, (2) the nature and extent of his or her property, and (3) the natural objects of his or her bounty and their claims on him or her, e.g., heirs, relatives, family members.

The mental health of the testator also will indicate whether he or she was in such a condition as to be subject to undue influence.

**D. Marriage.**  A marriage may be void or voidable if one of the parties was incapacitated because of mental illness such that he or she could not reasonably understand the nature and consequences of the transaction, i.e., consent.

**E. Guardianship.**  Guardianship involves a court proceeding for the appointment of a guardian if there is a formal adjudication of incompetence. The criterion is whether, by reason of mental illness, the person can manage his or her affairs.

## V. Legal issues in psychiatry and the criminal law

**A. Competence to stand trial.**  At any point in the criminal justice process, the psychiatrist may be called on to assess a defendant's present competence to be arraigned, be tried, take a plea, be sentenced, or be executed. The criteria for competence to be tried are whether in the presence of a mental disorder the defendant (1) understands the charges against him or her and (2) can assist in his or her defense.

The Supreme Court has set out a number of further standards. In the case of *Dusky v. U.S.* (1960), the court held that the criteria for competence to stand trial require more than a mere orientation and some recall of the event. The defendant must be able to consult with his or her lawyer "with a reasonable degree of rational understanding" and have a "rational as well as factual understanding of the proceedings against him." In *Pate v. Robinson* (1966), the court held that the psychiatric examination for competence to stand trial is a constitutional right. Finally, in *Jackson v. Indiana* (1972), the court held that a permanently incompetent person (in that case, a mentally retarded, deaf, and mute person) must be discharged from the criminal justice system.

**B. Criminal responsibility (the insanity defense).**   The legal issues of competence to stand trial and criminal responsibility (the insanity defense) are different in a number of respects and must not be confused. In contrast to competence to stand trial, the question of criminal responsibility involves a time in the past during which the criminal act was committed. The outcomes are different: finding of incompetence to stand trial usually only delays the legal proceedings, whereas a successful insanity plea results in exculpation in the form of a verdict of not guilty by reason of insanity. The underlying philosophical principles are different: competence to stand trial involves the integrity of the judicial process, whereas criminal responsibility relates to moral blameworthiness. In contrast to the criteria for competence to stand trial, the criteria for criminal responsibility involve two separate aspects: whether, at the time of the act, as a consequence of mental disorder, the defendant (1) did not know what he or she was doing or that it was wrong (a cognitive test) or (2) could not conform his or her conduct to the requirements of the law (a volitional test).

The most famous set of criteria for the insanity defense were developed by the House of Lords after the defendant was exculpated in the M'Naghten case (England, 1843). The M'Naghten rule states that the defendant is to be acquitted if "at the time of the committing of the act, the party accused was laboring under such a defect of reason, from disease of the mind, as not to know the nature and quality of the act he was doing, or, if he did know it, that he did not know he was doing what was wrong." The M'Naghten rule, therefore, is a cognitive test.

The American Law Institute (ALI) incorporates both a cognitive and a volitional test in its model penal code. The ALI rule has been adopted in a substantial number of states. The criteria for legal insanity set out in the rule is that "a person is not responsible for criminal conduct if at the time of such conduct he lacks substantial capacity either to appreciate the criminality (wrongfulness) of his conduct [the cognitive prong] or to conform his conduct to the requirements of the law [the volitional prong]."

To prevent the inclusion of antisocial personality disorder, the ALI rule adds, "As used in this article, the terms, 'mental disease or defect' do not include an abnormality manifested only by repeated criminal or otherwise antisocial conduct."

The ALI rule was used in the John Hinckley case (1983). Hinckley's acquittal raised a storm of protest. It seemed clear that the jury had decided that although Hinckley knew what he was doing when he attempted to murder President Ronald Reagan, he could not control himself, so they acquitted him by means of the volitional prong of the test. In response to powerful political demands, both the APA and the American Bar Association recommended a return to the M'Naghten rule, i.e., the cognitive test only. The American Medical Association went so far as to recommend abolishing the insanity defense altogether.

## VI. Conclusion

Implicit in this brief summary of the legal issues in the practice of psychiatry is that such matters require care and caution. Again, when there is any doubt, seek a consultation.

---

*For more detailed discussion of this topic, see Leong GB, Eth S: Medical-Legal Issues, Sec 49.8b, p 2642; Ross JW, Halpern J: Ethical Issues, Sec 49.8c, p 2648; Forensic Psychiatry, Chap 52, pp 2747–2776, in CTP/IV.*

# 27

## Laboratory Tests in Psychiatry

### I. General introduction

No psychiatric diagnosis can be based exclusively on a laboratory test. Laboratory tests are used to (1) screen for medical illnesses, (2) help with diagnosis, (3) determine whether a treatment can be given, and (4) evaluate the toxic and therapeutic effects of a treatment.

Occult medical problems may present initially as psychiatric syndromes. For example, thyroid disease and other endocrinopathies may present as a mood or psychotic disorder; cancer may present as depression; and infection and connective tissue diseases may present as acute changes in mental status. In addition, a range of organic and neurological conditions, e.g., multiple sclerosis, Parkinson's disease, Alzheimer's disease, Huntington's disease, dementia due to human immunodeficiency virus (HIV) disease, and temporal lobe epilepsy, may present initially to the psychiatrist. Any suspected medical or neurological condition should be thoroughly evaluated with appropriate laboratory tests and consultation.

The initial evaluation must always include a thorough assessment of the prescribed and over-the-counter medications that the patient is taking. Many psychiatric syndromes can be iatrogenically caused by medications, e.g., depression due to antihypertensives, delirium due to anticholinergics, and psychosis due to steroids. Often, if clinically possible, a washout of medications may aid diagnosis.

### II. Screening tests for medical illnesses

See Chapter 3.

**A. Outpatients.** Routine outpatient psychotherapy requires no specific tests, but obtain a thorough medical history and order tests if indicated. Suspected organicity warrants a neurological consultation.

**B. Inpatients.** Rule out organic causes for the psychiatric disorder. A thorough screening battery of laboratory tests given on admission may detect a significant amount of morbidity.

    **1. Routine admission workup**

        a. Complete blood count (CBC) with differential.

        b. Complete blood chemistries (including electrolytes, glucose, calcium, magnesium, hepatic and renal function tests).

        c. Thyroid function tests (TFTs).

        d. Rapid plasma reagin (RPR) or Venereal Disease Research Laboratory (VDRL).

        e. Urinalysis.

        f. Urine toxicology screen.

    g. Electrocardiogram (EKG).

    h. Chest x-ray (for patients over 35).

    i. Plasma levels of any drugs being taken, if appropriate.

## III. Psychiatric drugs

Before prescribing any psychotropic medication, take a detailed medical history, noting a previous response to specific drugs, family response to specific drugs, allergic reactions, renal or hepatic disease, and glaucoma (for any drugs that have anticholinergic activity).

**A. Benzodiazepines.** No special tests are needed before prescribing benzodiazepines, although liver function tests (LFTs) are often useful. These drugs are metabolized in liver by either oxidation or conjugation. Impaired hepatic function will increase the elimination half-life of benzodiazepines that are oxidized, but it will have less effect on benzodiazepines that are conjugated (oxazepam [Serax], lorazepam [Ativan], and temazepam [Restoril]). Benzodiazepines also can precipitate porphyria.

**B. Antipsychotics.** No special tests are needed, although it is good to have baseline LFTs and CBC. Antipsychotics are metabolized primarily in the liver, with metabolites excreted primarily in urine. Many metabolites are active. Peak plasma concentration usually is reached 2–3 hours after an oral dose. Elimination half-life is 12–30 hours, but may be much longer. Steady state requires at least 1 week at a constant dose (months at a constant dose of depot antipsychotics). With the exception of clozapine (Clozaril), all antipsychotics acutely cause elevation in serum prolactin (due to tuberoinfundibular activity). A normal prolactin level often indicates either noncompliance or nonabsorption. Side effects include leukocytosis, leukopenia, impaired platelet functioning, mild anemia (both aplastic and hemolytic), and agranulocytosis. Bone marrow and blood element side effects can occur abruptly even when dosage has remained constant. Low-potency antipsychotics are most likely to cause agranulocytosis, which is the most common bone marrow side effect. They also can cause EKG changes (not as frequently as with tricyclic antidepressants), including prolonged QT interval; flattened, inverted, or bifid T waves; and U waves. Dose-plasma concentration relations differ widely among patients. High plasma concentrations probably offer no clinical benefit and increase the risk of side effects.

Other side effects include hypotension, sedation, lowering of the seizure threshold, anticholinergic effects, tremor, dystonia, cogwheel rigidity, rigidity without cogwheeling, akathisia, akinesia, rabbit syndrome, and tardive dyskinesia.

**C. Cyclic antidepressants.** Baseline EKG and at least annual follow-up EKGs are needed—heart block is a relative contraindication. Baseline LFTs and CBC are useful. TFTs are also necessary because thyroid disease may present as depression. Also, antidepressants can have synergistic effects with thyroxine. Side effects include bone marrow depression; neurological (anticholinergic, in particular), hepatic, gastrointestinal, dermatological, and platelet dysfunction and other blood element side effects; and lowering of the seizure threshold. A common and possibly dangerous side effect is orthostatic hypotension, to which no tolerance develops. Nortriptyline

(Pamelor, Aventyl) is less likely to cause hypotension than imipramine (Tofranil), desipramine (Norpramin), and amitriptyline (Elavil). Congestive heart failure considerably increases the risk of hypotension. Patients with congestive heart failure who develop hypotension from tricyclic antidepressants should be treated with nortriptyline. Toxic EKG changes include prolonged PR interval (> 0.2 sec.), prolonged QRS interval (> 0.12 sec.), prolonged QT interval (> one third of R-R), sinus tachycardia (often due to hypotension), and heart block of all kinds (more likely in patients with preexisting conduction defects—the site of effect is thought to be the intraventricular bundle). At therapeutic levels, tricyclic antidepressants usually suppress arrhythmias, including premature ventricular contractions (PVCs), bigeminy, and ventricular tachycardia (V-tach) by a quinidinelike effect.

Trazodone (Desyrel), an antidepressant unrelated to the cyclic antidepressants, has been reported to cause ventricular arrhythmias, particularly in patients with underlying cardiac disease. Trazodone also has been associated with priapism, mild leukopenia, and neutropenia.

D. **Monoamine oxidase inhibitors (MAOIs).**  Record the normal blood pressure (BP) and follow BP during treatment, because MAOIs can cause hypertensive crisis if a tyramine-restricted diet is not followed. MAOIs also often cause orthostatic hypotension (a direct drug side effect unrelated to diet). Baseline TFTs are recommended. Relatively devoid of other side effects, although some patients may have insomnia or become irritable. May induce mania. A test used both in research and in current clinical practice involves correlating the therapeutic response with the degree of platelet monoamine oxidase inhibition.

E. **Lithium**
   1. Baseline TFTs, CBC, electrolytes, serum blood urea nitrogen and creatinine (BUN/Cr), and white blood cell count (WBC) are required.
   2. If serum BUN/Cr are abnormal, progress to 2-hour creatinine clearance and then to 24-hour creatinine clearance.
   3. Follow with regular serum lithium levels, electrolytes, especially in patients also on diuretics.
   4. Monitor thyroid and renal status—lithium can cause renal insufficiency, hypothyroidism, and rarely hyperthyroidism.
   5. Renal clearance parallels serum sodium ($Na^+$).
   6. Sodium depletion can cause toxic lithium levels.
   7. Low therapeutic index.
   8. Can cause leukocytosis.
   9. Baseline EKG is recommended. Lithium can cause reversible acute EKG changes, specifically flattening, isoelectricity, or inversion of T waves. Lithium also has been reported to be arrhythmogenic as well as causing various conduction defects (there is speculation that lithium substitutes for intracellular potassium).
   10. May have antipsychotic activity.
   11. Often used with antipsychotics for treatment of manic episodes with psychotic features.
   12. Direct antimanic effect may take up to 10–14 days.
   13. Lithium concentrations

a. Draw sample 8–12 hours after last dose, usually in the morning after a bedtime dose.
b. Measure the drug level at least 2 times a week while stabilizing the patient.
c. Half-life = 22 hours, excreted in urine (95%).

14. Therapeutic range
   a. 0.6–1.2 mEq/L for maintenance.
   b. 1,0–1.5 mEq/L for manic episodes. (Some patients may respond at lower levels, others may require higher levels—true therapeutic range may be wider, but a response at a level below 0.4 mEq/L is probably a placebo response).
   c. Toxic reactions may occur with levels over 2.0 mEq/L.

## IV. Laboratory Tests

### A. Dexamethasone suppression test (DST)

#### 1. Procedure
   a. Give dexamethasone, 1 mg orally at 11 PM.
   b. Measure plasma cortisol at 4 PM and 11 PM the next day (may also take 8 PM sample).
   c. Any plasma cortisol level above 5 μg/dL is abnormal (although the normal range should be adjusted according to the local assay so that 95% of normals are within the normal range).
   d. Baseline plasma cortisol level may be helpful.

#### 2. Indications
   a. To help confirm a diagnostic impression of major depressive disorder. If a patient is clinically depressed and has an abnormal DST, somatic treatment is required.
   b. To follow a depressed nonsuppressor through treatment of depression.
   c. To differentiate major depression from minor dysphoria.
   d. There is some evidence that depressed nonsuppressors are more likely to positively respond to treatment with electroconvulsive therapy (ECT) or tricyclic antidepressants.
   e. Proposed utility in predicting outcome of treatment, but DST may normalize before depression resolves.
   f. Proposed utility in predicting relapse in patients who are persistent nonsuppressors or whose DSTs revert to abnormal.
   g. Possible utility in differentiating delusional from nondelusional depression.
   h. Highly abnormal plasma cortisol results (>10 μg/dL) are more significant than mildly elevated levels.
   i. False-positive results—dementia, anorexia nervosa, bulimia nervosa, alcohol or barbiturate use, anticonvulsant treatment (particularly carbamazepine [Tegretol]), tricyclic antidepressant withdrawal, benzodiazepine withdrawal, recent weight loss, acute psychosis, diabetes mellitus, advanced age.
   j. Sensitivity of DST—45% in major depression; 70% in psychotic depressive disorders.
   k. Specificity of DST—90% compared with controls; 77% compared with other psychiatric diagnoses overall.

**B. Thyrotropin-releasing hormone (TRH) stimulation test.** Used to help diagnose hypothyroidism.
  **1. Procedure.**
    a. At 8 AM after an overnight fast, have patient lie down and explain that the patient may feel urge to urinate after the injection.
    b. Measure baseline thyroid-stimulating hormone (TSH) and $T_3$, $T_4$, $T_3$ resin uptake.
    c. Inject 500 μg of TRH intravenously.
    d. Measure TSH at 15, 30, 60, and 90 minutes.
  **2. Indications**
    a. Marginally abnormal thyroid tests or suspicion of subclinical hypothyroidism.
    b. Suspected lithium-induced hypothyroidism.
    c. Detection of patient who may require adjuvant L-triiodothyronine ($T_3$, Cytomel) with tricyclic antidepressant.
    d. Can often detect incipient hypothyroidism, of which depression is often the first symptom.
    e. 8% of all depressed patients have some thyroid disease.
  **3. Results**
    a. If TSH changes by:
      i. More than 35 μIU/mL → positive.
      ii. Between 20 and 35 μIU/mL → early hypothyroidism.
      iii. Less than 7 μIU/mL → blunted (may correlate with diagnosis of depression).
    b. Peak TSH should reach about double the baseline value in normals, i.e., 7–20 μ IU/mL.
    c. Does not distinguish well between hypothalamic and pituitary disease.
**C. Catecholamines**
  1. The amount of the serotonin metabolite 5-hydroxyindoleacetic acid (5-HIAA) in cerebrospinal fluid is low in some persons who are in a suicidal depression. Low cerebrospinal fluid 5-HIAA is associated with violence in general.
  2. Plasma catecholamines are elevated in pheochromocytoma, which is associated with anxiety, agitation, and hypertension.
  3. Some cases of chronic anxiety may share elevated blood norepinephrine and epinephrine levels. Some depressed patients have a low ratio of urinary norepinephrine to epinephrine.
  4. The norepinephrine metabolite 3-methoxy-4-hydroxyphenylglycol (MHPG) level is decreased in patients with severe depressive disorders, especially in those patients who attempt suicide.
**D. Renal function tests.** Creatinine clearance detects early kidney damage and can be serially monitored to follow the course of renal disease.
  1. Serum BUN/Cr are monitored in patients taking lithium.
  2. If the serum BUN or the creatinine is abnormal, the patient's 2-hour creatinine and ultimately the 24-hour creatinine clearance are tested.
**E. LFTs**
  1. Total and direct bilirubin are elevated in hepatocellular injury and intrahepatic bile stasis, which can occur with phenothiazine or tricyclic medication and with alcohol and other substance abuse.

2. Impaired hepatic function may increase the elimination half-lives of certain drugs, so that the drug may stay in the patient's system longer than it would under normal circumstances.

3. LFTs need to be routinely monitored when using certain drugs, such as carbamazepine (Tegretol) and valproate (Depakene).

## F. Electroencephalography (EEG)

1. First clinical application was by the psychiatrist Hans Berger in 1929.
2. Measures voltages between electrodes placed on skin.
3. Gives gross description of electrical activity of central nervous system (CNS) neurons.
4. Each person's EEG is unique, like a fingerprint.
5. For decades, researchers have attempted to correlate specific psychiatric conditions with characteristic EEG changes but have been unsuccessful.
6. Changes with age.
7. Normal EEG does not rule out seizure disorder or medical disease; yield is higher with sleep-deprived studies and with nasopharyngeal leads.
8. Indications
    a. General cognitive and medical workup; evaluation of delirium and dementia.
    b. Part of routine workup for any first-break psychosis.
    c. Can help diagnose some seizure disorders, e.g., epilepsy.
        i. Grand mal seizures—onset characterized by epileptic recruiting rhythm of rhythmic synchronous high-amplitude spikes between 8 and 12 Hz (cycles per second). After 15–30 seconds, spikes may become grouped and may be separated by slow waves (correlates with clonic phase). Finally, there is a quiescent phase of low-amplitude delta (slow) waves.
        ii. Petit mal seizures—sudden onset of bilaterally synchronous generalized spike and wave pattern with high amplitude and characteristic 3-Hz frequency.
    d. Helpful in diagnosing CNS lesions—space-occupying lesions, vascular lesions, and encephalopathies, among others.
    e. Detecting characteristic changes caused by specific drugs.
    f. EEG is exquisitely sensitive to drug changes.
    g. Diagnosing brain death.
9. EEG waves
    a. Beta 14–30 Hz.
    b. Alpha 8–13 Hz.
    c. Theta 4–7 Hz.
    d. Delta 0.5–3 Hz.

## G. Polysomnography

1. Records EEG during sleep; often used with EKG, electro-oculography (EOG), electromyography (EMG), chest expansion, and recordings of penile tumescence, blood oxygen saturation, body movement, body temperature, galvanic skin response (GSR), and gastric acid levels.
2. Indications—to assist in the diagnosis of
    a. Sleep disorders—insomnias, hypersomnias, parasomnias, sleep apnea, nocturnal myoclonus, and sleep-related bruxism.

b. Childhood sleep-related disorders—enuresis, somnambulism (sleep-walking), and sleep terror disorder (pavor nocturnus).

c. Other conditions—impotence, seizure disorders, migraine and other vascular headaches, substance abuse, gastroesophageal reflux, and major depressive disorder.

d. Comments:

  i. Rapid eye movement (REM) latency correlates with major depressive disorder, with the degree of decreased REM latency correlating with degree of depression.

  ii. Shortened REM latency as a diagnostic test for major depressive disorder seems to be slightly more sensitive than DST.

  iii. Use with DST or TRH stimulation test can improve sensitivity. Preliminary data indicate that depressed DST nonsuppressors are extremely likely to have shortened REM latency.

3. Polysomnographic findings in major depressive disorder

a. Most depressed patients (80–85%) show hyposomnia.

b. Depressed patients have decreased slow wave (delta wave) sleep and shorter sleep stages 3 and 4.

c. Depressed patients have a shortened time between onset of sleep and onset of the first REM period (REM latency).

d. Depressed patients have a greater percentage of their REM sleep early in the night (the opposite is true for nondepressed controls).

e. Depressed patients have been found to have more REMs over the entire night (REM density) than nondepressed controls do.

## H. Provocation of panic attacks with sodium lactate

### 1. Indications

a. Possible diagnosis of panic disorder.

b. Lactate-provoked panic confirms presence of panic attacks.

c. Up to 72% of panic patients will have a lactate-provoked attack.

d. Has been used to induce flashbacks in patients with posttraumatic stress disorder.

### 2. Procedure. Infuse 0.5 M racemic sodium lactate (total 10 mL/kg of body weight) over a 20-minute period or until panic occurs.

### 3. Physiological changes from lactate infusion. Include hemodilution, metabolic alkalosis (metabolized to bicarbonate), hypocalcemia (Ca bound to lactate), and hypophosphatemia (due to increased glomerular filtration rate [GFR]).

### 4. Comments

a. Effect is a direct, peripheral response to lactate or its metabolism.

b. Simple hyperventilation has not been as sensitive in inducing panic attacks.

c. Lactate-induced panic is not blocked by peripheral β-blockers, but is inhibited by alprazolam (Xanax) and by tricyclic antidepressants.

d. $CO_2$ inhalation precipitates panic attacks, but the mechanism is thought to be central and related to CNS concentrations of $CO_2$, possibly as a locus ceruleus stimulant ($CO_2$ crosses blood-brain barrier [BBB], whereas bicarbonate does not).

e. Lactate crosses BBB via an easily saturated active transport system.

f. L-Lactate is metabolized to pyruvate.

**I. Drug-assisted interview.** Common use of amobarbital (Amytal)—a medium half-life barbiturate with a half-life of 8–42 hours—led to popular name of "Amytal interview."

**1. Diagnostic indications.** Catatonia; supposed conversion disorder; unexplained muteness; differentiating functional and organic stupors (organic conditions should worsen, and functional conditions should improve because of decreased anxiety).

**2. Therapeutic indications.** As an interview aid for disorders of repression and dissociation.

a. Abreaction of posttraumatic stress disorder.

b. Recovery of memory in dissociative amnesia and fugue.

c. Recovery of function in conversion disorder.

**3. Procedure**

a. Have patient recline in an environment in which cardiopulmonary resuscitation is readily available should hypotension or respiratory depression develop.

b. Explain to patient that medication should help him or her to relax and feel like talking.

c. Insert a narrow-bore needle into peripheral vein.

d. Inject 5% solution of sodium amobarbital (500 mg dissolved in 10 mL of sterile water) at a rate no faster than 1 mL/min (50 mg/min).

e. Conduct interview beginning with neutral topics. Often it is helpful to prompt the patient with known facts about his or her life.

f. Continue infusion until either sustained lateral nystagmus or drowsiness is noted.

g. To maintain level of narcosis, continue infusion at a rate of 0.5–1.0 mL per 5 minutes (25–50 mg per 5 minutes).

h. Have the patient recline for at least 15 minutes after the interview is terminated and until the patient can walk without supervision.

i. Use the same method every time to avoid dosage errors.

**4. Contraindications**

a. Presence of upper respiratory infection or inflammation.

b. Severe hepatic or renal impairment.

c. Hypotension.

d. History of porphyria.

e. Barbiturate addiction.

**J. Tricyclic levels.** Should be routine when using imipramine, desipramine, or nortriptyline in the treatment of depression. Levels must also include measurement of active metabolites:

$$imipramine \rightarrow desipramine$$
$$amitriptyline \rightarrow nortriptyline$$

These assays are difficult to perform and interpret and are measuring extremely low concentrations. Active metabolites could contaminate the results. Reported data have been collected only on inpatients with nondelusional endogenous depression.

1. All tricyclics show complete gastrointestinal absorption, a high degree of tissue and plasma protein binding, a large volume of distribution, hepatic metabolism with prominent first-pass effect, and a plasma level directly correlated to brain level when at steady-state.

a. Imipramine (Tofranil)
  i. Favorable response correlates linearly with plasma level between 200 and 250 ng/mL.
  ii. Some patients may respond at a lower level.
  iii. At levels above 250 ng/mL, there is no improved favorable response and side effects increase.
b. Nortriptyline (Pamelor)
  i. Therapeutic window (therapeutic range) is between 50 and 150 ng/mL.
  ii. Response rate decreases at levels over 150 ng/mL.
c. Desipramine (Norpramin)
  i. Levels above 125 ng/mL correlate with a higher percentage of favorable response.
d. Amitriptyline (Elavil)
  i. Different studies show conflicting results.
2. Some patients are unusually poor metabolizers of tricyclic antidepressants and may have levels as high as 2,000 ng/mL while taking normal dosages. These patients may show a favorable response only at these extremely high levels, but must be monitored very closely for cardiac side effects. Patients with levels greater than 1,000 ng/mL are generally at risk for cardiotoxicity. Other patients have been reported with extremely high plasma levels at a normal dose who did not respond until the level was maintained somewhere between the usual therapeutic dose and their extremely high levels.
3. Procedure—draw a blood specimen 10–14 hours after the most recent dose. Usually, this is in the morning after a bedtime dose. The patient must have been on a stable daily dose for at least 5 days. Use an appropriate specimen container.
4. Indications
  a. Routine for patients receiving imipramine, desipramine, or nortriptyline.
  b. Poor response at a normal dose.
  c. High-risk patient for whom you want to maintain the lowest possible therapeutic level.

## K. Antipsychotic levels

1. In general, plasma level does not correlate with clinical response.
2. High plasma levels possibly correlate with toxic side effects (especially with chlorpromazine [Thorazine] and haloperidol [Haldol]).
3. Minimum therapeutic levels may be determined in the future but have been difficult to establish because of wide individual variation.
4. Radioreceptor assays measure serum dopamine blockade activity and can account for active metabolites, but a correlation with brain dopamine blockade is unclear.
5. No known relation between antipsychotic levels and tardive dyskinesia.
6. Conclusions
  a. Generally only useful to detect noncompliance or nonabsorption (but prolactin levels can also help).

TABLE 27-1
**THERAPEUTIC AND TOXIC BLOOD LEVELS**

| Drug | Therapeutic Level | Toxic Level |
|------|-------------------|-------------|
| Amitriptyline | >120 ng/mL | 500 ng/mL |
| Bromide | 20–120 mg/dL | 150 mg/dL |
| Carbamazepine | 8–12 μg/mL | 15 μg/mL |
| Desipramine | >125 ng/mL | 500 ng/mL |
| Imipramine | 200–250 ng/mL | 500 ng/mL |
| Lithium | 0.6–1.5 mEq/L | 2.0 mEq/L |
| Meprobamate | 10–20 μg/mL | 30–70 μg/mL |
| Nortriptyline | 50–150 ng/mL | 500 ng/mL |
| Phenobarbital | 15–30 μg/mL | 40 μg/mL |
| Phenytoin | 10–20 μg/mL | 30 μg/mL |
| Primidone | 5–12 μg/mL | 15 μg/mL |
| Propranolol | 40–85 ng/mL | >200 ng/mL |
| Valproic acid | 50–100 μg/mL | 200 μg/mL |

b. May be useful in identifying the nonresponder. Table 27–1 lists therapeutic and toxic blood levels for various drugs.

## L. Brain imaging

### 1. Computed tomography (CT) scan. (Formerly called computerized axial tomography [CAT] scan.)

a. Clinical indications—dementia or depression, general cognitive and medical workup, and routine workup for any first break psychosis.

b. Research:
   i. Differentiating subtypes of Alzheimer's disease.
   ii. Cerebral atrophy in alcohol abusers.
   iii. Cerebral atrophy in benzodiazepine abusers.
   iv. Cortical and cerebellar atrophy in schizophrenia.
   v. Increased ventricle size in schizophrenia.

### 2. Magnetic resonance imaging (MRI). Formerly called nuclear magnetic resonance.

a. Measures radio frequencies emitted by different elements in the brain following application of an external magnetic field and produces slice images.

b. Measures structure, not function.

c. Technique has been available to other sciences for 30 years.

d. Much higher resolution than CT scan, particularly in gray matter.

e. No radiation is involved; minimal or no risk to patients from strong magnetic fields.

f. Can image deep midline structures well.

g. Does not actually measure tissue density; measures density of particular nucleus being studied.

h. A major problem is the time needed to make a scan (5–40 minutes).

i. May offer information about cell function in the future, but stronger magnetic fields are needed.

j. The ideal technique for evaluating multiple sclerosis and other demyelinating diseases.

### 3. Positron emission tomography (PET) scan

a. Positron emitters, e.g., carbon-11 or fluorine-18, are used to label glucose, amino acids, neurotransmitter precursors, and many other molecules—particularly high-affinity ligands, which are used to measure receptor densities.

b. Can follow the distribution and fate of these molecules.

c. Produces slice images as the CT scan does.

d. Labeled antipsychotics can map out location and density of dopamine receptors.

e. It has been shown that dopamine receptors decrease with age (through PET scans).

f. Can assess regional brain function and blood flow.

g. 2-Deoxyglucose (a glucose analogue) is absorbed into cells as easily as glucose, but is not metabolized. Can be used to measure regional glucose uptake.

h. Measures brain function and physiology.

i. Potential for developing understanding of brain functioning and sites of action of drugs.

j. Research:
   i. Usually compare laterality, antero-posterior gradients, and cortical-subcortical gradients.
   ii. Findings reported in schizophrenia
      (a) Cortical hypofrontality (was also found in depressed patients).
      (b) Steeper subcortical to cortical gradient.
      (c) Decreased uptake in left compared with right cortex.
      (d) Higher activity in left temporal lobe.
      (e) Lower metabolism in left basal ganglia.
      (f) Higher density of dopamine receptors (needs replicated studies).
      (g) Higher increase in metabolism in anterior brain regions in response to unpleasant stimuli, but this finding not specific to patients with schizophrenia.

4. **Brain electrical activity mapping (BEAM)**

a. Topographic imaging of EEG and evoked potentials (EPs).

b. Shows areas of varying electrical activity in the brain through scalp electrodes.

c. New data processing techniques produce new ways of visualizing massive quantities of data produced by EEG and EP.

d. Each point on the map is given a numerical value representing its electrical activity.

e. Each value is computed by linear interpolation among the three nearest electrodes.

f. Some preliminary results show differences in schizophrenic patients. EPs differ spatially and temporally; asymmetric beta wave activity is increased in certain regions; delta wave activity is increased, most prominently in the frontal lobes.

5. **Regional cerebral blood flow (rCBF)**

a. Yields a two-dimensional cortical image, which represents blood flow to different brain areas.

b. Blood flow is believed to correlate directly with neuronal activity.

c. Xenon-133 (low energy γ-ray emitting radioisotope) is inhaled—crosses BBB freely but is inert.

TABLE 27-2
**DRUGS OF ABUSE THAT CAN BE TESTED IN URINE**

| Drug | Length of Time Detected in Urine |
|---|---|
| Alcohol | 7–12 hours |
| Amphetamine | 48 hours |
| Barbiturate | 24 hours (short-acting) |
| | 3 weeks (long-acting) |
| Benzodiazepine | 3 days |
| Cocaine | 6–8 hours (metabolites 2–4 days) |
| Codeine | 48 hours |
| Heroin | 36–72 hours |
| Marijuana (THC) | 3 days–4 weeks (depending on use) |
| Methadone | 3 days |
| Methaqualone | 7 days |
| Morphine | 48–72 hours |
| Phencyclidine (PCP) | 8 days |
| Propoxyphene | 6–48 hours |

    d. Detectors measure rate at which xenon-133 is cleared from specific brain areas and compare to calculated control, yielding a mean transit time for the tracer.
      i.  Gray matter—clears quickly.
      ii.  White matter—clears slowly.
    e. rCBF may have great potential in studying diseases that involve a decrease in the amount of brain tissue, e.g., dementia, ischemia, atrophy.
    f. Highly susceptible to transient artifacts, e.g., anxiety → hyperventilation → low $pCO_2$ → high CBF.
    g. Test is fast, equipment relatively inexpensive.
    h. Low radiation.
    i. Compared with PET, has less spatial resolution but better temporal resolution.
    j. Preliminary data show that schizophrenic patients may have decreased dorsolateral frontal lobe and increased left hemisphere CBF when activated, e.g., when subjected to the Wisconsin Card-Sorting Test.
    k. No differences have been found in resting schizophrenic patients.
    l. Still under development.
  **6. Single photon emission computed tomography (SPECT)**
    a. Adaptation of rCBF techniques to obtain slice tomograms rather than two-dimensional surface images.
    b. Presently can get tomograms at 2, 6, and 10 cm above and parallel to the canthomeatal line.

## V. Other laboratory tests

Drugs of abuse that can be tested in urine are listed in Table 27–2.

Laboratory tests listed in Table 27–3 are applied in clinical and research psychiatry. The reader is directed to a standard textbook of medicine to determine laboratory values. Always know the normal values of the particular laboratory performing the test, because these values vary from one laboratory to another. Two types of measurements currently are in use—the customary and the Système International (SI) units. The latter, now the more commonly accepted, is an

TABLE 27–3
**OTHER LABORATORY TESTS**

| Test | Major Psychiatric Indications | Comments |
|---|---|---|
| Acid phosphatase | Organic workup for cognitive disorders | Increased in prostate cancer, benign prostatic hypertrophy, excessive platelet destruction, bone disease |
| Adrenocorticotropic hormone (ACTH) | Organic workup | Increased in steroid abuse; may be increased in seizures, psychotic disorders, Cushing's disease, and in response to stress<br>Decreased in Addison's disease |
| Alanine aminotransferase (ALT) (formerly called serum glutamic-pyruvic transaminase (SGPT)) | Organic workup | Increased in hepatitis, cirrhosis, liver metastases<br>Decreased in pyridoxine (vitamine B₆) deficiency |
| Albumin | Organic workup | Increased in dehydration<br>Decreased in malnutrition, hepatic failure, burns, multiple myeloma, carcinomas |
| Aldolase | Eating disorders<br>Schizophrenia | Increased in patients who abuse ipecac (e.g., bulimic patients), schizophrenia (60–80%) |
| Alkaline phosphatase | Organic workup<br>Use of psychotropic medications | Increased in Paget's disease, hyperparathyroidism, hepatic disease, hepatic metastases, heart failure, phenothiazine use<br>Decreased in pernicious anemia (Vitamin B₁₂ deficiency) |
| Ammonia, serum | Organic workup | Increased in hepatic encephalopathy |
| Amylase, serum | Eating disorders | May be increased in bulimia nervosa |
| Antinuclear antibodies | Organic workup | Found in systemic lupus erythematosus (SLE) and drug-induced lupus (e.g., secondary to phenothiazines, anticonvulsants); SLE can be associated with delirium, psychotic disorders, mood disorders |
| Aspartate aminotransferase (AST) (formerly SGOT) | Organic workup | Increased in heart failure, hepatic disease, pancreatitis, eclampsia, cerebral damage, alcohol dependence<br>Decreased in pyridoxine (vitamin B₆) deficiency, terminal stages of liver disease |
| Bicarbonate, serum | Panic disorder<br>Eating disorders | Decreased in hyperventilation syndrome, panic disorder, anabolic steroid abuse<br>May be elevated in patients with bulimia nervosa, in laxative abuse, in psychogenic vomiting |
| Bilirubin | Organic workup | Increased in hepatic disease |

*(continued on next page)*

TABLE 27–3 (continued)
**OTHER LABORATORY TESTS**

| Test | Major Psychiatric Indications | Comments |
|---|---|---|
| Blood urea nitrogen (BUN) | Delirium | Elevated in renal disease, dehydration |
| | Use of psychotropic medications | Elevations associated with lethargy, delirium |
| | | If elevated, can increase toxic potential of psychiatric medications, especially lithium and amantadine (Symadine) |
| Bromide, serum | Dementia | Bromide intoxication can cause psychosis, hallucinations, delirium |
| | Psychosis | Part of dementia workup, especially when serum chloride is elevated |
| Caffeine level, serum | Anxiety | Evaluation of patients with suspected caffeinism |
| Calcium (Ca), serum | Organic workup | Increased in hyperparathyroidism, bone metastases |
| | Mood disorders | Increase associated with delirium, depression, psychosis |
| | Psychosis | Decreased in hypoparathyroidism, renal failure |
| | Eating disorders | Decrease associated with depression, irritability, delirium, long-term laxative abuse |
| Carotid ultrasound | Dementia | Occasionally included in dementia workup, especially to rule out vascular dementia |
| | | Primary value is in search for possible infarct causes |
| Catecholamines, urinary and plasma | Panic attacks | Elevated in pheochromocytoma |
| | Anxiety disorders | |
| Cerebrospinal fluid (CSF) | Organic workup | Increased protein and cells in infection, positive VDRL in neurosyphilis, bloody CSF in hemorrhagic conditions |
| Ceruloplasmin, serum; copper, serum | Organic workup | Low in Wilson's disease (hepatolenticular disease) |
| Chloride (Cl), serum | Eating disorders | Decreased in patients with bulimia nervosa and psychogenic vomiting |
| | Panic disorder | Mild elevation in hyperventilation syndrome, panic disorder |
| Cholecystokinin (CCK) | Eating disorders | Compared with controls, blunted in bulimic patients after eating meal (may normalize after treatment with antidepressants) |
| $CO_2$ inhalation; sodium bicarbonate infusion | Anxiety | Panic attacks produced in subgroup of patients |
| Coombs' test, direct and indirect | Hemolytic anemias secondary to psychotropic medications | Evaluation of drug-induced hemolytic anemias, such as those secondary to chlorpromazine, phenytoin, levodopa, and methyldopa |
| Copper, urine | Organic workup | Elevated in Wilson's disease |

| Test | Association | Description |
|---|---|---|
| Cortisol (hydrocortisone) | Organic workup; Mood disorders | Excessive level may indicate Cushing's disease associated with anxiety, depression, and a variety of other conditions |
| Creatine phosphokinase (CPK) | Use of antipsychotics; Use of restraints; Substance abuse | Increased in neuroleptic malignant syndrome, intramuscular injection, rhabdomyolysis (secondary to substance abuse), patients in restraints, patients experiencing dystonic reactions; asymptomatic elevations seen with use of antipsychotics |
| Creatinine, serum | Organic workup | Elevated in renal disease |
| Dopamine (DA) (L-dopa stimulation of dopamine) | Depression | Inhibits prolactin; Test used to assess functional integrity of dopaminergic system, which is impaired in Parkinson's disease, depression |
| Doppler ultrasound | Impotence; Organic workup | Carotid occlusion, transient ischemic attack (TIA), reduced penile blood flow in impotence |
| Echocardiogram (EKG) | Panic disorder | 10–40% of patients with panic disorder show mitral valve prolapse |
| Electroencephalogram (EEG) | Organic workup | Seizures, brain death, lesions; shortened REM latency in depression; High-voltage activity in stupor; low-voltage fast activity in excitement; in functional nonorganic cases (e.g., dissociative disorders), alpha activity is present in the background, which responds to auditory and visual stimuli; Biphasic or triphasic slow bursts seen in dementia of Creutzfeldt-Jakob disease |
| Epstein-Barr virus (EBV); cytomegalovirus (CMV) | Organic workup; Chronic fatigue; Mood disorders | Part of herpes virus group; EBV is causative agent for infectious mononucleosis, which can present with depression and personality change; CMV can produce anxiety, confusion, mood disorders; EBV associated with chronic mononucleosislike syndrome associated with chronic depression and fatigue; may be association between EBV and major depressive disorder |
| Erythrocyte sedimentation rate (ESR) | Organic workup | An increase in ESR represents a nonspecific test of infectious, inflammatory, autoimmune, or malignant disease; sometimes recommended in the evaluation of anorexia nervosa |

(continued on next page)

TABLE 27–3 *(continued)*
**OTHER LABORATORY TESTS**

| Test | Major Psychiatric Indications | Comments |
|---|---|---|
| Estrogen | Mood disorder | Decreased in menopausal depression and premenstrual syndrome; variable changes in anxiety |
| Ferritin, serum | Organic workup | Most sensitive test for iron deficiency |
| Folate (folic acid), serum | Alcohol abuse<br>Use of specific medications | Usually measured with vitamin $B_{12}$ deficiencies associated with psychotic disorders, paranoia, fatigue, agitation, dementia, delirium<br>Associated with alcohol dependence, use of phenytoin, oral contraceptives, estrogen |
| Follicle-stimulating hormone (FSH) | Depression | High normal in anorexia nervosa, higher values in postmenopausal women; low levels in patients with panhypopituitarism |
| Glucose, fasting blood (FBS) | Panic attacks<br>Anxiety<br>Delirium<br>Depression | Very high FBS associated with delirium<br>Very low FBS associated with delirium, agitation, panic attacks, anxiety, depression |
| Glutamyl transaminase, serum | Alcohol abuse<br>Organic workup | Increase in alcohol abuse, cirrhosis, liver disease |
| Gonadotropin-releasing hormone (GnRH) | Depression<br>Anxiety<br>Schizophrenia | Decrease in schizophrenia; increase in anorexia nervosa; variable in depression, anxiety |
| Growth hormone (GH) | Depression<br>Schizophrenia | Blunted GH responses to insulin-induced hypoglycemia in depressed patients; increased GH responses to dopamine agonist challenge in schizophrenic patients; increased in some cases of anorexia nervosa |
| Hematocrit (Hct); hemoglobin (Hb) | Organic workup | Assessment of anemia (anemia may be associated with depressive and psychotic disorders) |
| Hepatitis A viral antigen (HAAg) | Mood disorders<br>Organic workup | Less severe, better prognosis than hepatitis B; may present with anorexia, depression |
| Hepatitis B surface antigen (HBsAg); hepatitis Bc antigen (HBcAg) | Mood disorders<br>Organic workup | Active hepatitis B infection indicates greater degree of infectivity and of progression to chronic liver disease<br>May present with depression |
| Holter monitor | Panic disorder | Evaluation of panic disorder patients with palpitations and other cardiac symptoms |

| | | |
|---|---|---|
| Human immunodeficiency virus (HIV) | Organic workup | CNS involvement: AIDS dementia, personality change due to a general medical condition, mood disorder due to a general medical condition, acute psychotic disorders |
| 17-Hydroxycorticosteroid | Depression | Deviations detect hyperadrenocorticalism, which can be associated with major depressive disorder |
| | | Increased in steroid abuse |
| 5-Hydroxyindoleacetic acid (5-HIAA) | Depression<br>Suicide<br>Violence | Decrease in CSF in aggressive or violent patients with suicidal or homicidal impulses<br>May be indicator of decreased impulse control and predictor of suicide |
| Iron, serum | Organic workup | Iron-deficiency anemia |
| Lactate dehydrogenase (LDH) | Organic workup | Increased in myocardial infarction, pulmonary infarction, hepatic disease, renal infarction, seizures, cerebral damage, megaloblastic (pernicious) anemia, factitious elevations secondary to rough handling of blood specimen tube |
| Lupus anticoagulant (LA) | Use of phenothiazines | An antiphospholipid antibody, which has been described in some patients using phenothiazines, especially chlorpromazine |
| Lupus erythematosus (LE) test | Depression<br>Psychosis<br>Delirium<br>Dementia | Positive test associated with systemic LE, which may present with various psychiatric disturbances, such as psychotic disorders, depressive disorders, delirium, dementia; also tested for with antinuclear antibody (ANA) and anti-DNA antibody tests |
| Luteinizing hormone (LH) | Depression | Low in patients with panhypopituitarism; decrease associated with depression |
| Magnesium, serum | Alcohol abuse<br>Organic workup | Decreased in alcohol dependence; low levels associated with agitation, delirium, seizures |
| MAO, platelet | Depression | Low in depression |
| MCV (mean corpuscular volume) (average volume of a red blood cell) | Alcohol abuse | Elevated in alcohol dependence, vitamin $B_{12}$ folate deficiency |
| Melatonin | Mood disorder with seasonal pattern | Produced by light and pineal gland and decreased in mood disorder with seasonal pattern |

*(continued on next page)*

TABLE 27-3 (continued)
**OTHER LABORATORY TESTS**

| Test | Major Psychiatric Indications | Comments |
|---|---|---|
| Metal (heavy) intoxication (serum or urinary) | Organic workup | Lead—apathy, irritability, anorexia nervosa, confusion Mercury—psychosis, fatigue, apathy, decreased memory, emotional lability, "mad hatter" Manganese—manganese madness, Parkinson-like syndrome Aluminum—dementia Arsenic—fatigue, blackouts, hair loss |
| 3-Methoxy-4-hydroxyphenyglycol (MHPG) | Depression Anxiety | Most useful in research; decreases in urine may indicate decreases centrally |
| Myoglobin, urine | Phenothiazine use Substance abuse Use of restraints | Increased in neuroleptic malignant syndrome; in PCP, cocaine, or lysergic acid diethylamide (LSD) intoxication; in patients in restraints |
| Nicotine | Anxiety Nicotine addiction | Anxiety, smoking |
| Nocturnal penile tumescence | Impotence | Quantification of penile circumference changes, penile rigidity, frequency of penile tumescence Evaluation of erectile function during sleep Erections associated with rapid eye movement (REM) sleep Helpful in differentiation between organic and functional causes of impotence |
| Parathyroid (parathormone) hormone | Anxiety Organic workup | Low level causes hypocalcemia and anxiety Dysregulation associated with wide variety of cognitive disorders |
| Phosphorus, serum | Organic workup Panic disorder | Increased in renal failure, diabetic, acidosis, hypoparathyroidism, hypervitamin D Decreased in cirrhosis, hypokalemia, hyperparathyroidism, panic attack, hyperventilation syndrome |
| Platelet count | Use of psychotropic medications | Decreased by certain psychotropic medications (carbamazepine, clozapine, phenothiazines) |
| Porphobilinogen (PBG) | Organic workup | Increased in acute porphyria |
| Porphyria synthesizing enzyme | Psychosis Organic workup | Acute panic attack or a cognitive disorder can occur in acute porphyria attack, which may be precipitated by barbiturates, imipramine |

| Test | Conditions | Comments |
|---|---|---|
| Potassium (K), serum | Organic workup<br>Eating disorders | Increased in hyperkalemic acidosis; increase is associated with anxiety in cardiac arrhythmia<br>Decreased in cirrhosis, metabolic alkalosis, laxative abuse, diuretic abuse; decrease is common in bulimic patients and in psychogenic vomiting, anabolic steroid abuse |
| Prolactin, serum | Use of antipsychotic medications<br>Cocaine use<br>Pseudoseizures | Antipsychotics, by decreasing dopamine, increase prolactin synthesis and release, especially in women<br>Elevated prolactin levels may be seen secondary to cocaine withdrawal<br>Lack of prolactin rise after seizure suggests pseudoseizure |
| Protein, total serum | Organic workup<br>Use of psychotropic medications | Increased in multiple myeloma, myxedema, lupus<br>Decreased in cirrhosis, malnutrition, overhydration<br>Low serum protein can result in greater sensitivity to conventional doses of protein-bound medications (lithium is not protein-bound) |
| Prothrombin time (PT) | Organic workup | Elevated in significant liver damage (cirrhosis), patients with lupus coagulant, which can be found in certain patients receiving antipsychotic medications, especially chlorpromazine |
| Reticulocyte count (estimate of red blood cell production in bone marrow) | Organic workup<br>Use of carbamazepine | Low in megaloblastic or iron deficiency anemia and anemia of chronic disease<br>Must be monitored in patient taking carbamazepine |
| Salicylate, serum | Psychotic disorder due to a general medical condition with hallucinations<br>Suicide attempts | Toxic levels may be seen in suicide attempts and may cause psychotic disorder due to a general medical condition with hallucinations |

(continued on next page)

TABLE 27-3 (continued)
**OTHER LABORATORY TESTS**

| Test | Major Psychiatric Indications | Comments |
|---|---|---|
| Sodium (NA), serum | Organic workup | Decreased with water intoxication; SIADH<br>Increased with excessive salt intake; diabetes<br>Decreased in hypoadrenalism, myxedema, congestive heart failure, diarrhea, polydipsia, use of carbamazepine, anabolic steroids<br>Low levels associated with greater sensitivity to conventional dose of lithium |
| Testosterone, serum | Impotence<br>Hypoactive sexual desire disorder | Increase in anabolic steroid abuse<br>Follow-up of sex offenders treated with medroxyprogesterone<br>May be decreased in organic workup of impotence<br>Decrease may be seen in hypoactive sexual desire disorder<br>Decreased with medroxyprogesterone treatment |
| Thyroid function tests | Organic workup<br>Depression | Detection of hypothyroidism or hyperthyroidism<br>Abnormalities can be associated with depression, anxiety, psychosis, dementia, delirium |
| Urinalysis | Organic workup<br>Pretreatment workup of lithium<br>Drug screening | Provides clues to cause of various cognitive disorders (assessing general appearance, pH, specific gravity, bilirubin, glucose, blood, ketones, protein, etc.); specific gravity may be affected by lithium |
| Urinary creatinine | Organic workup<br>Substance abuse<br>Lithium use | Increased in renal failure, dehydration<br>Part of pretreatment workup for lithium |
| Venereal Disease Research Laboratory (VDRL) | Syphilis | Positive (high titers) in secondary syphilis (may be positive or negative in primary syphilis)<br>Low titers (or negative) in tertiary syphilis |
| Vitamin A, serum | Depression<br>Delirium | Hypervitaminosis A is associated with a variety of mental status changes |
| Vitamin B₁₂, serum | Organic workup<br>Dementia | Part of workup of megaloblastic anemia and dementia<br>$B_{12}$ deficiency associated with psychosis, paranoia, fatigue, agitation, dementia, delirium<br>Often associated with chronic alcohol abuse |
| White blood cell (WBC) | Use of psychotropic medications | Leukopenia and agranulocytosis associated with certain psychotropic medications, such as phenothiazines, carbamazepine, clozapine<br>Leukocytosis associated with lithium and neuroleptic malignant syndrome |

TABLE 27–4
**CONVERSION FACTORS**

| | | |
|---|---|---|
| 1 gram | = | 1,000 milligrams (mg) |
| 1 milligram (mg) | = | 1,000 micrograms (μg) |
| 1 microgram (μg) | = | 1,000 nanograms (ng) |
| *Blood concentrations:* | | |
| 1 microgram per mL | = | 100 micrograms per dL |
| | = | 1 milligram per liter |
| | = | 1,000 nanograms per mL |
| 100 mg per dL | = | 0.1 gram per dL |
| | = | 1,000 mg (1 gram) per liter |
| | = | 1.0 mg per mL |

international language of measurement calculated by multiplying the conventional unit by a number factor being adopted by many laboratories. The SI measurement system uses *moles* as the basic unit for the amount of a substance, *kilograms* for its mass, and *meters* for its length. Conversion factors are listed on Table 27–4.

---

*For a more detailed discussion of this topic, see Coppola R, Hyde T: Applied Electrophysiology, Sec 1.8, p 72; Innis RB, Malison RT: Principles of Neuroimaging; Cummings JL: Neuropsychiatry: Clinical Assessment and Approach to Diagnosis, Sec 2.1, p 167; Miller BL, Cummings JL, Mena I, Darcourt J: Neuroimaging in Clinical Practice, Sec 2.10, p 257; Rosse RB, Deutsch LH, Deutsch SI: Medical Assessment and Laboratory Testing in Psychiatry, Sec 9.7, p 601; Leuchter AF, Cook IA: Neuroimaging, Sec 49.5c, p 49.5c, in CTP/VI.*

# Index

# BOOKS BY HAROLD I. KAPLAN, M.D., AND BENJAMIN J. SADOCK, M.D.

*Published by Williams & Wilkins*

**Comprehensive Textbook of Psychiatry**
1st edition, 1967 (with A. M. Freedman)
2nd edition, 1975 (with A. M. Freedman)
3rd edition, 1980 (with A. M. Freedman)
4th edition, 1985
5th edition, 1989
6th edition, 1995

**Synopsis of Psychiatry**
1st edition, 1972 (with A. M. Freedman)
2nd edition, 1976 (with A. M. Freedman)
3rd edition, 1981
4th edition, 1985
5th edition, 1988
6th edition, 1991
7th edition, 1994 (with J. Grebb)

**Study Guide and Self-Examination Review for Synopsis of Psychiatry**
1st edition, 1983
2nd edition, 1985
3rd edition, 1989
4th edition, 1991
5th edition, 1994

**Comprehensive Group Psychotherapy**
1st edition, 1971
2nd edition, 1983
3rd edition, 1993

**The Sexual Experience**
1976 (with A. M. Freedman)

**Clinical Psychiatry**
1988

**Pocket Handbook of Clinical Psychiatry**
1st edition, 1990
2nd edition, 1996

**Comprehensive Glossary of Psychiatry and Psychology**
1991

**Pocket Handbook of Psychiatric Drug Treatment**
1st edition, 1993
2nd edition, 1996

**Pocket Handbook of Emergency Psychiatric Medicine**
1993

*Various editions of the above books have been translated and published in French, German, Greek, Indonesian, Italian, Japanese, Polish, Portuguese, Russian, Spanish, and Turkish. In addition, an International Asian edition has been published in English.*

*By other publishers*

**Studies in Human Behavior, 1–5**
1972 (with A. M. Freedman)
*Athenaeum*
   1. Diagnosing Mental Illness: Evaluation in Psychiatry and Psychology
   2. Interpreting Personality: A Survey of Twentieth-Century Views
   3. Human Behavior: Biological, Psychological, and Sociological
   4. Treating Mental Illness: Aspects of Modern Therapy
   5. The Child: His Psychological and Cultural Development
      Vol. 1: Normal Development and Psychological Assessment
      Vol. 2: The Major Psychological Disorders and their Treatment

**Modern Group Books   I–VI**
1972
*E.P. Dutton*
   I        Origins of Group Analysis
   II       Evolution of Group Therapy
   III      Groups and Drugs
   IV       Sensitivity Through Encounter and Motivation
   V        New Models for Group Therapy
   VI       Group Treatment of Mental Illness

**The Human Animal**
1974 (with A. M. Freedman)
*K.F.S. Publications*
   Vol. 1:   Man and His Mind
   Vol. 2:   The Disordered Personality

# ABOUT THE AUTHORS

**HAROLD IRWIN KAPLAN, M.D.,** is currently professor of psychiatry at New York University (NYU) School of Medicine, an appointment dating back to 1980. Since that time he has been an attending psychiatrist at Tisch Hospital (the University Hospital of the NYU Medical Center) and Bellevue Hospital of the NYU Medical Center. He is codirector of NYU Medical Center's Continuing Medical Education Program in Psychiatry and is consultant psychiatrist at Lenox Hill Hospital in New York City. From 1958 to 1980, he was professor of psychiatry at New York Medical College and director of Psychiatric Education, heading the undergraduate, residency, and continuing education programs in psychiatry, and he was a visiting psychiatrist at Metropolitan Hospital in New York City. He received his Bachelor of Arts degree from New York University. He received his M.D. from New York Medical College in 1949 at the age of 21, interned at Jewish Hospital of Brooklyn, and served his psychiatric residency training at Kingsbridge Bronx Veterans Administration Hospital, New York's Mount Sinai Hospital, and at Jewish Board of Guardians (in child psychiatry). He has received awards for academic excellence in psychiatry from the Alumni Association of New York Medical College (1983), the Distinguished Service Award in Psychiatry from the Association of Psychiatric Outpatient Centers of America and the NYU Post-Graduate Medical School (1982), and a Founders Day Award for Scholastic Achievement from NYU (1988). During his tenure at New York Medical College, he was the principal investigator of 10 educational grants in psychiatry from NIMH, several specializing in the psychiatric training of women physicians. He was a member of the Preparatory Commission on Psychiatric Education for NIMH and the American Psychiatric Association during 1973–1975. In 1957 he was certified in psychiatry by the American Board of Psychiatry and Neurology and has served as an Assistant and Associate Examiner of the American Board for 12 years. He received a Certificate of Commendation from the American Psychiatric Association for his work as chairman of their Committee on Education during 1973–1975. Professor Kaplan was certified in psychoanalysis in 1955 by New York Medical College. He has published many papers in numerous psychiatric journals and has authored and edited the books listed in this volume. He is a Life Fellow of the American Psychiatric Association, the American College of Physicians, the New York Academy of Medicine, and the American Orthopsychiatric Association. He is also a member of the Alpha Omega Alpha Honorary Medical Society and treasurer of the NYU-Bellevue Psychiatric Society. He presently makes his home in New York City, where he is married to actress Nancy Barrett. He has three children, Jennifer, Peter Mark, and Phillip. He maintains an active general psychiatric practice in Manhattan, which includes individual and group psychotherapy, psychiatric consultation, and psychoanalysis. In his leisure time he enjoys reading nonfiction, travel, and fine food.

**BENJAMIN JAMES SADOCK, M.D.,** is currently professor and vice chairman of the Department of Psychiatry at the New York University (NYU) School of Medicine. He graduated from Union College in 1955 and received his M.D. from New York Medical College in 1959. After an internship at Albany Hospital, he completed his residency at Bellevue Psychiatric Hospital and then entered military service, where he served as Assistant Chief and Acting Chief of Neuropsychiatry at Sheppard Air Force Base, Texas. He held faculty and teaching appointments at Southwestern Medical School and Parkland Hospital in Dallas and at New York Medical College, St. Luke's Hospital, the New York State Psychiatric Institute, and Metropolitan Hospital in New York City. He joined the faculty of the NYU School of Medicine in 1980 and served in various positions: director of Medical Student Education in Psychiatry, codirector of the Residency Training Program in Psychiatry, and director of Graduate Medical Education. Since 1980, Dr. Sadock has been director of Student Mental Health Services, psychiatric consultant to the Admissions Committee, and codirector of Continuing Education in Psychiatry at the NYU School of Medicine. He is on the staff of Bellevue Hospital and Tisch Hospital (the University Hospital of the NYU Medical Center) and is consultant psychiatrist at Lenox Hill Hospital. Dr. Sadock became a Diplomate of the American Board of Psychiatry and Neurology in 1966 and served as an assistant and associate examiner for the Board for over a decade. He is a Fellow of the American Psychiatric Association, the American College of Physicians, and the New York Academy of Medicine. He is also a member of the Alpha Omega Alpha Honor Society. He is active in numerous psychiatric organizations and is president and founder of the NYU-Bellevue Psychiatric Society. Dr. Sadock was a member of the National Committee on Continuing Education in Psychiatry of the American Psychiatric Association, served on the Ad Hoc Committee on Sex Therapy Clinics of the American Medical Association, was delegate to the Conference on Recertification of the American Board of Medical Specialists, and was a representative of the American Psychiatric Association's Task Force on the National Board of Medical Examiners and the American Board of Psychiatry and Neurology. In 1985 he received the Academic Achievement Award from New York Medical College. He is author or editor of more than 100 publications, including the books listed in this volume, and is a book reviewer for psychiatry journals. He is married to Virginia Alcott Sadock, M.D., Clinical Professor of Psychiatry and Director of Graduate Education in Human Sexuality at NYU Medical Center. They live in Manhattan and have an active private practice specializing in individual psychotherapy, group psychotherapy, sex and marital therapy, and pharmacotherapy. They have two children, James and Victoria. Dr. Sadock is an opera lover, a skier, and an avid fly fisherman.

or anxiolytic
dependence[a]

305.40 Sedative, hypnotic, or
anxiolytic abuse

**Sedative-, Hypnotic-,
or Anxiolytic-Induced
Disorders**

292.89 Sedative, hypnotic, or
anxiolytic intoxication

292.0 Sedative, hypnotic, or
anxiolytic withdrawal
*Specify if:* with
perceptual disturbances

292.81 Sedative, hypnotic, or
anxiolytic intoxication
delirium

292.81 Sedative, hypnotic, or
anxiolytic withdrawal
delirium

292.82 Sedative-, hypnotic-, or
anxiolytic-induced
persisting dementia

292.83 Sedative-, hypnotic-, or
anxiolytic-induced
persisting amnestic
disorder

292.xx Sedative-, hypnotic-, or
anxiolytic-induced
psychotic disorder

  .11 With delusions[I,W]

  .12 With hallucinations[I,W]

292.84 Sedative-, hypnotic-, or
anxiolytic-induced mood
disorder[I,W]

292.89 Sedative-, hypnotic-, or
anxiolytic-induced
anxiety disorder[W]

292.89 Sedative-, hypnotic-, or
anxiolytic-induced
sexual dysfunction[I]

292.89 Sedative-, hypnotic-, or
anxiolytic-induced sleep
disorder[I,W]

292.9 Sedative-, hypnotic-, or
anxiolytic-related
disorder NOS

**POLYSUBSTANCE-RELATED
DISORDER**

304.80 Polysubstance
dependence[a]

**OTHER (OR UNKNOWN)
SUBSTANCE-RELATED
DISORDERS**

**Other (or Unknown) Substance
Use Disorders**

304.90 Other (or unknown)
substance dependence[a]

305.90 Other (or unknown)
substance abuse

**Other (or unknown) substance-
Induced Disorders**

292.89 Other (or unknown)
substance intoxication
*Specify if:* with
perceptual disturbances

292.0 Other (or unknown)
substance withdrawal
*Specify if:* with
perceptual disturbances

292.81 Other (or unknown)
substance-induced
delirium

292.82 Other (or unknown)
substance-induced
persisting dementia

292.83 Other (or unknown)
substance-induced
persisting amnestic
disorder

292.xx Other (or unknown)
substance-induced
psychotic disorder

  .11 With delusions[I,W]

  .12 With hallucinations[I,W]

292.84 Other (or unknown)
substance-induced
mood disorder[I,W]

292.89 Other (or unknown)
substance-induced
anxiety disorder[I,W]

292.89 Other (or unknown)
substance-induced
sexual dysfunction[I]

292.89 Other (or unknown)
substance-induced sleep
disorder[I,W]

292.9 Other (or unknown
substance-related
disorder NOS)

**Schizophrenia and Other
Psychotic Disorders**

295.xx Schizophrenia
*The following classification of longi-
tudinal course applies to all subtypes of schizophrenia:*

Episodic with interepisode residual
symptoms (*specify if:* with prominent negative symptoms)/episodic
with no interepisode residual symp-
toms/continuous (*specify if:* with
prominent negative symptoms)

Single episode in partial remission
(*specify if:* with prominent negative
symptoms)/single episode in full
remission

Other or unspecified pattern

  .30 Paranoid type

  .10 Disorganized type

  .20 Catatonic type

  .90 Undifferentiated type

  .60 Residual type

295.40 Schizophreniform
disorder
*Specify if:* without good
prognostic features/with
good prognostic features

295.70 Schizoaffective disorder
*Specify type:* bipolar
type/depressive type

297.1 Delusional disorder
*Specify type:* erotomanic
type/grandiose type/
jealous type/persecutory
type/somatic type/mixed
type/unspecified type

298.8 Brief psychotic disorder
*Specify if:* with marked
stressor(s)/without
marked stressor(s)/with
postpartum onset

297.3 Shared psychotic
disorder

293.xx Psychotic disorder due
to . . . *[indicate the
general medical
condition]*

  .81 With delusions

  .82 With hallucinations

\_\_\_ . \_\_ Substance-induced
psychotic disorder (*refer
to substance-related
disorders for substance
specific codes*)
*Specify if:* with onset
during intoxication/with
onset during withdrawal

298.9 Psychotic disorder NOS

**Mood Disorders**
*Code current state of major depress-
ive disorder or bipolar I disorder in
fifth digit:*

  1 = mild

  2 = moderate

  3 = Severe without psychotic
features

  4 = Severe with psychotic
features
*Specify:* mood-congruent
psychotic features/mood-
incongruent psychotic features

  5 = in partial remission

  6 = in full remission

  0 = unspecified

*The following specifiers apply (for
current or most recent episode) to
mood disorders as noted:*

[a]Severity/psychotic remission
specifiers/[b]chronic/[c]with catatonic features/[d]with melancholic
features/[e]with atypical features/
[f]with postpartum onset

*The following specifiers apply to
mood disorders as follows:*

[g]With or without full interepisode
recovery/[h]with seasonal pattern/
[i]with rapid cycling

## DEPRESSIVE DISORDERS

296.xx   Major depressive disorder
.2x   Single episode[a,b,c,d,e,f]
.3x   Recurrent[a,b,c,d,e,f,g,h]
300.4   Dysthymic disorder
    *Specify if:* early onset/ late onset
    *Specify:* with atypical features
311   Depressive disorder NOS

## BIPOLAR DISORDERS

296.xx   Bipolar I disorder
.0x   Single manic episode[a,c,f]
    *Specify if:* mixed
.40   Most recent episode hypomanic[g,h,i]
.4x   Most recent episode manic[a,c,f,g,h,i]
.6x   Most recent episode mixed[a,c,f,g,h,i]
.5x   Most recent episode depressed[a,b,c,d,e,f,g,h,i]
.7   Most recent episode unspecified[g,h,i]
296.89   Bipolar II disorder[a,b,c,d,e,f,g,h,i]
    *Specify (current or most recent episode):* hypomanic/depressed
301.13   Cyclothymic disorder
296.80   Bipolar disorder NOS

293.83   Mood disorder due to . . . *[indicate the general medical condition]*
    *Specify type:* with depressive features/with major depressivelike episode/with manic features/with mixed features
___.__   Substance-induced mood disorder *(refer to substance-related disorders for substance-specific codes)*
    *Specify type:* with depressive features/with manic features/with mixed features
    *Specify if:* with onset during intoxication/with onset during withdrawal

296.90   Mood disorder NOS

### Anxiety Disorders

300.1   Panic disorder without agoraphobia

300.21   Panic disorder with agoraphobia
300.22   Agoraphobia without history of panic disorder
300.29   Specific phobia
    *Specify type:* animal type/natural environment type/blood-injection-injury type/situational type/other type
300.23   Social phobia
    *Specify if:* generalized
300.3   Obsessive-compulsive disorder
    *Specify if:* with poor insight
309.81   Posttraumatic stress disorder
    *Specify if:* acute/chronic
    *Specify if:* with delayed onset
308.3   Acute stress disorder
300.02   Generalized anxiety disorder
293.89   Anxiety disorder due to . . . *[indicate the general medical condition]*
    *Specify if:* with generalized anxiety/with panic attacks/with obsessive-compulsive symptoms
___.__   Substance-induced anxiety disorder *(refer to substance-related disorders for substance-specific codes)*
    *Specify if:* with generalized anxiety/with panic attacks/with obsessive-compulsive symptoms/with phobic symptoms
    *Specify if:* with onset during intoxication/with onset during withdrawal
300.00   Anxiety disorder NOS

### Somatoform Disorders

300.81   Somatization disorder
300.81   Undifferentiated somatoform disorder
300.11   Conversion disorder
    *Specify type:* with motor symptom or deficit/with sensory symptom or deficit/with seizures or convulsions/with mixed presentation
307.xx   Pain disorder
.80   Associated with psychological factors
.89   Associated with both psychological factors and a general medical condition
    *Specify if:* acute/chronic
300.7   Hypochondriasis
    *Specify if:* with poor insight
300.7   Body dysmorphic disorder
300.81   Somatoform disorder NOS

### Factitious Disorders

300.xx   Factitious disorder
.16   With predominantly psychological signs and symptoms
.19   With predominantly physical signs and symptoms
.19   With combined psychological and physical signs and symptoms
300.19   Factitious disorder NOS

### Dissociative Disorders

301.12   Dissociative amnesia
301.13   Dissociative fugue
301.14   Dissociative identity disorder
300.6   Depersonalization disorder
300.15   Dissociative disorder NOS

### Sexual and Gender Identity Disorders

#### SEXUAL DYSFUNCTIONS
*The following specifiers apply to all primary sexual dysfunctions:*
    Lifelong type/acquired type
    Generalized type/situational type
    Due to psychological factors/due to combined factors

#### Sexual Desire Disorders
302.71   Hypoactive sexual desire disorder
302.79   Sexual aversion disorder

#### Sexual Arousal Disorders
302.72   Female sexual arousal disorder
302.72   Male erectile disorder

#### Orgasmic Disorders
302.73   Female orgasmic disorder
302.74   Male orgasmic disorder
302.75   Premature ejaculation

## Sexual Pain Disorders
302.76   Dyspareunia (not due to a general medical condition)

306.51   Vaginismus (not due to a general medical condition)

## Sexual Dysfunction Due to a General Medical Condition

625.8   Female hypoactive sexual desire disorder due to . . . *[indicate the general medical condition]*

608.89   Male hypoactive sexual desire disorder due to . . . *[indicate the general medical condition]*

607.84   Male erectile disorder due to . . . *[indicate the general medical condition]*

625.0   Female dyspareunia due to . . . *[indicate the general medical condition]*

608.89   Male dyspareunia due to . . . *[indicate the general medical condition]*

625.8   Other female sexual dysfunction due to . . . *[indicate the general medical condition]*

608.89   Other male sexual dysfunction due to . . . *[indicate the general medical condition]*

___ . ___   Substance-induced sexual dysfunction *(refer to substance-related disorders for substance-specific codes)*
*Specify if:* with impaired desire/with impaired arousal/with impaired orgasm/with sexual pain
*Specify if:* with onset during intoxication

302.70   Sexual dysfunction NOS

## PARAPHILIAS
302.4   Exhibitionism
302.81   Fetishism
302.89   Frotteurism
302.2   Pedophilia
*Specify if:* Sexually attracted to males/sexually attracted to females/sexually attracted to both
*Specify if:* limited to incest
*Specify type:* exclusive type/nonexclusive type
302.83   Sexual masochism
302.84   Sexual sadism

302.3   Transvestic fetishism
*Specify if:* with gender dysphoria
302.82   Voyeurism
302.9   Paraphilia NOS

## GENDER IDENTITY DISORDERS
302.xx   Gender identity disorder
  .6   in children
  .85   in adolescents or adults
*Specify if:* sexually attracted to males/sexually attracted to females/sexually attracted to both/sexually attracted to neither

302.6   Gender identity disorder NOS

302.9   Sexual disorder NOS

---

### Eating Disorders

307.1   Anorexia nervosa
*Specify type:* restricting type; binge-eating/purging type

307.51   Bulimia nervosa
*Specify type:* purging type/nonpurging type

307.50   Eating disorder NOS

---

### Sleep Disorders

## PRIMARY SLEEP DISORDERS

**Dyssomnias**
307.42   Primary insomnia
307.44   Primary hypersomnia
*Specify if:* recurrent
347   Narcolepsy
780.59   Breathing-related sleep disorder
307.45   Circadian rhythm sleep disorder
*Specify type:* delayed sleep phase type/jet lag type/shift work type/unspecified type
307.47   Dyssomnia NOS

**Parasomnias**
307.47   Nightmare disorder
307.46   Sleep terror disorder
307.46   Sleepwalking disorder
307.47   Parasomnia NOS

## SLEEP DISORDERS RELATED TO ANOTHER MENTAL DISORDER
307.42   Insomnia related to . . . *[indicate the Axis I or Axis II disorder]*

307.44   Hypersomnia related to . . . *[indicate the Axis I or Axis II disorder]*

## OTHER SLEEP DISORDERS
780.xx   Sleep disorder due to . . . *[indicate the general medical condition]*
  .52   Insomnia type
  .54   Hypersomnia type
  .59   Parasomnia type
  .59   Mixed type

___ . ___   Substance-induced sleep disorder *(refer to substance-related disorders for substance-specific codes)*
*Specify type:* insomnia type/hypersomnia type/parasomnia type/mixed type
*Specify if:* with onset during intoxication/with onset during withdrawal

---

### Impulse-Control Disorders Not Elsewhere Classified

312.34   Intermittent explosive disorder
312.32   Kleptomania
312.33   Pyromania
312.31   Pathological gambling
312.39   Trichotillomania
312.30   Impulse-control disorder NOS

---

### Adjustment Disorders

309.xx   Adjustment disorder
  .0   With depressed mood
  .24   With anxiety
  .28   With mixed anxiety and depressed mood
  .3   With disturbance of conduct
  .4   With mixed disturbance of emotions and conduct
  .9   Unspecified
*Specify if:* acute/chronic

---

### Personality Disorders

*Note:* These are coded on Axis II.
301.0   Paranoid personality disorder
301.20   Schizoid personality disorder
301.22   Schizotypal personality disorder
301.7   Antisocial personality disorder
301.83   Borderline personality disorder
301.50   Histrionic personality disorder

| 301.81 | Narcissistic personality disorder |
|---|---|
| 301.82 | Avoidant personality disorder |
| 301.6 | Dependent personality disorder |
| 301.4 | Obsessive-compulsive personality disorder |
| 301.9 | Personality disorder NOS |

**Other Conditions That May Be a Focus of Clinical Attention**

## PSYCHOLOGICAL FACTORS AFFECTING MEDICAL CONDITION

| 316 | . . . [Specified psychological factor] Affecting . . . [indicate the general medical condition] Choose name based on nature of factors: Mental disorder affecting medical condition Psychological symptoms affecting medical condition Personality traits or coping style affecting medical condition Maladaptive health behaviors affecting medical condition Stress-related physiological response affecting medical condition Other or unspecified psychological factors affecting medical condition |
|---|---|

## MEDICATION-INDUCED MOVEMENT DISORDERS

| 332.1 | Neuroleptic-induced parkinsonism |
|---|---|
| 333.92 | Neuroleptic malignant syndrome |
| 333.7 | Neuroleptic-induced acute dystonia |
| 333.99 | Neuroleptic-induced acute akathisia |
| 333.82 | Neuroleptic-induced tardive dyskinesia |
| 333.1 | Medication-induced postural tremor |
| 333.90 | Medication-induced movement disorder NOS |

## OTHER MEDICATION-INDUCED DISORDER

| 995.2 | Adverse effects of medication NOS |
|---|---|

## RELATIONAL PROBLEMS

| V61.9 | Relational problem related to a mental disorder or general medical condition |
|---|---|
| V61.20 | Parent-child relational problem |
| V61.1 | Partner relational problem |
| V61.8 | Sibling relational problem |
| V62.81 | Relational problem NOS |

## PROBLEMS RELATED TO ABUSE OR NEGLECT

| V61.21 | Physical abuse of child (code 995.5 if focus of attention is on victim) |
|---|---|
| V61.21 | Sexual abuse of child (code 995.5 if focus of attention is on victim) |
| V61.21 | Neglect of child (code 995.5 if focus of attention is on victim) |
| V61.1 | Physical abuse of adult (code 995.81 if focus of attention is on victim) |
| V61.1 | Sexual abuse of adult (code 995.81 if focus of attention is on victim) |

## ADDITIONAL CONDITIONS THAT MAY BE A FOCUS OF CLINICAL ATTENTION

| V15.81 | Noncompliance with treatment |
|---|---|
| V65.2 | Malingering |
| V71.01 | Adult antisocial behavior |
| V71.02 | Child or adolescent antisocial behavior |
| V62.89 | Borderline intellectual functioning |

*Note: This is coded on Axis II.*

| 780.9 | Age-related cognitive decline |
|---|---|
| V62.82 | Bereavement |
| V62.3 | Academic problem |
| V62.2 | Occupational problem |
| 313.82 | Identity problem |
| V62.89 | Religious or spiritual problem |
| V62.4 | Acculturation problem |
| V62.89 | Phase of life problem |

**Additional Codes**

| 300.9 | Unspecified mental disorder (nonpsychotic) |
|---|---|
| V71.09 | No diagnosis or condition on Axis I |
| 799.9 | Diagnosis or condition deferred on Axis I |
| V71.09 | No diagnosis on Axis II |
| 799.9 | Diagnosis deferred on Axis II |

**Multiaxial System**

| Axis I | Clinical disorders Other conditions that may be a focus of clinical attention |
|---|---|
| Axis II | Personality disorders Mental retardation |
| Axis III | General medical conditions |
| Axis IV | Psychosocial and environmental problems |
| Axis V | Global assessment of functioning |

# DSM-IV Classification

© Copyright 1994, American Psychiatric Association

NOS = Not otherwise specified.

An x appearing in a diagnostic code indicates that a specified code number is required.

An ellipsis (. . .) is used in the names of certain disorders to indicate that the name of a specific mental disorder or general medical condition should be inserted when recording the name (e.g., 293.0 delirium due to hypothyroidism).

If criteria are currently met, one of the following severity specifiers may be noted after the diagnosis:
Mild
Moderate
Severe

If criteria are no longer met, one of the following specifiers may be noted:
In partial remission
In full remission
Prior history

---
**Disorders Usually First Diagnosed in Infancy, Childhood, or Adolescence**
---

## MENTAL RETARDATION
*Note: These are coded on Axis II.*
| | |
|---|---|
| 317 | Mild mental retardation |
| 318.0 | Moderate mental retardation |
| 318.1 | Severe mental retardation |
| 318.2 | Profound mental retardation |
| 319 | Mental retardation, severity unspecified |

## LEARNING DISORDERS
| | |
|---|---|
| 315.00 | Reading disorder |
| 315.1 | Mathematics disorder |
| 315.2 | Disorder of written expression |
| 315.9 | Learning disorder NOS |

## MOTOR SKILLS DISORDER
| | |
|---|---|
| 315.4 | Developmental coordination disorder |

## COMMUNICATION DISORDERS
| | |
|---|---|
| 315.31 | Expressive language disorder |
| 315.31 | Mixed receptive-expressive language disorder |
| 315.39 | Phonological disorder |
| 307.0 | Stuttering |
| 307.9 | Communication disorder NOS |

## PERVASIVE DEVELOPMENTAL DISORDERS
| | |
|---|---|
| 299.00 | Autistic disorder |
| 299.80 | Rett's disorder |
| 299.10 | Childhood disintegrative disorder |
| 299.80 | Asperger's disorder |
| 299.80 | Pervasive developmental disorder NOS |

## ATTENTION-DEFICIT AND DISRUPTIVE BEHAVIOR DISORDERS
| | |
|---|---|
| 314.xx | Attention-deficit/hyperactivity disorder |
| .01 | Combined type |
| .00 | Predominantly inattentive type |
| .01 | Predominantly hyperactive-impulsive type |
| 314.9 | Attention-deficit/hyperactivity disorder NOS |
| 312.8 | Conduct disorder *Specify type:* childhood-onset type/adolescent-onset type |
| 313.81 | Oppositional defiant disorder |
| 312.9 | Disruptive behavior disorder NOS |

## FEEDING AND EATING DISORDERS OF INFANCY OR EARLY CHILDHOOD
| | |
|---|---|
| 307.52 | Pica |
| 307.53 | Rumination disorder |
| 307.59 | Feeding disorder of infancy or early childhood |

## TIC DISORDERS
| | |
|---|---|
| 307.23 | Tourette's disorder |
| 307.22 | Chronic motor or vocal tic disorder |
| 307.21 | Transient tic disorder *Specify type:* nocturnal only/diurnal only/nocturnal and diurnal |
| 307.20 | Tic disorder NOS |

## ELIMINATION DISORDERS
| | |
|---|---|
| —.— | Encopresis |
| 787.6 | With constipation and overflow incontinence |
| 307.7 | Without constipation and overflow incontinence |
| 307.6 | Enuresis (not due to a general medical condition) *Specify type:* nocturnal only/diurnal only/nocturnal and diurnal |

## OTHER DISORDERS OF INFANCY, CHILDHOOD, OR ADOLESCENCE
| | |
|---|---|
| 309.21 | Separation anxiety disorder *Specify if:* early onset |
| 313.23 | Selective mutism |
| 313.89 | Reactive attachment disorder of infancy or early childhood *Specify type:* inhibited type/disinhibited type |
| 307.3 | Stereotypic movement disorder *Specify if:* with self-injurious behavior |
| 313.9 | Disorder of infancy, childhood, or adolescence NOS |

---
**Delirium, Dementia, and Amnestic and Other Cognitive Disorders**
---

## DELIRIUM
| | |
|---|---|
| 293.0 | Delirium due to . . . *[indicate the general medical condition]* |
| —.— | Substance intoxication delirium *[refer to substance-related disorders for substance-specific codes]* |
| —.— | Substance withdrawal delirium *[refer to substance-related disorders for substance-specific codes]* |
| —.— | Delirium due to multiple etiologies *(code each of the specific etiologies)* |
| 780.09 | Delirium NOS |

## DEMENTIA
| | |
|---|---|
| 290.xx | Dementia of the Alzheimer's type, with early onset *(also code 331.0 Alzheimer's disease on Axis III)* |

| | |
|---|---|
| .10 | Uncomplicated |
| .11 | With delirium |
| .12 | With delusions |
| .13 | With depressed mood |
| | Specify if: with behavioral disturbance |

290.xx Dementia of the Alzheimer's type, with late onset (also code 331.0 Alzheimer's disease on Axis III)

| | |
|---|---|
| .0 | Uncomplicated |
| .3 | With delirium |
| .20 | With delusions |
| .21 | With depressed mood |
| | Specify if: with behavioral disturbance |

290.xx Vascular dementia

| | |
|---|---|
| .40 | Uncomplicated |
| .41 | With delirium |
| .42 | With delusions |
| .43 | With depressed mood |
| | Specify if: with behavioral disturbance |

294.9 Dementia due to HIV disease (also code 043.1 HIV infection affecting central nervous system on Axis III)

294.1 Dementia due to head trauma (also code 854.00 head injury on Axis III)

294.1 Dementia due to Parkinson's disease (also code 332.0 Parkinson's disease on Axis III)

294.1 Dementia due to Huntington's disease (also code 333.4 Huntington's disease on Axis III)

290.10 Dementia due to Pick's disease (also code 331.1 Pick's disease on Axis III)

290.10 Dementia due to Creutzfeldt-Jakob disease (also code 046.1 Creutzfeldt-Jakob disease on Axis III)

294.1 Dementia due to . . . [indicate the general medical condition not listed above] (also code the general medical condition on Axis III)

—.— Substance-induced persisting dementia (refer to substance-related disorders for substance specific codes)

—.— Dementia due to multiple etiologies (code each of the specific etiologies)

294.8 Dementia NOS

## AMNESTIC DISORDERS

294.0 Amnestic disorder due to . . . [indicate the general medical condition]
Specify if: transient/chronic

—.— Substance-induced persisting amnestic disorder (refer to substance-related disorders for substance-specific codes)

294.8 Amnestic disorder NOS

## OTHER COGNITIVE DISORDERS

294.9 Cognitive disorder NOS

---

**Mental Disorders Due to a General Medical Condition Not Elsewhere Classified**

293.89 Catatonic disorder due to . . . [indicate the general medical condition]

310.1 Personality change due to [indicate the general medical condition]
Specify type: labile type/disinhibited type/aggressive type/apathetic type/paranoid type/other type/combined type/unspecified type

293.9 Mental disorder NOS due to . . . [indicate the general medical condition]

---

**Substance-Related Disorders**

[a] The following specifiers may be applied to substance dependence:
With physiological dependence/without physiological dependence
Early full remission/early partial remission/sustained full remission/sustained partial remission
On agonist therapy/in a controlled environment

The following specifiers apply to substance-induced disorders as noted:

[I] With onset during intoxication/
[W] With onset during withdrawal

## ALCOHOL-RELATED DISORDERS

**Alcohol Use Disorders**

| | |
|---|---|
| 303.90 | Alcohol dependence[a] |
| 305.00 | Alcohol abuse |

**Alcohol-Induced Disorders**

| | |
|---|---|
| 303.00 | Alcohol intoxication |
| 291.8 | Alcohol withdrawal |
| | Specify if: With perceptual disturbances |
| 291.0 | Alcohol intoxication delirium |
| 291.0 | Alcohol withdrawal delirium |
| 291.2 | Alcohol-induced persisting dementia |
| 291.1 | Alcohol-induced persisting amnestic disorder |
| 291.x | Alcohol-induced psychotic disorder |
| .5 | With delusions[I,W] |
| .3 | With hallucinations[I,W] |
| 291.8 | Alcohol-induced mood disorder[I,W] |
| 291.8 | Alcohol-induced anxiety disorder[I,W] |
| 291.8 | Alcohol-induced sexual dysfunction[I] |
| 291.8 | Alcohol-induced sleep disorder[I,W] |
| 291.9 | Alcohol-related disorder NOS |

## AMPHETAMINE (OR AMPHETAMINELIKE)-RELATED DISORDERS

**Amphetamine Use Disorders**

| | |
|---|---|
| 304.40 | Amphetamine dependence[a] |
| 305.70 | Amphetamine abuse |

**Amphetamine-Induced Disorders**

| | |
|---|---|
| 292.89 | Amphetamine intoxication |
| | Specify if: with perceptual disturbances |
| 292.0 | Amphetamine withdrawal |
| 292.81 | Amphetamine intoxication delirium |
| 292.xx | Amphetamine-induced psychotic disorder |
| .11 | With delusions[I] |
| .12 | With hallucinations[I] |
| 292.84 | Amphetamine-induced mood disorder[I,W] |
| 292.89 | Amphetamine-induced anxiety disorder[I] |
| 292.89 | Amphetamine-induced sexual dysfunction[I] |

292.89   Amphetamine-induced sleep disorder[i,W]

292.9   Amphetamine-related disorder NOS

## CAFFEINE-RELATED DISORDERS

### Caffeine-Induced Disorders
305.90   Caffeine intoxication
292.89   Caffeine-induced anxiety disorder[i]
292.89   Caffeine-induced sleep disorder[i]

292.9   Caffeine-related disorder NOS

## CANNABIS-RELATED DISORDERS

### Cannabis Use Disorders
304.30   Cannabis dependence[a]
305.20   Cannabis abuse

### Cannabis-Induced Disorders
292.89   Cannabis intoxication
    *Specify if:* with perceptual disturbances
292.81   Cannabis intoxication delirium
292.xx   Cannabis-induced psychotic disorder
  .11     With delusions[i]
  .12     With hallucinations[i]
292.89   Cannabis-induced anxiety disorder[i]

292.9   Cannabis-related disorder NOS

## COCAINE-RELATED DISORDERS

### Cocaine Use Disorders
304.20   Cocaine dependence[a]
305.60   Cocaine abuse

### Cocaine-Induced Disorders
292.89   Cocaine intoxication
    *Specify if:* with perceptual disturbances
292.0   Cocaine withdrawal
292.81   Cocaine intoxication delirium
292.xx   Cocaine-induced psychotic disorder
  .11     With delusions[i]
  .12     With hallucinations[i]
292.84   Cocaine-induced mood disorder[i,W]
292.89   Cocaine-induced anxiety disorder[i]
292.89   Cocaine-induced sexual dysfunction[i]

292.89   Cocaine-induced sleep disorder[i,W]

292.9   Cocaine-related disorder NOS

## HALLUCINOGEN-RELATED DISORDERS

### Hallucinogen Use Disorders
304.50   Hallucinogen dependence[a]
305.30   Hallucinogen abuse

### Hallucinogen-Induced Disorders
292.89   Hallucinogen intoxication
292.89   Hallucinogen persisting perception disorder (flashbacks)
292.81   Hallucinogen intoxication delirium
292.xx   Hallucinogen-induced psychotic disorder
  .11     With delusions[i]
  .12     With hallucinations[i]
292.84   Hallucinogen-induced mood disorder[i]
292.89   Hallucinogen-induced anxiety disorder[i]

292.9   Hallucinogen-related disorder NOS

## INHALANT-RELATED DISORDERS

### Inhalant Use Disorders
304.60   Inhalant dependence[a]
305.90   Inhalant abuse

### Inhalant-Induced Disorders
292.89   Inhalant intoxication
292.81   Inhalant intoxication delirium
292.82   Inhalant-induced persisting dementia
292.xx   Inhalant-induced psychotic disorder
  .11     With delusions[i]
  .12     With hallucinations[i]
292.84   Inhalant-induced mood disorder[i]
292.89   Inhalant-induced anxiety disorder[i]

292.9   Inhalant-related disorder NOS

## NICOTINE-RELATED DISORDERS

### Nicotine Use Disorders
305.10   Nicotine dependence[a]

### Nicotine-Induced Disorder
292.0   Nicotine withdrawal
292.9   Nicotine-related disorder NOS

## OPIOID-RELATED DISORDERS

### Opioid Use Disorders
304.00   Opioid dependence[a]
305.50   Opioid abuse

### Opioid-Induced Disorders
292.89   Opioid intoxication
    *Specify if:* with perceptual disturbances
292.0   Opioid withdrawal
292.81   Opioid intoxication delirium
292.xx   Opioid-induced psychotic disorder
  .11     With delusions[i]
  .12     With hallucinations[i]
292.84   Opioid-induced mood disorder[i]
292.89   Opioid-induced sexual dysfunction[i]
292.89   Opioid-induced sleep disorder[i,W]

292.9   Opioid-related disorder NOS

## PHENCYCLIDINE (OR PHENCYCLIDINELIKE)-RELATED DISORDERS

### Phencyclidine Use Disorders
304.90   Phencyclidine dependence[a]
305.90   Phencyclidine abuse

### Phencyclidine-Induced Disorders
292.89   Phencyclidine intoxication
    *Specify if:* with perceptual disturbances
292.81   Phencyclidine intoxication delirium
292.xx   Phencyclidine-induced psychotic disorder
  .11     With delusions[i]
  .12     With hallucinations[i]
292.84   Phencyclidine-induced mood disorder[i]
292.89   Phencyclidine-induced anxiety disorder[i]
292.9   Phencyclidine-related disorder NOS

## SEDATIVE-, HYPNOTIC-, OR ANXIOLYTIC-RELATED DISORDERS

### Sedative, Hypnotic, or Anxiolytic Use Disorders
304.10   Sedative, hypnotic,

*(continued on page 403)*